Nutrition for Women

THE COMPLETE GUIDE

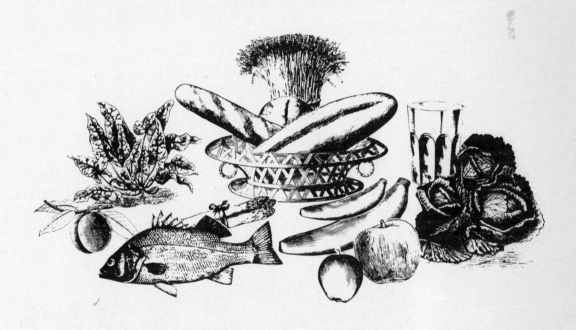

ELIZABETH SOMER, M.A., R.D.

A HENRY HOLT REFERENCE BOOK

Henry Holt and Company

New York

Henry Holt and Company, Inc.
Publishers since 1866
115 West 18th Street
New York, New York 10011

Henry Holt® is a registered trademark
of Henry Holt and Company, Inc.

Published in Canada by Fitzhenry & Whiteside Ltd.,
195 Allstate Parkway, Markham, Ontario L3R 4T8.

The figures in Part III are here reprinted with the permission of
Slawson Communications, 165 Vallecitos de Oro,
San Marcos, CA 92069

Library of Congress Cataloging-in-Publication Data
Somer, Elizabeth.
Nutrition for women : the complete guide /
Elizabeth Somer.—1st ed.
p.   cm.
Includes index.
1. Women—Nutrition.   2. Women—Health and hygiene.   I. Title.
RA778.S647   1993

613.2'082—dc20   93-27486
                                                          CIP

ISBN 0-8050-2389-5
ISBN 0-8050-3563-X (An Owl Book: pbk.)

Henry Holt books are available for special promotions
and premiums. For details contact: Director, Special Markets.

First published in hardcover in 1993 by
Henry Holt Reference Books.

First Owl Book Edition—1995

Designed by Kate Nichols

Printed in the United States of America
All first editions are printed on acid-free paper.∞

3   5   7   9   10   8   6   4
1   3   5   7   9   10   8   6   4   2
(pbk.)

Every woman needs remarkable women in her life.
I have been surrounded by many,
including my mother, Miriam,
my sisters Gayle and Lovey, and
my lifelong friend Sandra.

A woman is lucky to find one good man.
I have two:
my father, Rolly,
and my husband, Patrick.

This book is dedicated to them.

Contents

Foreword

Do you know what is the single most important nutrient in your diet? Many of us don't. Furthermore, we fail to realize that our health doesn't just happen. Life-style choices, including diet, influence our body's health and risk for disease, as well as its aging process.

With today's fast pace, maintaining a healthy life-style can seem overwhelming. The demands from home, work, and family can make bettering your health and your life a difficult priority, unless you find the resources and support that can help.

Noted nutrition expert Elizabeth Somer has compiled an indispensable guide to help you understand current research and fine-tune your diet. Based on her summary of more than two thousand nutrition studies related to women's health, *Nutrition for Women* is among the most definitive research-based tools for exploring your nutritional needs. Step-by-step, you can test your knowledge, analyze your diet and eating habits, and learn to make healthier, more nutritious food choices.

Furthermore, you can easily access information you've been looking for, including that *water* is the most important nutrient in your diet. Want to know why? Read on. The book's a treasure chest.

—Barbara Harris,
Editor in Chief, *Shape* magazine

Preface

"One source tells me vegetable oils increase my risk for breast cancer, while another says fat has no effect. Which one should I believe?"

"Whenever I mentioned the mood swings and bloating I experienced just before my period, I was told it was all in my head. I finally stopped talking about it."

"One report claims that the only way to make sure I get enough [nutrients] is to supplement my diet; someone else says supplements are useless and possibly harmful. How can I make sense out of such different opinions?"

For fifteen years I have listened to the frustration in women's voices. They wanted to know what to believe, how to cut through the nutrition hype to reach the facts, and where to get accurate nutrition information. They were willing to make changes in their diets to improve their health and the quality of their lives, but they were confused and sometimes overwhelmed at the conflicting news. That is why I wrote this book.

FINALLY, NUTRITION INFORMATION YOU CAN TRUST

Nutrition for Women is an easy-to-read reference guide for and about women. It is the first book of its kind to provide a bottom-line summary of scientific nutrition research from more than two thousand studies on the issues pertinent to women's health. *Nutrition for Women* distills scientific jargon into simple, understandable terms. It dispels the myths and presents the facts.

I WISH SOMEONE WOULD JUST TELL ME HOW TO EAT

"Everywhere I turn I hear different advice."

"I'm concerned about osteoporosis, but if I include dairy products in my diet for calcium, won't the fat in these foods increase my risk for heart disease?"

"I've thrown in the towel on fad diets. I just wish there was a diet I could live with that also would help me lose weight."

For many women, nutrition is more than a bit confusing. Diets abound, from the antiheart–disease diet to the PMS diet to the hundreds of weight-loss diets. Women want to simplify this nutrition puzzle and combine the best advice into one diet.

Nutrition for Women has done just that. This book includes the Healthy Woman's Diet, a diet plan that combines the nutritional advice for many of the disorders unique to women. The Healthy Woman's Diet takes into account how the dietary guidelines to prevent one illness, such as heart disease, might interact with the advice for another disorder, such as cancer, food cravings, or osteoporosis, and applies this combined advice to dietary recommendations for women throughout the many stages of their lives.

BUSY LIVES, QUICK REFERENCE

"With my busy life-style, I don't have time to sift through volumes of nutrition texts looking for answers. I need a source where I can get the truth fast."

Women juggling family, work, social, and other commitments don't have time to waste. Since most women don't have wives, secretaries, or maids, they must squeeze their own health concerns into their few fleeting moments of "free" time during the week.

Nutrition for Women is a quick-reference guide. Part I presents the Healthy Woman's Diet and all the skills necessary to adapt your habits to a more healthful eating style. In this section you will also find ten keys for successfully making changes and staying motivated. Part II presents the latest research on the role nutrition plays in the many stages of a woman's life, including weight management, pregnancy, exercise, menopause, and the senior years. Part III presents easy-to-read summaries and dietary recommendations based on current research for each disorder from AIDS to yeast infections.

SIMPLE ANSWERS TO COMPLEX ISSUES

Nutrition is a new and evolving science. While women want absolute answers, often only limited information is available for making dietary recommendations. It is this battlefield between incomplete supply and high demand that is fertile ground for misinformation.

For this book to be an accurate source deserving of your trust, I have made every effort to weigh the scientific literature and present the facts when there are facts, and possibilities when there are no facts. For this reason, take the word "might" seriously when it is used to link any aspect of nutrition with the possible prevention or treatment of a disease.

Researching and writing this book on and for women has been a joy. I hope it serves you well.

—Elizabeth Somer, M.A., R.D.

Introduction

It's Not "All in Your Head"

For centuries women's health complaints have been dismissed as being "all in their heads." Insecurity, depression, and irritability the week before menstruation signaled emotionalism; a craving for sweets, lack of willpower. Reporting these symptoms to a physician, husband, or friend was often met with only a gentle smile and a not-so-soothing recommendation to take it easy. Because of inherently vague symptoms such as lethargy, depression, mood swings, headaches, and even fluid retention, these conditions were poorly understood by the medical community.

Times are changing. Numerous emotional and physical symptoms that at one time went undiagnosed are now recognized as stemming from specific metabolic processes, many of which are affected by diet. The mood swings, food cravings, and anxiety many women experience before their periods now have a name—Premenstrual syndrome (PMS)—and can be partially alleviated by changes in diet and exercise. Poor concentration, memory problems, and fatigue could be a result of something as simple as iron deficiency. Other mood and emotional problems have been linked to sugar, vitamin deficiencies, and even caffeine consumption.

Until recently many diseases were considered the inevitable consequence of growing old. The frail, stooped old lady with the protruding abdomen was a woman's destiny. Now researchers acknowledge that this condition—osteoporosis—can be prevented or at least dramatically slowed by exercise and increasing dietary intake of calcium. Numerous age-related conditions from cataracts and skin aging to bowel disorders, heart disease, and many of the emotional and physical changes related to menopause also might be prevented, or the symptoms reduced, by a few changes in diet. With regular exercise there is every reason to feel vibrant, radiant, and youthful in your sixties, seventies, and beyond.

REPROGRAMMING THE AGING PROCESS

You cannot avoid growing old, but there is no reason you must succumb to the aging process. The belief that you are at the mercy of Mother Nature stems from the era when we didn't understand the alternatives. Many conditions associated with aging and ill health result from faltering defenses that could be strengthened by a low-fat, nutrient-dense diet plus regular exercise.

For example, consuming ample amounts of the antioxidant nutrients, including beta carotene, vitamin C, vitamin E, and selenium, strengthens one of the body's basic defense systems against aging. Optimal intake of the trace minerals iron, zinc, and copper, and many of the vitamins builds the body's immune system and protects against colds, infections, premature aging, and many diseases, including cancer and arthritis.

By staying fit, that is, by eating a low-fat, nutrient-dense diet and moving daily, you can reprogram your body's aging process. Basically, what you eat and how much you move can make the difference between feeling and looking great or, at best, just getting by while the aging process advances toward disease and disability.

ROOM FOR IMPROVEMENT

Your diet must work with you rather than against you to maximize your health potential. While there is always room for improvement, the good news is that it is never too late to start.

As recently as five years ago, preventing clinical nutrient deficiencies was considered the extent of a woman's nutritional concerns. That consensus is changing. Even if women did consume "balanced diets," which they don't, those diets might not be good enough to prevent certain degenerative diseases or emotional problems.

Research has repeatedly shown that women's diets have a long way to go. Granted, we consume less whole milk and beef, and consequently less saturated fat and cholesterol, than women did ten years ago. The 29 percent decrease in heart disease reflects these dietary changes. However, intakes of polyunsaturated fats, such as vegetable oils and margarine, have skyrocketed, and the average fiber intake is still only one-third the recommended amount (that is, 10 grams versus 30+ grams). Women are eating more chicken than beef, but the chicken is fried. (There is the equivalent of five pats of butter in one serving of Chicken McNuggets.) In an effort to lose weight, we are eating more salads, but those salads are smothered in high-fat dressings. Despite recommendations to increase complex carbohydrate foods, such as bread, rice, pasta, and cereals, women still consume less than one-half the amount of these foods that their grandmothers did in 1910. Today, women consume more French fries, sugar, cake, and doughnuts than pasta. These food choices increase the intake of fat and sugar and jeopardize the nutritional adequacy of the diet.

FOOD AND MOOD

Women tend to choose food to meet needs other than health. More than half of all women eat to relax, and nearly as many turn to sweets when they are depressed. In fact, two of the top three sources of carbohydrates in the typical American woman's diet are sugar and soft drinks. (Soft drinks supply two and a half times more of total calories than does low-fat milk.)

Women are also much more likely than men to have a specific "comfort" food, such as chocolate. Research now shows that these cravings might be a way of self-regulating mood, since these foods alter brain chemistry, produce a calming effect, and temporarily relieve depression. (See pages 349–56 for more information on food and mood.)

WHY AREN'T WOMEN GETTING ENOUGH?

It is no surprise that women's diets are low in many essential nutrients. A woman's special physiology makes her more vulnerable than a man to nutrient deficiencies during different stages of her life, such as puberty, pregnancy, and menopause. One out of every two women consumes less than two-thirds the Recommended Dietary Allowance (RDA) for folic acid, vitamin E, iron, zinc, calcium, magnesium, copper, vitamin A, vitamin D, and many of the B vitamins. (See pages 19–23 for more information on the RDAs.) Many of these deficiencies are caused by eating too many processed foods, fast foods, and convenience items that are high in fat and sugar and low in nutrients. For example, the average woman consumes 13 teaspoons of sugar daily or 265 calories from foods that supply little or no nutritional quality.

Women also diet. The average daily calorie intake for women in the United

States ranges from 1,400 to 1,800 calories. In comparison, men usually consume more than 2,500 calories daily. It is virtually impossible to meet even RDA levels of all vitamins and minerals when food intake is restricted to these amounts.

Women do not consume even minimal amounts of the recommended foods to prevent clinical deficiencies, let alone the amounts needed to prevent cancer, heart disease, premature aging, and other conditions such as PMS and osteoporosis. For example, women on average consume 5 IU (International Units) to 10 IU of vitamin E daily. The RDA for vitamin E is 12 IU, which seems paltry in comparison to the 200 IU to 400 IU used in most research studies on cancer prevention. Other nutrients, such as beta carotene and vitamin C, needed in greater amounts than previously recognized, can be obtained from the diet if a woman consumes at least five servings of fruits and vegetables each day. In short, women are not consuming enough of the right foods.

LESS IS MORE

Despite busy life-styles, careers, and family and social responsibilities, women must take time to take care of themselves. Health does not just happen. Your body will automatically deteriorate, and with increasing speed, unless you take an active role in keeping it fine-tuned.

The habits that support a healthy body are simple and in most cases require only minor adjustments in an otherwise healthful life-style. However, they are not instinctive. Your body cannot automatically choose nutritious foods, especially in light of modern distractions and highly sophisticated marketing and advertising techniques. Consequently, you must make a conscious effort to treat it well by eating nutritious food.

The most important dietary change you can make for your health, waistline, and appearance is to eat less fat and more minimally processed, fiber-rich foods. Less fat means more nutrients consumed for each spoonful of food. Less fat means more food can be eaten at a lower calorie cost. Less fat means a lower body weight and risk for diseases, from heart disease to cancer. Less fat means a longer and healthier life.

As the population ages, women are becoming more serious about eating for health and sorting through the conflicting claims to find diets they can live with. They also are standing up for their rights. A growing army of diet-weary women are abandoning their bathroom scales and saying "Enough," and rightfully so. In the past several decades, women have fallen prey to every get-thin-quick product, from the sublime to the ridiculous. At best, diets don't work, and at worst, they may compromise health, disease resistance, and life spans. A new movement is rising out of the ashes of burned weight-loss books, pills, and programs—one that for the first time focuses on health, not hips, thighs, or pocketbooks.

BECOMING YOUR OWN NUTRITION ADVOCATE

On the one hand, it is a relief to know that many of the ills women have faced are not "all in their heads," that there are physical and possibly nutritional bases for many of these conditions. On the other hand, this means you are at least partially responsible for taking charge of your health and nutritional status in an effort to achieve and maintain your healthiest self.

The best way to be your own nutrition advocate is to stay informed. You need to understand nutrition basics and then design an individualized diet and supplement plan based on a review of the current nutrition and medical research. (See table on page 6.)

Nutrition Basics

Most of the chemicals and compounds needed to maintain health are manufactured in the body. In many cases, the body makes one nutrient from other nutrients. The B vitamin niacin, for example, can be manufactured from an amino acid called tryptophan, or one amino acid (the building blocks for protein) can be made from another.

More than forty-five substances cannot be manufactured either in sufficient quantities or at all and therefore must be obtained from the diet. These include protein, carbohydrates, fat, vitamins, minerals, and water. Protein, carbohydrate, and fat supply energy or calories, while the other nutrients do not. These six categories of nutrients can be obtained from a variety of foods in a wide variety of combinations and calorie intakes.

The essential nutrients work in teams, with each of the millions of metabolic processes in the body requiring two or more nutrients for normal function. For example, most women know they need iron to build red blood cells. However, red blood cells also need calories, protein, vitamin E, vitamin C, most of the B vitamins, copper, zinc, and other minerals to function properly. Poor dietary intake of one or more of these nutrients, even if iron intake is adequate, will reduce the formation or activity of red blood cells and compromise health.

Rating Your Health

Total your score on the following quiz twice a year to monitor your health behavior and keep yourself "on track."

1. Do you eat a variety of fresh fruits and vegetables, whole grains, legumes, nonfat dairy products, and extra-lean meats?
   Always 5
   Usually 3
   Sometimes 0
2. Do you purchase low-fat foods, prepare foods without fat, and order low-fat foods in restaurants?
   Always 5
   Usually 3
   Sometimes 0
3. How often do you use refined sugars, including honey?
   Seldom 2
   Sometimes 1
   Often . . . . −1
4. Do you limit the amount of salt in cooking and at the table and avoid salty processed foods?
   Always 1
   Usually 0
   Sometimes . . . . −1
5. Are you at or close to your desirable weight?
   I'm 11 pounds or more below my desirable weight . . . . −3
   I'm within 10 pounds of my desirable weight 6
   I'm 11 to 15 pounds above my desirable weight . . . . −1
   I'm 16 to 30 pounds above my desirable weight . . . . −3
   I'm more than 30 pounds above my desirable weight . . . . −6
   Most of my excess fat is in my abdomen and chest . . . . −3
6. Have you frequently dieted in the past?
   No 1
   Yes . . . . −2
7. How much time do you spend in physical activity, that is, walking, bicycling, running, or other structured activity?
   60 minutes or more/5 days a week 13

30 to 59 minutes/at least 4 days a week 10
15 to 29 minutes/at least 4 days a week 5
Less than 1 hour per week 0

8. Do you take time to stretch before and after exercise?
Yes, always 1
Yes, but only sometimes 0
No, never . . . . −1

9. Do you overdo it and sometimes exercise despite pain or fatigue?
No 0
Yes . . . . −3

10. Do you smoke or are you frequently around smokers?
No 4
Yes . . . . −5

11. Do you drink alcohol?
No, or less than one drink a day 1
Yes, about two drinks a day 0
Yes, often, and I frequently get drunk . . . . −5

12. Do you use illegal drugs?
No 2
Yes . . . . −5

13. Do you use prescription or nonprescription drugs?
Seldom, and only as directed 2
Yes, but I don't follow directions . . . . −1

14. How well do you sleep?
I sleep soundly for 7 to 8 hours nightly 2
I sometimes have restless nights or often sleep less than 6 hours . . . . −1

15. How stressful is your life?
Seldom experience stress, and when I do, it is only mild tension 2
I frequently experience tension or anxiety . . . . −2
I am constantly under stress . . . . −5

16. Do you like your job and your home life?
Yes, I am very happy with both work and home 3
I have my good days and bad days 1
I hate my job, home, or both . . . . −3

Rating Your Health *(continued)*

17. Do you like who you are?

I like myself and am confident about my future and capabilities 3

I am somewhat comfortable with who I am but have doubts about my future 1

I don't like who I am . . . . −3

18. How much control do you feel you have over your life and your health?

I have considerable control 3

I have some control 0

I have little control . . . . −3

19. How often do you have medical checkups?

Regularly, once or twice a year 2

Every 4 to 5 years . . . . −1

I seldom have checkups . . . . −2

20. Do you give yourself monthly breast self-exams?

Yes 2

No . . . . −2

Total your score to obtain a rough idea of your health status:

Score of 40 to 60: You take excellent care of yourself and deserve a pat on the back for a job well done.

Score of 20 to 39: You take good care of your health.

Score of 0 to 19: Your health care practices are marginal and could use improvement.

Score of −15 to −1: Your health may be in jeopardy.

Score less than −15: Take action to improve your health habits since you are in the "red zone" for disease down the road.

THE CALORIE-CONTAINING NUTRIENTS: PROTEIN, CARBOHYDRATE, AND FAT

The nutrients that supply calories are protein, carbohydrate, and fat. Although alcohol supplies calories, it is not considered a nutrient since it is not necessary for life and is harmful to health when consumed in excess. Consuming too much of any calorie-containing food, not just fat, can result in weight gain.

Calorie-dense foods are foods that supply a large amount of calories for relatively few nutrients. These foods are usually high in sugar or fat and include butter and oils, fatty cheese, avocados, fatty cuts of meat, fatty or sugary desserts, and many processed foods. In contrast, nutrient-dense foods supply large amounts of nutrients for relatively few calories. Examples of nutrient-dense foods include fresh fruit and vegetables, cooked dried beans and peas, nonfat milk, whole grain breads and cereals, fish, extra-lean meat, and chicken without the skin.

Protein: Proteins are composed of large strings of amino acids, eight to ten of which cannot be manufactured in the body and must be supplied in the diet. Consequently, they are called the "essential" amino acids, not because they are more important than the other thirteen to fifteen amino acids but because they must be supplied regularly from food. Most foods contain at least some protein, with the exception of fruit, sugar, and oils or fats; however, the best sources include extra-lean meat, chicken, fish, low-fat milk products, and cooked dried beans and peas combined with whole grain breads and cereals.

Protein is essential for tissue repair, maintenance, and growth. Many essential body compounds are composed of protein, including hemoglobin in red blood cells, many hormones, all enzymes (the body's catalysts for all metabolic reactions), and antibodies in the immune system. Other proteins maintain the fluid balance in the body or buffer against changes in the acid-base balance. In a pinch, protein can also be broken down for energy when carbohydrate and fat intakes are low.

Too little protein can result in severe damage to most body processes; however, most American women typically consume too much. The overemphasis on protein and planning menus around meat has led to a protein excess, with most people consuming two to four times as much protein as they need. For example, a breakfast of eggs, bacon, toast, and milk provides almost the entire day's requirement for protein. A bowl of oatmeal, toast, and milk provides more than a third of the day's protein allotment. Even athletes trying to build muscle do not need to increase protein intake. Since their diets typically contain more protein than is required, there is no need for protein powders or extra servings of protein-rich foods. (See pages 191–93 for more information on protein and bodybuilding.)

Carbohydrates: Carbohydrates are supplied as simple sugars in fruits, honey, and sugar, and as complex carbohydrates or starches in grains, beans, and vegetables. Processed foods high in simple sugars usually are calorie-dense, nutrient-poor selections, even if they have been arbitrarily fortified with a handful of nutrients. In contrast, the simple sugars in fruits come packaged with fiber, vitamins, minerals, and water, and are considered nutrient-dense inclusions in the diet. Minimally processed complex carbohydrates, from whole grain bread to potatoes, also supply ample amounts of vitamins, minerals, fiber, and protein, and are considered the mainstay of a low-fat, nutrient-dense diet.

Carbohydrate-rich foods supply the body with its primary source of fuel—glucose. Glucose is the form of sugar in the blood, is stored in the muscles, and is the main fuel source for the nervous system, including the brain. Carbohydrates are also essential for the efficient burning of body fat and for sparing protein for use in building muscles and other protein-rich tissues.

Fats: Dietary fats include a variety of compounds that are insoluble in water, including cholesterol, saturated and unsaturated fats, and linoleic acid. Cholesterol is manufactured by the body and is not required in the diet. Although it supplies no calories, this form of fat is associated with an increased risk for developing heart disease. Triglycerides are the primary fat in the diet and in the blood, and are the storage form of fat in the body. They can be either saturated or unsaturated. If they are unsaturated, they can be either monounsaturated, as is olive oil and canola oil, or polyunsaturated, as is safflower oil or corn oil.

Saturated and unsaturated fats are the most concentrated source of energy, supplying more than twice the calories per ounce of carbohydrate and protein. In addition, the body prefers to store dietary fat as body fat rather than converting it to energy. Consequently, this calorie source is associated with weight problems. Excess fat intake also increases the risk of cancer, heart disease, diabetes, and many other degenerative disorders.

Linoleic acid is a component of polyunsaturated fats and is the only fat the body cannot manufacture. It therefore is called the "essential" fatty acid and can be obtained from polyunsaturated fats found in vegetable oils, nuts, seeds, and wheat germ. Lecithin is a type of fat called a phospholipid, which means it contains water-soluble and fat-soluble sides. It is a source of choline, is manufactured in the body, and does not supply calories.

The body needs some dietary fat to ensure adequate intake of linoleic acid and to help in the absorption of the fat-soluble vitamins—A, E, D, and K. However, other than personal preference and taste, there is no benefit to eating a diet that has more than 20 percent of its calories from fat; currently, most Americans consume 37 percent or more, almost twice as much as is needed or even healthful.

DIETARY SOURCES OF THE CALORIE NUTRIENTS
Most foods contain a mixture of protein, carbohydrate, and fat, although the combination varies greatly from one food to another. For example, nuts are primarily

A Summary of the Vitamins, Their Functions, and Toxic Effects*

NUTRIENT	FUNCTIONS	TOXIC EFFECTS
Vitamin A (RDA: 4,000 IU)	Eyesight, healthy tissues, bone growth, immunity, reproduction, anticancer agent, skin	More than 50,000 IU causes joint pain, hair loss, itching, dry skin, weakness, fatigue
Beta carotene (RDA: none)	Same as vitamin A	No toxicity symptoms except possibility of menstrual problems with long-term excessive intake
Vitamin D (RDA: 200–400 IU)	Strong bones, muscles, nerves, hearing, immunity, possibly anticancer agent	More than 10,000 IU causes nausea, vomiting, loss of appetite, headache, bone pain. More than 1,200 IU may cause kidney stones or calcification of soft tissue
Vitamin E (RDA: 12 IU)	Antioxidant against cancer, heart disease, eye disorders, aging, diabetes, arthritis	No adverse symptoms with doses under 800 IU
Vitamin K (RDA: 55–65 mcg)	Blood clotting	Large doses cause anemia, jaundice in infants
Vitamin B1 (RDA: 1.0–1.5 mg)	Energy metabolism, nerve function, converts excess calories to fat	Large doses (5,000–10,000 mg) cause headaches, irritability, rapid pulse, weakness
Vitamin B2 (RDA: 1.2–1.3 mg)	Energy metabolism, growth and development, hormones, red blood cells, possible antiprostate cancer agent	No toxicity symptoms reported
Niacin (RDA: 13–15 mg)	Energy metabolism, hormones, red blood cells, detoxification of drugs, lowers blood	Nicotinic acid: More than 100 mg causes flushing, tingling, itching. Long-term effects in-

(continues)

NUTRIENT	FUNCTIONS	TOXIC EFFECTS
	cholesterol, improves some psychiatric disorders	clude nausea, diarrhea, ulcers at 100–300 mg. Niacinamide: More than 300 mg causes headache and nausea. More than 3,000 mg causes fatigue, hives, and sore mouth
Vitamin B6 (RDA: 1.4–1.6 mg)	Energy, protein, and fat metabolism; asthma; improves depression, irritability, insomnia; carpal tunnel syndrome; premenstrual syndrome; heart disease; immunity; kidney disorders	More than 500 mg: Potentially irreversible nerve damage, including impaired walking, numbness, tingling, poor sense of touch
Vitamin B12 (RDA: 2.0 mcg)	Energy, protein, and fat metabolism; nerve function; red blood cells; maintains genetic code	No toxic effects reported
Folic Acid (RDA: **400 mcg)	Maintains genetic code; red blood cells; growth and development of all cells; helps prevent cervical cancer	May mask a vitamin B12 deficiency at doses of more than 1,000 mcg. May interfere with anticonvulsant medications
Biotin (RDA: 30–100 mcg)	Energy, protein, and fat metabolism	No toxic effects reported
Pantothenic Acid (RDA: 4–7 mg)	Energy, protein, and fat metabolism; helps manufacture cholesterol, bile, vitamin D, red blood cells, and some hormones; stimulates wound healing	More than 200 mg might cause diarrhea, fluid retention, memory loss, drowsiness, depression, nausea

A Summary of the Vitamins, Their Functions, and Toxic Effects* *(continued)*

NUTRIENT	FUNCTIONS	TOXIC EFFECTS
Vitamin C (RDA: 60 mg)	Formation of collagen, antiallergy agent, anticancer agent, anticataract agent, prevention of heart disease, immunity, stress	More than 1,000–2,000 mg might cause impaired immunity, kidney stones

*Values are for nonpregnant, non-breast-feeding women.
**Previous RDA values are used here because the most recent RDAs were decreased despite extensive research showing that more, not less, of this nutrient might improve health indicators.

fat but also contain protein. Meat is considered a protein-rich food but also supplies fat. Cooked dried beans and peas are excellent sources of both protein and carbohydrate, with little fat. Milk contains protein, carbohydrate (as lactose or milk sugar), and varying amounts of fat depending on whether it is nonfat, low-fat, or whole milk. One guideline for balancing these nutrients is to consume approximately 12 percent to 15 percent of calories from protein, no more than 30 percent (preferably less) from fat, and the rest from carbohydrate (primarily complex and minimally processed sources).

VITAMINS AND MINERALS

Vitamins and minerals are consumed in much smaller amounts than the calorie-counting nutrients, but they are just as important for health. Many substances have been touted as "vitamins"; however, a substance must be essential for normal body functioning and create deficiency symptoms when removed from the diet in order to qualify as a vitamin. Consequently, vitamin B15, pangamic acid, the bioflavonoids, and vitamin P, promoted as "essential nutrients" in the popular press, are not true vitamins.

Vitamins are either fat- or water-soluble. The fat-soluble vitamins include A, D, E, and K. The water-soluble vitamins include the B vitamins—B1, B2, B6, B12, folic acid, pantothenic acid, biotin, and niacin—and vitamin C. In the past only the fat-soluble vitamins were thought to be stored in the body and capable of reaching toxic levels if consumed in excess. In recent years some of the water-soluble vitamins, such as vitamin B6, also have shown toxicity symptoms when consumed in excess for long periods of time. Exceptions to this rule are vitamins C, E, and beta carotene, which show relatively no harmful effects even when consumed in amounts several times the recommendation. (See table on page 11.)

Some vitamins can be manufactured in the body but not always in sufficient amounts to ensure health, so dietary sources remain essential. These vitamins include vitamin D and niacin. Vitamin K, biotin, and other B vitamins are manufactured by bacteria in the intestines, and appreciable amounts are absorbed into the body.

Essential minerals are inorganic substances (that is, they do not contain carbon) required in small amounts to sustain life and promote health. Twenty minerals and mineral-related compounds are recognized as essential. They include the following:

calcium	fluoride	molybdenum	silicon
chloride	iodine	nickel	sodium
chromium	iron	phosphorus	sulfur
cobalt	magnesium	potassium	vanadium
copper	manganese	selenium	zinc

These minerals function interdependently; consequently, optimal dietary intake requires a delicate balance among them. Many minerals compete in the intestine for absorption, so overconsumption of one mineral could reduce absorption of another and result in what is called a "secondary deficiency." For example, large supplemental doses of iron reduce zinc absorption, and excessive calcium intake impairs magnesium absorption.

The proper balance between minerals also enhances their use in the body. Copper and iron work together in the formation of red blood cells. Magnesium and calcium work jointly in the regulation of muscle contraction, nerve function, and bone formation. The bottom line is that diet is the best source of minerals since a wide variety of foods supplies the best balance of minerals. If supplements are used, they should be chosen wisely to maximize mineral use and reduce the risk of developing secondary deficiencies. (See pages 111–16 for guidelines in choosing a supplement.) (See table on page 15.)

Selected Minerals, Their Functions, and Toxic Effects*

NUTRIENT	FUNCTIONS	TOXIC EFFECTS
Calcium (RDA: 800–1,200 mg)	Bones and teeth, blood clotting, anticancer agent, lowers blood pressure, muscle contraction, nerve transmission	More than 3,000 mg might cause nausea, diarrhea, calcification of soft tissue, reduced zinc and iron absorption, impaired vitamin K metabolism, loss of calcium from bones
Chromium (RDA: 50–200 mcg)	Blood sugar regulation, lowers blood cholesterol, protein synthesis	No known toxic effects reported
Copper (RDA: 1.5 mg–3.0 mg)	Enzymes, hormones, red blood cells, hair and skin color, antioxidant, possible anticancer agent, blood sugar regulation, bone formation	Toxicity is rare. More than 20 mg causes nausea, vomiting
Iron (RDA: **18 mg)	Red blood cells, oxygen transport within cells, immunity	More than 25 mg might cause constipation or diarrhea. Excess intake (more than 100 mg) causes iron overload characterized by abdominal and joint pain, weight loss, fatigue, excess thirst, hunger, yeast infections. Women with underlying genetic predisposition or kidney disorders develop toxic symptoms at lower doses
Magnesium (RDA: **300 mg)	Energy, protein, and fat metabolism; removes toxic waste	More than 600 mg might cause diarrhea. More than 1,700 mg

*Values are for nonpregnant, non-breast-feeding women.
**Previous RDA values are used here because the most recent RDAs were decreased despite extensive research showing that more, not less, of this nutrient might improve health indicators.

(continues)

NUTRIENT	FUNCTIONS	TOXIC EFFECTS
	products; muscle relaxation; nerve transmission; heart-beat; helps prevent heart disease; premenstrual syndrome; reduces pain of intermittent claudication; helps prevent high blood pressure	might cause low blood pressure, drowsiness, slurred speech, nausea
Manganese (RDA: 2.5–5.0 mg)	Connective tissue, fat metabolism, blood clotting, protein formation and digestion	Excessive intake might cause secondary deficiency of iron
Molybdenum (RDA: 75–250 mg)	Formation of uric acid, iron metabolism, normal growth and development	Toxicity varies with age group. More than 10 mg might cause goutlike symptoms, including pain and joint swelling
Selenium (RDA: 50–55 mcg)	Antioxidant against cancer, heart disease, aging, and arthritis	More than 2,400 mcg causes brittle hair and fingernails, dizziness, fatigue, jaundice, nausea, diarrhea, discolored skin
Zinc (RDA: 12 mg)	Numerous enzymes, detoxification of alcohol, protein synthesis, bone growth, protein digestion, energy metabolism, insulin regulation, genetic code, taste, wound healing, vitamin A blood levels, immunity, hormones, blood pressure, heart rate, oil glands of the skin, anorexia, anticancer agent	More than 50 mg might cause secondary deficiency of copper. More than 80 mg might lower HDL (good) cholesterol. More than 150 mg might impair immune function

WATER: THE MOST IMPORTANT NUTRIENT

Water is the most important and yet often the most likely forgotten nutrient. The body of a 135-pound woman contains 81 pounds of water, while the remaining 54 pounds come from a combination of fat, protein, carbohydrate, and minerals. Water is essential for all body processes. It surrounds and fills all cells and tissues, helps regulate body temperature, lubricates joints, and transports oxygen and nutrients to all the tissues. Water cushions the organs and protects them against injury, helps maintain the proper acidity of the body, and keeps the skin moist. Adequate intake of water helps prevent fluid retention and the fatigue and faulty regulation of body temperature associated with dehydration.

People who are only moderately active should consume at least six to eight glasses of water daily. More active people should consume more than eight glasses. Since thirst is a poor indicator of water needs, you should consume twice as much water as it takes to quench thirst. Other fluids such as coffee, tea, or caffeinated colas, certain medications, and alcohol act as diuretics and increase daily water requirements.

FIBER

Fiber is an umbrella term for a family of compounds that are indigestible. Dietary fiber adds bulk to the stool and helps move waste through the intestine but is not absorbed by the body. Insoluble fibers such as cellulose are found in wheat bran, celery, and other vegetables, and are associated with a reduced risk for developing intestinal cancers and digestive tract disorders such as constipation and diverticulosis. Soluble fibers, such as pectin in fruit, oat bran, and the fiber in cooked dried beans and peas, are associated with a reduced risk for developing heart disease and diabetes.

No single food supplies all the soluble and insoluble fiber needed for health, so a wide variety of minimally processed, high-fiber foods is needed in the diet. Studies linking fiber to a reduced risk for disease have investigated naturally occurring fiber-rich foods, such as vegetables, fruits, beans, and whole grain breads. There is no evidence that fabricated fiber foods such as bran flakes protect against disease. Other processed fiber foods such as commercial bran muffins are often high in sugar, fat, or salt.

In general, the less processed a food, the greater its fiber content. The average American woman consumes less than 10 grams of fiber daily, while intakes of 27 grams to 35 grams are considered optimal. Excessive fiber intake—50 grams or more a day—could irritate the intestinal lining, cause diarrhea, or even reduce

The United States Recommended Daily Allowances *(U.S. RDAs)*

NUTRIENTS THAT MUST APPEAR ON THE LABEL	U.S. RDA	NUTRIENTS THAT MAY APPEAR ON THE LABEL	U.S. RDA
Vitamin A	5,000 IU	Vitamin D	400 IU
Vitamin C	65 mg	Vitamin E	30 IU
Vitamin B1	1.5 mg	Vitamin B6	2 mg
Vitamin B2	1.7 mg	Folic Acid	400 mcg
Niacin	20 mg	Vitamin B12	6 mcg
Calcium	1,000 mg	Phosphorus	1,000 mg
Iron	18 mg	Iodine	150 mg
		Magnesium	400 mg
		Zinc	15 mg
		Copper	2 mg
		Biotin	300 mcg
		Pantothenic Acid	10 mg

the absorption of certain minerals. The recommended daily amount of fiber can be obtained from the following foods:

5 servings of fruits and vegetables	12–23 grams
6 servings of whole grain breads/cereals	13
1 cup cooked dried beans and peas	9
Total	34–45 grams

STORING NUTRIENTS IN THE BODY

The body requires a constant supply of all the essential nutrients, but fortunately it has developed complex systems for storing most nutrients for later use. For example, the bones accumulate calcium, the liver stores vitamin A and other nutrients, the muscles store glucose, fat tissues reserve extra calories as fat, and every cell in the body has a backup supply of iron. As long as the weekly diet is optimal, these stores are maintained and are readily available when dietary intake is temporarily inadequate. However, repeated poor food choices, especially during times of increased need, can drain many of the body's nutrient stores, jeopardize health, and reduce resistance to disease.

Minimally processed foods contain a wide variety of nutrients, but no one food supplies all forty-five-plus of the essential nutrients. Although milk is an excellent source of protein, vitamin D, calcium, magnesium, and vitamin B2, it contains little iron. Extra-lean meat is an excellent source of protein, iron, B vitamins, and zinc but contains little or no calcium and vitamin D. The need to combine a variety of foods in the diet for optimal nutrient intake (as defined by the Recommended Dietary Allowances or RDAs) has led to the concept of the "balanced diet."

The Recommended Dietary Allowances (RDAs)

As with any profession, the science of nutrition needs standards. Among these standards are the Recommended Dietary Allowances—or RDAs—that were developed by a panel of experts at the National Research Council's Food and Nutrition Board. The RDAs list appropriate nutrient intakes for people based on age and gender. When this panel feels there is insufficient evidence to set a specific RDA for a nutrient, then a range of desirable intakes called the "Estimated Safe and Adequate Daily Dietary Intakes" is developed.

A separate set of recommendations called the U.S. Recommended Daily Allowances or U.S. RDAs have been developed by the Food and Drug Administration (FDA) and are extrapolations from the RDAs. The U.S. RDAs are used specifically for labeling food products and supplements. Unlike the National Research Council's RDAs, the U.S. RDAs do not vary with age and gender. Usually the highest value from the RDA is used as the standard for the U.S. RDA. For example, the highest RDA for vitamin A for any age or gender is 5,000 IU, so that is the value used for the U.S. RDAs. (See table on page 18).

THE RDAS: THE PROS AND CONS

There are several important aspects of the RDAs to consider. First, they are recommendations, not requirements, that are revised every five years based on a review of the research. Usually they contain a "margin of safety" so that a person's nutritional needs are met even when less than the RDA is consumed.

Second, they are recommendations for healthy people and are not designed to meet the additional needs of people who are ill, stressed, taking medications, or have other conditions that might increase nutrient needs.

Third, they represent an estimated range within which most healthy people's nutrient needs should fall. Because individual needs can vary as much as two hundredfold, so may individual RDA requirements.

Fourth, they were originally developed in 1941 for quantity food production in the military, not for planning and evaluating individual daily intake. The RDAs are therefore best used as "averages" for large groups of people, and their usefulness in assessing the nutritional adequacy of one woman's diet is limited. In short, the RDAs are used mostly because they are the only guidelines available.

Fifth, the RDAs are designed for the average woman (5 feet 4 inches to 5 feet 5 inches) with an average weight (120 to 143 pounds), body fat percentage (approximately 18 percent to 25 percent body fat), nutrient absorption and excretion rate, stress level, and hereditary pattern. The RDAs must be adjusted when data falls outside any one of these parameters.

HOW ACCURATE ARE THE RDAS?

The RDAs, once considered the nutritional Ten Commandments, are currently a controversial topic in the nutrition community. They were first designed to prevent clinical nutrient deficiency diseases such as scurvy and beriberi. The recommended amounts were based on minimum needs plus a little extra to prevent these disorders.

Recent research has uncovered numerous other nutrient-disease links that far exceed these original clinical deficiencies. Chromium is now suspected to lower heart disease and diabetes risk. Magnesium and calcium help prevent and control hypertension. Vitamin C and vitamin E are useful in the prevention of certain forms of cancer. Vitamin B6 might help in the treatment of mild depression. Iron, zinc, and numerous other nutrients strengthen the immune system. The antioxidant nutrients, including beta carotene, vitamin E, selenium, and vitamin C, are implicated in the prevention of many diseases, from heart disease to cataracts, and in the prevention of premature aging. Folic acid helps prevent neural tube defects and possibly cervical cancer. The RDA for vitamin A is based on its ability to prevent xerophthalmia (a rare eye disorder), but does not recognize this vitamin's link to cancer prevention. In fact, none of these associations were considered when developing the RDAs. It now appears that an RDA that simply prevents clinical deficiencies is not necessarily the optimal daily recommendation for promoting the best possible health.

Even within the limits of the RDAs, some researchers question whether recommendations are high enough. Researchers at the Medical College of Wisconsin in Milwaukee investigated the vitamin C recommendation of 100 mg to determine if it was adequate to maintain optimal vitamin C status for smokers. Their results showed that smokers require twice this amount of vitamin C, or 200 mg daily, to attain and maintain blood vitamin C levels similar to nonsmokers.

Researchers at the U.S.D.A. Human Nutrition Research Center in North Dakota report that the RDA for zinc, which is based on the assumption that at least 40 percent of the mineral is absorbed, is inadequate. Their study showed that as little as 17.6 percent of dietary zinc actually enters the bloodstream and is available for metabolic processes, indicating that the RDA would need to be doubled to meet even basic recommendations.

One reason for the discrepancies between research studies and the RDAs is that many of the RDAs were established based on typical, not optimal, dietary intakes. For example, the recommendations for folic acid and iron were reduced in the most recent version of the RDAs primarily because it is difficult for women to consume higher amounts. The adult RDAs for vitamin E (8 mg to 10 mg) are based primarily on "normal" dietary intakes and blood levels of the vitamin in "normal" individuals. In the support text for the RDAs, the authors state that daily intakes range from 7 mg to 11 mg for people consuming balanced diets of 2,000 to 3,000 calories. However, national nutrition surveys report that women's caloric intake falls below these figures and that they do not regularly consume a balanced diet.

RDAS VERSUS ODIS

A standard for optimal dietary intakes (ODIs) is needed. Unfortunately, there is insufficient information to make definitive ODI recommendations at this time. Until more is known about optimal nutrient intakes, it is best to strive for 100 percent of the RDA for all nutrients, including protein, vitamins, and minerals. Some nutrients, such as vitamin C, beta carotene, and vitamin E, might provide additional benefits at larger than RDA levels, while other nutrients can be toxic, such as vitamin A and vitamin D, and amounts should be limited to no more than 300 percent of the RDA.

Minerals work in critical ratios to one another, and excessive intake of one mineral could offset another. Minerals should therefore be consumed in 1-to-1 RDA ratios. For example, for iron the RDA is 18 mg, and for zinc it is 12 mg. If iron intake is doubled to 36 mg, then zinc intake should also be increased to 24 mg to maintain the 1-to-1 RDA ratio, which should help prevent secondary mineral deficiencies.

It is likely that the RDAs will undergo major revisions. Researchers at Louisiana State University speculate that recommendations eventually will be more precisely geared to different disorders. In the future, Level One of the RDA might propose 75 percent or more of the current recommendations for conditions that are completely prevented or cured with small amounts of a nutrient, much as clinical nutrient deficiency diseases are reversed with even minimal intakes.

Level Two of the RDA may suggest larger amounts of a nutrient, possibly 100 percent of the current RDA, to protect against certain conditions, with intakes less than this showing measurably greater disease risk. Level Three of the RDA could introduce amounts far in excess of current RDA levels for the prevention or treatment of more resistant disorders. For example, improvements in immunity are noted with increasingly greater amounts of vitamin E to levels much higher than 100 percent of current RDAs.

This approach to nutritional adequacy would allow people to design diet and supplement plans tailored to individual needs and could potentially make great strides in the prevention and treatment of many major diseases.

The "Balanced Diet"

Most people have been taught to equate nutrition with a "balanced diet." Nutritionists tell women to consume their nutrients from a balanced diet rather than from vitamin-mineral supplements. Mothers are concerned when their children do not eat a balanced diet. Teenage girls are told that soda pop is not part of a balanced diet, while the family meal planner worries about preparing at least one balanced meal for the family each day. People are supposed to know instinctively the components of a "balanced diet," but more often than not, this term brings more confusion than nutrition to the dinner table. Just what is a balanced diet, anyway?

THE BALANCED DIET IS BORN

The first evidence of a balanced diet dates possibly from the sixth century B.C. when a physician named Ho divided all known diseases into six categories. Each was thought to be caused by an imbalance in one of the six aspects of Ch'i, the breath of life. These aspects included fire, water, air, earth, wood, and metal, and eventually formed the basis of yin (moist-cool or feminine) and yang (dry-hot or masculine). A balance of yin and yang became the foundation of diet planning in the Far East.

The concept of a balanced diet was transported across Europe by the Crusaders and became popular because it promoted a longer life and an extension of youth. The concept of a balance between air, fire, water, and earth was translated into body humors called blood, bile, phlegm, and black bile, and the goal of a balanced diet was to maintain an equilibrium among these humors. Dietary advice, such as hot foods prescribed for a water-phlegm imbalance, flourished for centuries until a more advanced understanding evolved of the human body and the development of disease.

The balanced diet has come a long way since early history. Today, it provides all of the more than forty-five essential nutrients in sufficient quantities and in the proper proportion to each other to assure optimal nutritional health. A strict interpretation of this definition implies that a balanced diet would differ based on each person's age and unique genetic, biochemical, and environmental makeup. For practical purposes, however, a balanced diet must be simple and easy to follow as well as nutritious.

THE BASIC FOUR FOOD GROUPS PLAN

There are as many ways to obtain all the essential nutrients as there are cultures and food traditions in the world. The most widely used guideline in the United States is the Basic Four Food Groups Plan. This plan consists of four basic categories of foods and suggests that they be included in the daily menu in the following proportions: approximately one-third fruits and vegetables, one-third breads and cereals, one-sixth milk products, and one-sixth protein-rich foods such as meat, chicken, fish, and cooked dried beans and peas. The Basic Four Food Groups Plan is designed so the variety and quantity of nutrients consumed approximates the amounts specified by the Recommended Dietary Allowances (RDAs). The U.S. Department of Agriculture's "Food Guide Pyramid," published in 1992, is an improvement on the Basic Four, but it makes little mention of the saturated fats in meat and dairy products and mistakenly groups dried beans (a low-fat protein) with red meat.

The foods in the Basic Four Food Groups Plan are categorized according to their specific nutrient content. Meat is a good source of protein, B vitamins, zinc, and iron, while fruit and vegetables are reliable sources of vitamin C, beta caro-tene, fiber, and folic acid.

Avoiding one food group could jeopardize your nutritional status by increas-ing the risk of developing deficiencies of the nutrients supplied by that food group. For example, the milk group supplies more than 40 percent of a woman's need for vitamin B2 and calcium, and is the only reliable dietary source of vitamin D. Avoidance of milk products would require careful menu planning to ensure these nutrients were supplied in adequate amounts.

Certain women are at particular risk of nutrient deficiencies if a food group is avoided. Pregnant or breast-feeding women would have an especially difficult time meeting the RDAs for calcium if milk products were avoided. Zinc defi-ciency is common in vegetarians who avoid meat, chicken, and fish, the best dietary sources for this trace mineral. And it is nearly impossible to obtain accept-able amounts of beta carotene or vitamin E if a meat lover avoids fresh fruits and vegetables.

THE BASIC FOUR SHORTCOMINGS

The Basic Four Food Groups Plan is not without its faults. Its nutrient adequacy is dependent on specific food choices; therefore a diet based on the Basic Four can fall below the RDAs for any or all nutrients. For example, white bread contains a fraction of the trace minerals, fiber, and several vitamins found in 100 percent whole wheat bread. A hot dog barely meets the qualifications to be in the high-protein group and is considerably higher in fat and lower in vitamins and minerals than other lean selections such as chicken breast or fish. French-fried potatoes are a nutrient-poor alternative to broccoli, which is high in vitamin A, vitamin C, calcium, iron, folic acid, and other nutrients. Yet, according to national nutrition surveys, these nutrient-poor food selections are common.

Another shortcoming of the Basic Four is that it does not stipulate the type of food preparation. Frying or other methods that use fat or oil contribute consid-erably more calories than do steaming and broiling. For example, fried chicken contains more than twice the calories of broiled chicken but the same amount of protein, vitamins, and minerals. Broiled chicken is nutrient-dense, while fried chicken is not.

Processing has much to do with why the Basic Four cannot guarantee opti-mal nutrition. The nutrients that are low in typical American diets are also those that are removed during processing, such as vitamin B6, vitamin C, folic acid, chromium, zinc, selenium, fiber, and magnesium. Random fortification of some processed foods, such as ready-to-eat cereals, does not offset these poor nutrient intakes.

If followed to the letter, the Basic Four supplies about 1,200 to 1,500 calories. But optimal intake of many nutrients cannot be guaranteed on less than 2,000 to 3,000 calories daily. For example, a well-planned "balanced" diet supplies about 6 grams of iron for every 1,000 calories. Thus, in order to meet the daily recommendation for this mineral (18 mg) you must consume 3,000 calories. The average calorie intake for women, however, is between 1,421 and 1,607 calories. It comes as no surprise that data gathered from the U.S.D.A. Nationwide Food Consumption Survey found that a third of the population consumes below 70 percent of the RDA for iron.

Even qualified nutrition experts have difficulty planning diets that meet the RDA for all nutrients when energy intake is less than 1,600 to 2,000 calories, which is still hundreds of calories more than the Basic Four provides. In fact, the Basic Four does not supply adequate amounts of all nutrients to ensure the RDAs are met. An analysis of diets based on this plan shows that people eating the "balanced diet" would be low in vitamin E, vitamin B1, vitamin B6, folic acid, magnesium, zinc, fiber, and iron.

The Healthy Woman's Diet

The Healthy Woman's Diet resembles the Basic Four Food Groups Plan but comes much closer to an ideal balanced diet. This eating plan ensures optimal intake of all vitamins and minerals, and doing so reduces the risk of developing disease and aging prematurely. It can be tailored to personal preferences, tastes, and time demands.

The most important guideline in this low-fat, nutrient-dense diet is to limit dietary fat intake to less than 30 percent of total calories, saturated fat to less than 10 percent of calories, cholesterol to less than 300 mg per day, salt to slightly more than one teaspoon per day, and to consume between 25 and 35 grams of fiber each day.

While cutting the fat, you should increase consumption of fresh fruits and vegetables, especially dark orange or green vegetables and citrus fruits, to at least five servings daily. Whole grain breads and cereals should be increased to at least six servings daily. At least three to four calcium-rich foods should be included in the daily menu, including nonfat milk or yogurt, low-fat cheeses, dark green leafy vegetables, tofu, or canned salmon with the bones.

Consume at least 2,000 calories of the above nutrient-dense foods and select less nutritious foods only after all other nutrient needs for the day have been met. Limit sugar intake to less than 10 percent of calories. Consider a moderate-dose vitamin/mineral supplement when calorie intake drops below 2,000 calories. Make sure to balance calorie intake with exercise to maintain a desirable weight, and avoid repeated, unsuccessful attempts at weight loss.

As part of this low-fat, nutrient-dense eating plan, you should limit alcohol to five drinks or less each week. Pregnant women or women considering getting pregnant should avoid all alcoholic beverages until after the baby is born. Finally, divide the day's total food intake into several small meals and snacks throughout the day. Skills for applying these guidelines to menu planning, shopping, and food preparation are discussed in detail in chapters 1 and 2.

OTHER BALANCED DIETS

The balanced diet common in the United States is not typical fare in other countries. Many American diets emphasize meat and plan the menu around the protein-laden entrée. By contrast, the food habits of populations in less industrialized countries resemble the Healthy Woman's Diet by emphasizing grains and vegetables and using meats as a condiment in the meal. Whole grains constitute the bulk of the diet in many nonindustrialized cultures, followed by cooked fresh vegetables, dried beans, and raw vegetables. Vitamin B12–containing foods, such as meat, chicken, fish, and milk products, are consumed in smaller quantities. A diet based on these five food categories (whole grains, legumes, vegetables, raw vegetables, and vitamin B12–containing foods) can meet the RDAs for all vitamins, minerals, and protein, and fit within the guidelines of the Healthy Woman's Diet.

There are three general guidelines for diet planning:

1. A balanced diet should contain a wide variety of foods. Eating a variety of foods will improve the likelihood of an adequate intake of all the nutrients necessary for health and growth.
2. Moderation is important. Severe diets, such as the macrobiotic diet

and many of the restrictive weight-loss diets, serve little purpose other than to increase the likelihood of nutrient deficiencies and compromised health.

3. Making changes in the diet takes time. Too many dietary changes made too rapidly often result in failure and frustration. Identifying one habit that is easy to change and successfully accomplishing your goal is encouraging and helps motivate you to stick with it. (See chapter 4 for information on how to successfully change eating habits.)

Marginal Nutrient Deficiencies

In the days of scurvy, beriberi, and goiter, everyone thought that even minute amounts of a vitamin or mineral could cure the clinical signs of these classic nutrient-deficiency diseases and that a diet based on the Basic Four Good Groups would more than meet this minimum requirement.

Nutritional status was based primarily on a visual inspection. If a woman looked well, if her gums did not bleed, if the number and size of her red blood cells were normal, and if she did not suffer from severe dermatitis or hair loss, she was considered nutritionally healthy.

THE FIVE STAGES OF DEFICIENCY

Researchers now recognize that nutritional depletion develops much like other disorders, such as cancer, arthritis, and the common cold. A person starts out well and slowly succumbs to disease over the course of days, weeks, months, or years.

Like health status, nutritional status is a continuum from optimal health to overt disease. Marginal deficiencies are the middle ground on this continuum. Clinical deficiency symptoms such as anemia and scurvy are actually the final stages in the development of nutrient deficiencies. Preceding this are nonspecific symptoms that include fatigue, stress, irritability, insomnia, poor memory, and mood swings. Because these symptoms can result from numerous problems, the diagnosis is difficult.

Nutrient deficiencies are now classified into five stages that begin with a preliminary, then a biochemical deficiency, where the nutrient concentration in some tissues is progressively reduced. If the diet remains marginal, the next stage is called the physiological stage, where enzymes, hormones, and other critical body processes dependent on the nutrient are slowly lost. Up to this point these marginal deficiency symptoms are nonspecific, but if ignored, suppressed immune processes could increase a person's susceptibility to disease, or the deficiency itself will progress to even more serious levels. (See pages 244–49 for more information on nutrition and the immune system.)

This border between marginal and clinical disease is called subclinical (because the symptoms usually go undetected) or borderline deficiency. The last stages, called the clinical and anatomical stages, are where obvious signs of disease have set in that are detectable by a visual inspection. Death also can occur at the fifth (anatomical) stage if immediate action is not taken to correct the deficiency.

Marginal deficiency symptoms are at best vague because depletion of nutrients from the tissues is a gradual process. Consequently, prior to overt disease, a woman may experience reduced resistance to infection and disease, loss of appetite, personality changes, irritability, insomnia, or lethargy without realizing these symptoms are a result of poor diet. For example, a vitamin B1–deficient diet can cause personality changes, such as increased depression, anxiety, and nausea, well before the clinical signs of beriberi or tissue damage appear.

These symptoms are often ignored since the person is not ill enough to seek medical help. Marginal deficiency symptoms often go unnoticed in otherwise healthy individuals, but when combined with the added stress of illness, they can impair wound healing, increase the likelihood of secondary infections, interfere with recovery, and set the stage for clinical nutrient deficiencies.

HOW COMMON ARE MARGINAL DEFICIENCIES?

National diet surveys repeatedly show that the American diet does not meet the Recommended Dietary Allowances (RDA) for several nutrients. The likelihood of nutritional inadequacy is further compounded by the wide fluctuations in individual nutrient requirements that can vary as much as two hundredfold.

Even when nutrient intake is within the guidelines of the RDAs, a marginal deficiency can develop. A number of life situations, including disease, stress, smoking, and exposure to air pollution, increase nutrient needs above typical recommendations. Studies of women who use birth control pills show that blood levels of several nutrients, including vitamins B1, B2, B6, B12, and folic acid, are low despite adequate intake. People who abuse alcohol are highly susceptible to marginal deficiencies of vitamins B1, B6, and folic acid.

Many diseases once thought to be inevitable consequences of aging, such as osteoporosis, cataracts, and heart disease, are now suspected to be at least partially a result of marginal nutrient deficiencies. In short, a marginal deficiency of one or more nutrients could have far-reaching effects on a woman's health today and in the future. Consuming an optimal, not just an adequate, diet that is low in fat and rich in all the vitamins and minerals is essential to maintain health and avoid the subtle effects of marginal nutrient deficiencies.

PART ONE

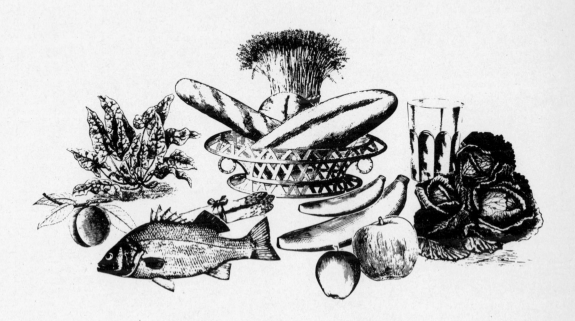

The Healthy Woman's Diet

Introduction

How's Your Diet?

How nutrition relates to health, disease, and aging is often poorly understood. The guidelines for nourishing the body however, are simple and straight-forward.

Basically, you should eat less fat and more minimally processed foods of plant origin. Women have reduced their fat intake from more than 40 percent of calories to 36 percent of calories, but their fiber intake still remains low—only 10 grams a day versus the recommended 27 to 35 grams. Women continue to eat too many pastries (high in fat); too much beef, eggs, fatty cheeses, cream, regular salad dressings, and butter; and not enough fruits, vegetables, whole grain breads and cereals, and cooked dried beans and peas. The good news is that you can change your eating habits.

How does your diet rate? First, take a detailed look at your diet and current nutritional status (see page 36). From the information gathered you can tailor your current eating habits to better match your individual nutritional needs within the framework of the Healthy Woman's Diet.

Standard nutrition guidelines such as the Four Food Groups Plan, the Food Guide Pyramid, and the Recommended Dietary Allowances (RDAs) are useful for general diet planning but do not address the unique biochemical needs of each individual. Wide variations in all body processes, including body weight and size, enzyme activity, nerve transmission and response, hormone levels, and immune function, result in differing nutritional needs even between identical twins. Individualized genetic makeup is accentuated by the specific combination of life-style and environmental factors peculiar to each person. (See page 19 for more information on the RDAs and the Balanced Diet.)

Each body has one or more "weak health links" that vary in severity and many times can be modified or strengthened by life-style choices. For example, high blood cholesterol levels and heart disease are common in some families and rare in others. A woman in a high-risk family may or may not develop heart disease depending on her health habits, including tobacco use, alcohol consumption, diet, stress, and exercise.

DETERMINING NUTRITIONAL STATUS

Many techniques for determining nutritional status are available; however, only a few are credible and accurate. A general physical examination is a starting point and can detect clinical vitamin or mineral deficiencies such as scurvy and beriberi. (See table on page 35.)

Another type of physical measurement of nutritional status is called an anthropometric measurement or a measurement of the body. Anthropometric measurements include height, weight, upper arm circumference, waist-to-hip ratio (WHR), fatfold thickness, and head circumference. Assessment of body measurements and interpretation of results should be conducted by a trained health professional such as a physician, a registered nurse, or a registered dietitian.

Laboratory tests of blood, urine, or tissues can detect vitamin or mineral deficiencies at an earlier stage than can a physical examination. Measurements of red blood cell volume, serum ferritin, hemoglobin, or total iron-binding capacity (TIBC) provide information on the presence of nutritional anemia or low tissue stores associated with iron. Blood levels of various enzymes are also indicators of nutritional status.

Other laboratory tests, such as the Schilling test for vitamin B12, detect the absorption of certain nutrients. Immune function assessment measures the type and amount of white blood cells in the blood, which provides an indicator of the body's nutritional status and resistance to disease. However, most laboratory tests, other than hematocrit and hemoglobin, are often too cumbersome and expensive to conduct on a routine basis.

ALTERNATIVE TESTS

Many unorthodox tests for nutritional status are inaccurate and unreliable. Hair analysis is a convenient measure of toxic metal concentrations in the body, such as

Physical Signs of Severe Nutrient Deficiencies Include the Following

1. General appearance (indicators of general nutritional status, including protein, calories, vitamin B1, vitamin B2, iron, and zinc): apathy; muscle or tissue wasting; excessive irritability; underweight, undersized, underdeveloped for age; paleness and loss of color of the skin, nail beds, lips, or hair

2. Hair (indicators of protein, zinc, or general nutritional status): dry, wiry, stiff, brittle, loss of color, easily pulled out

3. Nails (indicators of iron or general nutritional status): spoon-shaped, brittle, ridged

4. Skin (indicators of protein, essential fatty acid, vitamin A, vitamin K, vitamin C, niacin, vitamin B2, other B vitamins, or iron): cracks, scales, fluid retention and edema, dermatitis, flakiness, small hemorrhages or bruises (petechial hemorrhages), gooseflesh, rough patches, reddened, irregular pigmentation

5. Eyes (indicators of high blood fat levels, vitamin A, vitamin B2, or iron): Small, circular, grayish or yellowish gray, dull, dry, or foamy irritations on the surface of the eye (Bitot's spots); inflammation of the eyelids; softening or thickening of the outer surface of the eye; loss of night vision or adaptation from dark to light

6. Face (indicators of protein, vitamin B2, iron, or general nutritional status): irritations at the corners of the mouth (cheilosis); greasy scaling around nose or mouth

7. Mouth (indicators of excessive sugar consumption, vitamin C, niacin, vitamin B2, folic acid, vitamin B12, or general nutritional status): smooth, reddened, shiny, swollen, or dry tongue; swollen or bleeding gums; excessive tooth decay; reduced taste sensation

8. Skeleton (indicators of protein, vitamin A, vitamin D, vitamin C, calcium, magnesium, phosphorus, or general nutritional status): bowlegged, enlarged joints, shortening of stature, humped posture called Dowager's hump, rickets, osteoporosis

mercury, lead, arsenic, aluminum, and cadmium, but it is an unreliable test for nutrient status. Numerous environmental factors such as tobacco, smoke, water, sweat, shampoos, and hair sprays alter the mineral composition of hair and disqualify hair analysis as an accurate measurement.

Cytotoxic testing is promoted as a means of identifying and treating disorders by testing the blood for food allergies. The information obtained from cytotoxic testing and other tests that promise a simple and complete analysis of a person's nutritional status is often unreliable and misleading. No proof exists that

Analyzing Your Diet

Where do you stand diet-wise? The following checklist can help you stay on track. Your goals should be a passing grade of 70—not a perfect score—with a plan to keep getting better.

There are no partial scores; you either score all the points for a question if you answer "yes," or you score no points for that question if you answer "no." Recheck yourself periodically to monitor your progress.

	TOTAL POINTS	YOUR POINTS

General Diet

	TOTAL POINTS	YOUR POINTS
1. Are you within 10% of your ideal body weight?	10	_____
2. Do you avoid "quick weight loss" diets and dramatic fluctuations in weight?	10	_____
3. Do you consume at least 2,000 calories daily of low-fat, nutrient-dense foods?	10	_____
4. Do you feel, look, act, and function at your best?	10	_____
SUBTOTAL . . . . **40** points		*20*

Fruits and Vegetables

	TOTAL POINTS	YOUR POINTS
5. Do you consume daily at least 5 servings of unsweetened fruits or vegetables?	5	_____
6. Is at least one serving a vitamin C–rich selection, such as a citrus fruit?	2	*2*
7. Is at least one serving a dark green or orange selection? (See pages 69–70 for suggested serving sizes.)	2	_____
8. Do you eat cruciferous vegetables such as broccoli, cabbage, asparagus, Brussels sprouts, and kohlrabi at least 3 times a week?	1	_____
SUBTOTAL . . . . **10** points		*2*

Grains and Other Carbohydrates

	TOTAL POINTS	YOUR POINTS
9. Do you consume daily at least 6 servings of breads and cereals, most of which are 100% whole grains?	5	_____
10. Do you use half the sugar/honey required in recipes or limit desserts?	3	_____
SUBTOTAL . . . . **8** points		_____

(continues)

TOTAL POINTS   YOUR POINTS

Iron, Calcium, and Other Minerals

11. Do you consume 2 servings each day of extra-lean meat (that is, 9% fat by weight), chicken without the skin, or fish, and 2 servings of cooked dried beans and peas? If you are a vegetarian, do you consume daily at least 4 servings of cooked dried beans and peas?   5   _____

12. Do you limit your daily red meat intake to no more than 6 ounces?   1   _1_

13. Do you consume 3 or more servings each day of low-fat or nonfat milk and milk products, including low-fat or nonfat yogurt, milk, or cheese, or other foods high in calcium?   5   _____

SUBTOTAL . . . . **11** points   _1_

Fat Intake

14. Do you almost always bake, steam, broil, poach, or grill food, rather than fry, sauté, or use sauces and gravies that contain fat?   2   _____

15. Do you sauté in water, broth, herbs, or other no-fat liquids?   2   _____

16. Do you use tomato-based or no-fat sauces on pasta rather than creamy sauces or sauces with fatty meats?   2   _2_

17. Do you use salad dressing sparingly (that is, 2 teaspoons of safflower oil–based dressing or less per salad)?   2   _1_

18. Do you eat at fast-food restaurants or order fatty foods in restaurants less than once a week?   2   _____

19. Do you avoid or strictly limit intake of butter, margarine, oils, whipping cream, sour cream, whipped toppings, ice cream, whole milk, salad dressings, mayonnaise, and shortening?   2   _2_

20. Do you use no-fat alternatives to high-fat items such as nonfat sour cream, nonfat tartar sauce, nonfat cheese, or no-fat salad dressings?   2   _____

(continues)

TOTAL POINTS   YOUR POINTS

21. Do you read food labels and usually select foods that contain 3
grams of fat or less for every 100 calories?   2   _____

                                                                               5

SUBTOTAL . . . . **16** points

Cholesterol

22. Do you limit whole egg (or yolk) consumption to three eggs or
less per week?   2

SUBTOTAL . . . . **2** points   2

Salt, Fluids, and Caffeine

23. Do you drink at least 6 glasses of water each day?   2   _____
24. Do you limit intake of salty foods and avoid using salt in food
preparation or at the table?   2   _____
25. Do you limit soft drink intake to less than 5 servings a week?   2   _____
26. Do you limit coffee or caffeinated beverages to no more than 2
servings per day?   2   _____

SUBTOTAL . . . . **8** points   _____

Junk Foods

27. Do you limit intake of snack items such as potato chips, crackers,
doughnuts, French fries, and corn chips to less than 5 servings
a week?   2   _____
28. Do you limit intake of alcohol to less than 5 drinks a week? (One
drink is a 6-ounce glass of wine, 1 ounce of hard liquor, or a   3
12-ounce can of beer.)   3   _____

SUBTOTAL . . . . **5** points   _____

TOTAL POINTS POSSIBLE . . . . **100**   _____

these assessments provide anything useful in the identification of nutritional problems. The only reliable means of determining nutritional status include a comprehensive review of a woman's overall health and analysis of her dietary intake. (See table on page 36).

Putting It All Together

Before any dietary change is made, you should first accurately and thoroughly review your current eating habits, preferences, and health status. This information is essential to making decisions regarding nutritional needs, dietary choices, and vitamin or mineral supplementation. The guidelines for purchasing, planning, and preparing the low-fat, nutrient-dense meals outlined in the Healthy Woman's Diet or ordering these meals in restaurants are described in detail in chapters 1 and 2.

CHAPTER ONE

The Healthy Woman's Diet

Fortunately, the guidelines for developing a low-fat, nutrient-dense diet that will reduce the risk for most degenerative disease, help prevent premature aging, and strengthen the body's fundamental defenses against infection and disease are simple and straightforward.

The health benefits of the Healthy Woman's Diet include the following:

- improved resistance to colds and infection
- reduced risk of developing heart disease, cancer, diabetes, high blood pressure, and osteoporosis
- increased resistance to stress and stress-related disorders
- maintenance of a feeling of well-being
- help in the prevention of premature aging
- increased energy to enjoy life and complete work
- improved emotional and mental health

The Eight Guidelines

A healthful diet can be assured if the eight simple steps in the Healthy Woman's Diet are followed:

(See pages 69–70 for specific portions.)

1. Limit dietary fat intake to less than 30 percent of total calories, saturated fat to less than 10 percent of calories, and cholesterol to less

than 300 mg per day. Consume between 25 grams and 35 grams of fiber each day.

2. Consume at least five daily servings of fresh fruits and vegetables, especially dark orange or green vegetables and citrus fruits.

3. Consume at least six servings of whole grain breads and cereals each day.

4. Consume at least three to four calcium-rich foods daily, including nonfat milk.

5. Consume at least 2,000 calories of the above nutrient-dense foods. Select less nutritious foods only after all other nutrient needs for the day have been met, and limit sugar intake to less than 10 percent of calories. Include a moderate-dose vitamin-mineral supplement when calorie intake drops below 2,000 calories. The supplement should include fluoride if the drinking water is not fluoridated.

6. Balance calorie intake with exercise to maintain a desirable weight. Avoid repeated, unsuccessful attempts at weight loss.

7. Limit alcohol to five drinks or less each week. Pregnant women or women considering getting pregnant should avoid all alcoholic beverages until after the baby is born. Limit salt intake to less than 1 teaspoonful per day. Drink at least six glasses of water per day.

8. Divide the total day's food intake into several small meals and snacks.

The Most Important Dietary Advice: Cut the Fat

The most important dietary change you can make for your waistline and health is to reduce dietary fat. Dietary fat, especially saturated fat, increases your risk of heart disease, cancer, diabetes, obesity, and possibly high blood pressure. Americans have already cut fat consumption from 42 percent to 37 percent of total calories, which is one reason the incidence of heart disease has decreased by 33 percent in the last few years.

However, every national health organization that has published dietary guidelines, from the American Heart Association and the American Cancer Society to the Food and Nutrition Board of the National Academy of Sciences, recommends that everyone except infants and toddlers under two years old cut total fat intake to less than 30 percent and saturated fat to less than 10 percent of calories.

Dietary cholesterol also increases your risk of developing heart disease by

TABLE 1-1 Fiber: Highs and Lows

HIGH-FIBER FOODS

The following foods are high-fiber (3 grams or more of fiber), low-fat selections.

Food	Quantity	Fiber Content (grams)
Crackers		
Wasa Fiber Plus Crispbread	2	5.5
Manischewitz Whole Wheat Matzos with bran	1	4
Ryvita High Fiber Crispbread	2	4
Bread		
Arnold's Bran'nola Original	2 slices	6
Arnold's Bran'nola Hearty Wheat	2 slices	6
Roman Meal Light Seven Grain	2 slices	5.8
Pita bread, whole wheat	1	4.4
Earth Grains Gold and Bran	2 slices	4.2
100% whole wheat bread	2 slices	4
Pepperidge Farm Whole Wheat, thinly sliced	2 slices	4
Grains		
Bulgur (cracked wheat)	1 cup cooked	8.1
Whole wheat spaghetti	1 cup cooked	5.9
Near East couscous	1 cup cooked	3.9
Buckwheat pancake mix	3 pancakes	5.0
Popcorn, air-popped	3 cups	3.9
Brown rice	1 cup cooked	3.3
Cereals		
Kellogg's All Bran with Extra Fiber	½ cup	14.0
General Mills Fiber One	½ cup	13.0
Wheat bran	½ cup	12.6
Nabisco 100% Bran	½ cup	10.0

TABLE 1-1 Fiber: Highs and Lows *(continued)*

Food	Quantity	Fiber Content (grams)
Ralston Bran Chex	⅔ cup	6.1
Kellogg's Fruitful Bran	⅔ cup	5.0
Post Fruit & Fiber	½ cup	5.0
Oat bran	⅔ cup	4.0
Nabisco Shredded Wheat 'N Bran	⅔ cup	4.0
Kellogg's Nutri-Grain Wheat	⅔ cup	3.0
Post Grape-Nuts	¼ cup	3.0
Beans		
Campbell's Old-Fashioned Beans	¾ cup cooked	14.7
Pinto beans	¾ cup cooked	14.2
Kidney beans	¾ cup cooked	13.8
Campbell's Pork & Beans	¾ cup cooked	13.0
Black-eyed peas	¾ cup cooked	12.3
Green Giant Chili Beans	¾ cup cooked	11.0
Split pea soup	10 ounces	10.4
Van Camp's Pork & Beans	¾ cup cooked	7.4
Vegetables		
Baked potato with skin	1 medium	4.2
Sweet potato without skin	1 medium	3.4
Brussels sprouts	½ cup cooked	3.3
Salsa, homemade	½ cup	3.0
Fruits		
Figs, dried	3	5.3
Guava	1	5.3
Pear	1	4.3
Apricots, dried	10	3.6
Prunes, dried	5	3.5
Orange	1	3.1

(continues)

TABLE 1-1 **Fiber: Highs and Lows** *(continued)*

Food	Quantity	Fiber Content (grams)
Nuts and Seeds		
Almonds	¼ cup	3.8
Pistachios	¼ cup	3.8

MODERATE-FIBER FOODS

The following foods are moderate-fiber (1.5 to 2.9 grams of fiber) selections.

Food	Quantity	Fiber Content (grams)
Crackers		
Ryvita Rye Crispbread	2	2.6
Ryvita Sesame Crispbread	2	2.8
Finn Crisp Original Rye Crispbread	1	2.0
Breads		
Continental Baking Co. Lite White Fiber Bread	2 slices	2.8
Rainbo Country Meal	2 slices	2.6
Roman Meal Multibran	2 slices	2.4
Corn tortilla	one 6-inch	2.4
Pepperidge Farm Dijon Mustard Rye	2 slices	2.0
Grains		
Barley	½ cup cooked	2.2
Corn grits	½ cup cooked	2.2
Spaghetti or macaroni	1 cup cooked	2.1
Cereals		
Quaker Oatmeal	⅔ cup cooked	2.7
Cheerios	1¼ cup	2.0
Grape-Nuts Flakes	⅞ cup	2.0

TABLE 1-1   Fiber: Highs and Lows *(continued)*

Food	Quantity	Fiber Content (grams)
Vegetables		
Winter squash	½ cup cooked	2.9
Peas	½ cup	2.9
Carrot, raw	1	2.3
Spinach	½ cup cooked	2.0
Broccoli	½ cup cooked	2.0
Fruits		
Nectarine	1	2.7
Orange	1	2.6
Banana	1	2.4
Blueberries	½ cup	2.0
Cantaloupe	½ cup	2.0
Nuts and Seeds		
Peanuts	¼ cup	2.9
Tahini (sesame butter)	2 tablespoons	2.8
Peanut butter	2 tablespoons	2.0
Sunflower seeds	¼ cup	1.8

LOW-FIBER FOODS

The following foods are low-fiber (less than 1.5 grams of fiber) selections.

Food	Quantity	Fiber Content (grams)
Crackers		
Nabisco Oat Thins	8	1.0
Quaker Rice Cakes	2	0.6

(continues)

TABLE 1-1 Fiber: Highs and Lows *(continued)*

Food	Quantity	Fiber Content (grams)
Nabisco Triscuits	3	0.5
Saltines	4	0.3
Breads		
Continental Baking Co. Home Pride Butter Top White	2 slices	1.4
Continental Baking Co. Wonder Italian or French	2 slices	1.4
Hamburger or hot dog bun	1	1.2
Tortilla, flour	one 8-inch	1.1
Croissant	1	1.1
Grains		
Rice-A-Roni Spanish Style Rice	1 cup cooked	1.4
Millet	½ cup cooked	1.3
Uncle Ben's Converted White Rice	1 cup cooked	1.0
Graham crackers	4	1.0
Cereals		
Corn Chex	1 cup	1
Product 19	1 cup	1
Cream of Wheat	¾ cup	1
Cream of Rice	¾ cup	0
Beans		
Tofu	4 ounces	1.4
Vegetables		
Cauliflower	½ cup cooked	1.4
Spinach, raw	1 cup	1.4
Olives	10	1.4
Bok choy, cabbage	1 cup shredded	1.2
Jicama	1 cup	1.0

TABLE 1-1   Fiber: Highs and Lows (continued)

Food	Quantity	Fiber Content (grams)
Celery, raw	½ cup	1.0
Tomato	½ cup	0.8
Green pepper	½ cup	0.6
Mushrooms	½ cup	0.5
Fruits		
Pineapple	½ cup	1.1
Grapefruit juice	6 ounces	0.8
Grapes, seedless	20	0.6

raising blood cholesterol levels, even though saturated fats remain the primary culprit. Therefore, limit high-cholesterol items such as eggs, liver, and red meat so that the day's total cholesterol intake is below 300 mg.

More Fruits, Vegetables, and Grains

You should consume daily at least five servings of fresh fruits and vegetables, and six or more servings of other complex carbohydrates such as whole grain breads and cereals, potatoes, and legumes. (Legumes are also excellent sources of protein.) More is even better. These foods are low-fat, high-fiber, nutrient-dense "gold stars" for any menu.

Fiber intake should range between 25 and 35 grams and should come from a variety of wholesome foods, such as fresh fruits and vegetables, whole grain breads and cereals, nuts, and cooked dried beans and peas. Do not depend on processed fiber foods as the primary source of fiber in your diet. Research shows a strong association between fiber-rich foods, not fiber itself, and the prevention of cancer, heart disease, and diabetes. It might be that other components of these foods, perhaps in combination with fiber, reduce the risk of disease. (See table 1-1.)

The days when meals revolved around the pork chop or the meatloaf are past. The Healthy Woman's Diet is planned around pasta, rice, and bean dishes, with meat, chicken, and fish serving as a condiment. Examples include spaghetti with meatballs (made from extra-lean beef or ground turkey), Chinese or East Indian dishes of vegetables and grain with small amounts of meat, and stews and soups made with small amounts of meat. The consumption of extra-lean meat, poultry, and seafood should be limited to no more than 6 ounces a day, or two 3-ounce servings.

A Healthy Weight Is Best

Women concerned about their health should maintain a desirable body weight. Overweight—or, more accurately, excessive body fat above the waist—is associated with an increased risk of developing heart disease, diabetes, breast cancer, osteoarthritis, gallbladder disease, high blood pressure, and other diseases. Attaining and maintaining a desirable weight is best achieved by combining the Healthy Woman's Diet with daily exercise.

Repeated attempts at quick weight loss that result in dramatic fluctuations in weight are more harmful than maintaining a slightly overweight figure. Attempt weight loss only if you are determined to lose the weight gradually and maintain the loss. More important, focus on healthful eating and life-style habits and deemphasize weight loss as the ultimate goal. (See chapter 7 for guidelines on how to lose weight and keep it off.)

Is Alcohol Safe or Harmful?

Popular literature can be confusing when it comes to alcohol. Some studies report that moderate alcohol consumption is associated with a reduced risk of developing heart disease, while other studies show alcohol consumption increases cardiovascular risk. In either case, alcohol is not recommended as a way to prevent this disease. No safe level for alcohol during pregnancy has been identified, and a woman planning to get pregnant should refrain from all alcohol until after the baby is born.

Go Easy on the Salt Shaker

Few women recognize their susceptibility to high blood pressure. The typical American diet often contains as much as twenty-five times the recommended dietary levels of salt. Since reducing this excessive salt intake has no harmful side effects, national dietary recommendations agree that all Americans would benefit by limiting salt to no more than 6 grams per day (which is slightly more than a teaspoonful). Further reductions to 4 grams or less are even healthier. Keep in mind that salt (sodium chloride) is 40 percent sodium, so this recommendation is the equivalent of 2.4 grams of sodium.

The Calcium Connection

You should include several servings a day of calcium-rich foods throughout life for the prevention of osteoporosis. A high-calcium diet helps build bone mass during childhood and early adulthood. Optimal calcium intake helps maintain bone density during the middle years and slows bone loss later in life. High blood pressure and possibly heart disease have also been linked to inadequate calcium intake.

A woman should consume the equivalent of three to four glasses of milk or yogurt each day (there is approximately 300 mg of calcium in an 8-ounce serving), and make it nonfat.

Dairy products supply more than 40 percent of your daily need for calcium and vitamin B2. Eliminating these foods would require major changes in eating habits to ensure optimal nutrition. For example, it takes 1½ cups of broccoli to supply the same amount of calcium in a 1-ounce slice of cheese. Cheese also is a source of vitamin B12, zinc, and high-quality protein for women who are reducing their intake of red meat.

Low-Fat, No-Fat Cheeses
On the other hand, between 70 percent and 75 percent of the calories in most cheeses are from fat, and they contain about 25 mg to 30 mg of cholesterol per serving. The milk fat in cheese is a major contributor to the development of heart disease, probably because of its high saturated fat content. It seems you can't live with and can't live without dairy products.

In an effort to solve this dilemma, manufacturers have developed a line of no-fat and low-fat cheeses by replacing the grease with skim milk, whey (the watery protein- and vitamin-rich portion of milk), and harmless vegetable gums such as guar gum, locust bean gum, or carrageenan. These products contain little or no fat and cholesterol while maintaining a high calcium, vitamin B2, and protein content. However, many of the "light," "reduced-fat," or "part skim" cheeses still may have a fat content comparable to conventional cheeses. To identify a truly low-fat cheese, ignore the label on the front and go straight to the grams of fat on the back. A low-fat cheese will have either 3 grams of fat or less per serving or no more than 3 grams per ounce. Moderate-fat cheeses have 4 to 5 grams of fat per ounce, while high-fat items contain 6 grams or more. Also, check the serving size; some packaged slices are "lighter" only because they weigh less than an ounce (compared to the full-ounce slice of other brands).

Supplementation: When and Why

If you do not consume at least 2,000 calories and the recommended number of servings of foods listed above, consider a moderate-dose vitamin-mineral supplement to ensure optimal nutrient intake. In addition, fluoridated water ensures a beautiful smile and healthy teeth, so if your water supply is not fluoridated, consider fluoride supplements. (See chapter 5 for more information on how to select a well-balanced supplement.)

Snacking Versus the Three Square Meals

Food intake should be divided into several (that is, four or more) small meals and snacks throughout the day. Eating every four hours or so is more likely to help you maintain a desirable weight and a lower risk of disease than is skipping meals, fasting, or eating most of the day's food in three or fewer meals.

The good news is that the guidelines for the Healthy Woman's Diet are simple and require, in most cases, only moderate changes in current eating habits.

The Supermarket Survival Guide

The following guidelines can make the supermarket experience a nutritious one:

- Plan ahead.
- Learn how to read labels.
- Choose minimally processed foods.
- Increase awareness of the fat, cholesterol, and sugar content of foods.

Plan Ahead

Careful planning prior to shopping can save time and improve the nutrient content of any nutrition plan. A list based on a thorough check of the cupboards, refrigerator, and freezer for needed items and a plan for the week's meals and snacks can help the shopper stay "on track." A list posted on the refrigerator is handy for jotting down needed items and organizing the shopping list according to the sections of the grocery store.

At the store, the most important rule is to be "fat conscious." Shop primarily around the periphery of the grocery store, where most of the minimally processed, low-fat foods are located. The fruit and vegetable section, milk section, meat and fish department, and bakery usually line the side walls and the back of the store. Other nutritious foods such as whole grain cereals, noodles, canned and frozen vegetables, and dried beans and peas are located on a few aisles, while the greatest percentage of shelf space is devoted to processed and convenience foods. If the grocery store does not carry some nutritious items such as 100 percent whole grain bread, ask the grocery store manager to stock these items, or purchase them from a local health food store.

Planning ahead helps avoid the marketing techniques used by the grocery store that entice people to purchase unnecessary or high-priced items. Impulse foods are often placed at eye level, at the end of aisles, out of place, or at the checkout counter. Hunger reduces your resistance to these impulse foods, so eat something before shopping to curb your appetite. Mothers should be aware that shopping with small children can also result in unnecessary food purchases unless they plan ahead of time what foods are nutritionally acceptable.

In addition, you should take advantage of advertised sales, coupons, and specials only if they are compatible with the guidelines for a low-fat, nutrient-dense diet. You may also find it useful to bring a calculator to estimate the cost per serving, the fat content of foods based on label information, or to maintain a running total of the food bill.

Read Labels

A label provides information on the nutrient composition of a food, including the calories and grams of protein, fat, and carbohydrates per serving. This information can be particularly useful in determining the percentage of calories supplied by fat (that is, the fat calories). The Healthy Woman's Diet contains less than 30 percent fat calories. Although some foods can be higher in fat than others and still meet this quota, a good general rule is to choose items that contain no more than 3 grams of fat for every 100 calories. (Each gram of fat supplies 9 calories, so the grams of fat in a serving multiplied by 9, divided by the total number of calories, and multiplied by 100 equals the percentage of fat calories.)

Labeling is confusing when it comes to fat. For example, comparing grams of protein or carbohydrate to grams of fat is deceptive since a gram of fat has more than twice the calories of a gram of carbohydrate or protein. Consequently, a product that contains fewer grams of fat than grams of carbohydrate and protein still might contain more than 30 percent fat calories. In addition, foods are often labeled according to the percentage of fat by weight, not by calories. Ground beef labeled "less than 22 percent fat" is actually as high as 60 percent fat calories. Whole milk labeled as 3.5 percent fat (by weight) is actually 50 percent fat calories. In short, seldom do foods disclose the fat calories, so you must calculate this from information provided on the label.

Women who are concerned about their weight can use the calorie information provided on a label to compare different foods or to tally their daily calorie intake. A 1-cup serving of whole milk, for example, supplies 160 calories, while the same serving of nonfat milk contains only 90. They both contain equal amounts of all other nutrients, including calcium, protein, vitamin B2, vitamin D, and magnesium, but the whole milk has a higher fat and calorie count.

The sugar content and nutrient density of a food can also be determined by labels that provide detailed information on the sugar and complex carbohydrate content of the food item. For easy reference, 4 grams of sugar equals 1 teaspoon, and 12 grams of sugar equals 1 tablespoon. A ready-to-eat cereal that contains 13 grams of sugar (more than 1 tablespoon) could have more than 50 percent of its calories from sugar. Most labels, however, only disclose the total carbohydrates, lumping all starch and sugars into one category.

Food labels also provide information on nutrient density. In general, a food that contains at least 10 percent of the U.S. RDA (United States Recommended Daily Allowance) for three or more nutrients and also is low in fat (that is, less than 30 percent fat calories) and sugar is probably a nutrient-dense food.

The ingredients list on a label provides another indication of the nutrient content of a food. Foods are listed in descending order according to weight, so the ingredients listed first are present in the greatest amount. A food is likely to be high in calories and low in nutrients if fats or sugars are listed in the first three ingredients. All fat—whether it is polyunsaturated, monounsaturated, saturated, or a fatty acid, or listed as vegetable oil, milk fat, or hydrogenated vegetable oil— contains the same amount of calories.

Sugar is disguised by a variety of names, such as dextrose, sucrose, fructose, "natural sweeteners," honey, brown sugar, corn sweeteners, and corn syrup, and may appear more than once in an ingredient list. It is the total amount of all sugars that is important to note.

Label Lingo

The language on labels is designed to promote sales, not nutrition. Labels have become so deceptive and confusing that in 1990 Congress passed the National Labeling and Education Act, which attempts to simplify label lingo and protect the consumer against fraud. Enforcement of this act begins in 1993, and over the next few years the look of labels will be changing to comply. In the meantime, beware of the following:

1. "Wheat flour" does not mean whole wheat flour. Most breads are made from wheat flour; however, most of this flour is refined white wheat flour. If a product doesn't state "100% whole wheat," it probably contains primarily refined flour.
2. An ingredient list on a label that reads "vegetable oil" could contain either saturated fats, such as coconut oil or palm oil, or unsaturated fats, such as safflower oil or corn oil. Hydrogenated vegetable oils found in shortening, margarine, crackers, French fries, and many

snack foods also contain saturated fat and polyunsaturated trans fatty acids. These altered polyunsaturated fats act more like saturated fats in the body and are linked to an increased risk of heart disease and possibly cancer.

3. Products that claim to be low in cholesterol still might be high in fat, salt, or other unhealthful ingredients. For example, a peanut butter that claims "no cholesterol" is deceiving since no peanut butters contain cholesterol. The product contains the same amount of fat and calories as any other peanut butter on the grocery store shelf.

4. Note the wording of ingredients. "Beef flavoring" is flavoring, not beef. A soup titled "Noodles and Chicken" contains more noodles than chicken, whereas another soup titled "Chicken and Noodles" contains more chicken.

   The words "diet" or "dietetic" do not necessarily provide fewer calories. A diet product is defined as any food that is lower in sodium, cholesterol, protein, or other food components; the calories may be the same, higher, or lower than a comparable product.

5. The word "sodium" in the name of any ingredient, such as monosodium glutamate (MSG), bisodium carbonate, or sodium nitrite, is the same sodium found in sodium chloride or table salt.

6. More than half of all Americans think "natural foods" are more nutritious than other foods. Terms such as natural, organic, and health food in many cases have been legally meaningless. The most important considerations when choosing nutritious foods are that they are fresh, wholesome, and minimally processed.

7. Other potentially deceptive terminology includes the following:
   A. Fruit beverages: "Fruit-flavored drinks" and "fruit drinks" contain little or no real fruit juice. "Fruit juice" is 100 percent fruit juice. Many mixed fruit juices now contain "white grape juice" as their primary ingredient. However, white grape juice concentrate is a refined product of grapes containing almost exclusively sugar.
   B. Sugar: "Sugar-free" or "sugarless" means the food contains no sucrose (table sugar); however, other sugars such as honey or corn syrup can be included.

C. Additives: Foods that claim "no preservatives" still may contain sweeteners, fat, emulsifiers, stabilizers, flavorings, colorings, and other additives. Foods flavored with "natural flavors" may also contain synthetic flavor enhancers.

"Enriched" and "Fortified" Foods

Many convenience foods, from bread and rice to milk and fruit drinks, are either enriched or fortified with vitamins or minerals.

"Enriched" refers to the addition of vitamins or minerals to the level found before the food was processed. For example, bread is made with white flour enriched with three vitamins (vitamin B1, vitamin B2, and niacin) and one mineral (iron) to replace the loss of these nutrients during the refining process. The term "enriched" is deceiving since it implies extra nutritional benefits when in reality many more nutrients and fiber were removed than have been replaced. "Enriched" products are actually poor nutritional substitutes for their original, unprocessed, wholesome foods.

The term "fortified" means that one or more vitamins or minerals have been added to levels greater than were originally found in the unprocessed food. Fortifying some foods has been beneficial, such as the fortification of milk with vitamin D, which reduced the incidence of rickets in children, and the fortification of salt with iodine, which reduced the risk of developing goiter.

Fortification is misused when random amounts of vitamins or minerals are added to otherwise nutrient-poor, highly processed foods, such as high-sugar breakfast cereals, fruit drinks, and granola bars. The original, minimally processed food is always more nutritious than the processed and fortified product since convenience foods are never fortified with all the nutrients, fiber, and other essential dietary factors at the same level as found in the original food. (See table 1-2.)

Convenience Foods: What Is the Nutritional Cost?

Foods prepared at home have given way to a relatively modern concept—convenience foods, or foods partially or entirely manufactured outside the home. The number of convenience foods has increased rapidly since the 1940s and includes the following:

TABLE 1-2   A Sample Shopping List

Use the following shopping list as a guide for purchasing low-fat, nutrient-dense foods.

BREADS AND CEREALS

Bakery

100% whole wheat bread
Whole wheat bagels
English muffins
French bread
Cornbread
Pumpernickel
Whole wheat pita bread
Whole wheat rolls
Corn tortillas
French bread

Crackers and Snacks

Akmak, Ry-Krisp, or other low-fat whole wheat crackers
Corn chips, low salt
Rice cakes
Graham crackers
Tortilla chips
Pretzels
Popcorn, air popped

Cereals

Nutri-Grain cereal (ready-to-eat)
Grape-Nuts
Shredded wheat
Puffed wheat and puffed rice
Whole grain hot cereal such as oatmeal
Wheat germ
Kasha

Noodles, Rice, and Other Grains

Whole wheat noodles
Spinach noodles
"Enriched" noodles
Long-grain or short-grain brown rice
Wild rice
Millet
Cracked wheat or bulgur
Barley
Tabouli mix, rice pilaf, wheat pilaf, Spanish rice (omit packets if sodium is a concern)

Flour

Whole wheat
Rye
Oat
Unbleached white flour (less nutritious than the whole grain varieties)

_____

_____

_____

FRUITS AND VEGETABLES

Fruits

All fresh fruits
Fruits canned in their own juices
All 100% fruit juice, canned, bottled, or frozen concentrate

Vegetables

All fresh or plain frozen vegetables except avocados and olives
All 100% vegetable juices
Tomato sauce
Tomato paste
Marinara sauce such as Healthy Choice spaghetti sauce

TABLE 1-2   A Sample Shopping List (continued)

Salsa

Artichoke hearts canned in water

_____

_____

_____

Beans and Peas

All dried beans and peas, including kidney, black, garbanzo, navy, soybean, lentils, split peas, and lima

Canned cooked dried beans and peas (beans in "dishes" such as chili or baked beans should be chosen on an individual basis by their fat content)

Packaged bean mixes such as hummus and lentil pilaf

Peanut butter (in small quantities; choose major brand names to ensure low levels of aflatoxin)

_____

_____

_____

Meat, Chicken, and Fish

Chicken (remove the skin before cooking)

Extra-lean beef, that is, less than 9% fat by weight

Extra-lean pork

Turkey (remove the skin before cooking)

Canned tuna packed in water

All fresh and frozen unprocessed fish

_____

_____

_____

Milk and Eggs

No-fat cheeses, including no-fat cream cheese, cheddar, American, mozzarella, and Monterey Jack

Low-fat mozzarella cheese

Nonfat or 1% fat plain yogurt

Nonfat or 1% fat milk

Nonfat or 1% fat buttermilk

Nonfat, low-fat, or dry curd cottage cheese

Low-fat Parmesan cheese

Partially skimmed Swiss and ricotta

Eggs (use 1 to 2 each week or use only the egg white)

_____

_____

_____

ADDITIONAL FOOD ITEMS

Beverages

Mineral water

Diet soda

Tea

Decaf coffee

Decaf tea

Spices and Flavorings

Garlic powder

Selected spices and herbs, including dill

Mustard

(continues)

TABLE 1-2　A Sample Shopping List *(continued)*

Sugar substitute
Clam juice
Pimento

Oils and Fats

Low-calorie margarine
No-fat salad dressing
Low-calorie mayonnaise
Safflower oil
Dry roasted nuts such as almonds
Sunflower seeds

Sweets and Desserts

Jam (preferably all-fruit, no-sugar variety)
Angel food cake
Sherbet
Vanilla wafers
Dole frozen fruit bar
Dole Fruit Ice
Healthy Choice ice cream

_____

_____

_____

- ready-to-eat cereals (that is, cold breakfast cereals)
- frozen foods (frozen waffles, vegetables, egg substitutes, or fruit juice)
- frozen entreés or breakfast foods
- pre-prepared meals and desserts that require the addition of one or more ingredients such as water, milk, eggs, or nuts
- canned or packaged foods (that is, vegetables, soups, noodle dishes, bread, seasoning mixes for meat, or gravy packets)
- powdered or condensed beverages (that is, fruit punch mix or condensed milk)

Some convenience foods are minimally processed versions of natural foods, such as 100 percent whole wheat bread or pure frozen orange juice. These selections retain most of the original nutrient content while supplying relatively few calories. Most convenience foods, however, are highly processed, refined, enriched, fortified, condensed, tenderized, powdered, freeze-dried, or precooked to varying degrees. They often contain additives or have lost much of their original vitamin, mineral, and fiber content.

In general, the more processed a food, the higher its content of fat, salt, sugar, calories, or cholesterol, and the lower the content of vitamins, minerals, and fiber. For example, 100 percent whole wheat bread is a minimally processed product that contains the grain's original content of fiber, B vitamins, and minerals, including chromium, iron, magnesium, manganese, selenium, and zinc. "Enriched" white bread is more processed and contains significantly less fiber and other nutrients except for three vitamins and one mineral added back in the "enrichment" process.

Unless you read the labels, the nutrient and calorie content of convenience foods can deceive you. Fresh or frozen vegetables are low in calories and high in nutrients, whereas frozen vegetables in a cream sauce are high in fat, calories, salt, and possibly cholesterol. Another example are whole grain crackers; unless the package states 100 percent whole wheat and low fat, the first ingredient is probably enriched white flour, and the product probably contains too much fat.

When purchasing convenience foods, you should choose minimally processed products that contain whole grains, plain fruits and vegetables packaged in their own juice, nonfat or low-fat dairy products, and chicken, fish, legumes, and lean cuts of meat. Ignore the label claims and go straight to the nutrition information on the back. Purchase only convenience foods that contain 3 grams or less of fat for every 100 calories. For example, many luncheon meats that advertise that they are 80 percent fat free actually contain as much as 12 grams of fat in two slices, or the equivalent of almost three teaspoons of fat.

Turkey is the latest low-fat buzzword, but when you calculate the fat calories in turkey hot dogs, you will find they contain 50 percent fat calories or more even though the label reads 82 percent fat free. Read labels and purchase only those products that contain 3 grams or less of fat per 100 calories.

Frozen entreés labeled as "light" are not always low in fat, so read the label to calculate the fat percentage. "Low calorie" does not mean "low fat," and an entreé that provides only 300 calories might derive more than 50 percent of those calories from fat, not to mention the cholesterol content. Some best bets include the Healthy Choices entreés and the Stouffer's Right Course entreés.

Fake Fats and Artificial Sweeteners

The thought of eating French fries, doughnuts, and fudge without having to worry about waistlines and heart disease sounds too good to be true. However, the new fat substitutes, such as NutraSweet's Simplesse, promise to be the answer to some people's prayers.

Simplesse is made with egg and milk protein and can be used in any food not fried or baked. Currently, this "fake fat" is found in the frozen dessert Simple Pleasures, but it soon will be available in salad dressings and mayonnaise products. So far no adverse effects from its use or ingestion have been noted.

Other fake fats, such as olestra, are still in the investigative stages of development. Initial requests from its manufacturer, Procter and Gamble, for FDA approval were denied because laboratory animals developed cancer, liver damage, and other serious problems after ingestion of olestra.

Food products containing fake fats are not panaceas for weight problems, just as the sugar substitutes, such as aspartame (NutraSweet) have not slowed the progressive increase in obesity. Until more is known about the safety of fake fats, consumption of foods containing them should be moderate.

Non-nutritive sweeteners, in particular aspartame, have contributed to the skyrocketing sales of diet soft drinks. Despite the popular belief that consuming these no-calorie beverages will help a woman lose weight, research shows that diet soft drinks at best have no effect on appetite and food consumption. At worst, they might encourage weight gain. Even when aspartame-containing beverages are shown to decrease appetite, researchers report that artificial sweetener users are no more likely than nonusers to lose weight. There is no conclusive evidence that aspartame reduces appetite or aids in weight control.

In addition, although it is composed of "natural" substances and sanctioned by the FDA, some researchers are not convinced that aspartame is safe. Some studies report moodiness, nausea, headaches, and seizures in women who consume large quantities of aspartame. However, even more evidence exists that aspartame is safe in moderate to large doses.

To be safe, pregnant women and people with a metabolic disorder called phenylketonuria should avoid foods and beverages that contain aspartame. Women who experience any uncomfortable side effects when consuming the sweetener should also avoid foods that contain it. For those who choose to include aspartame in their diet, moderate to low consumption appears to have few or no harmful effects, but it should not be counted on as an effective weight-loss aid.

Designer Foods and New Foods

Increasing awareness of food factors that promote health has resulted in a new category of foods called designer foods or neutraceuticals. Although only in the developmental stage, these foods are genetically engineered to contain higher amounts of health-enhancing, naturally occurring substances.

For example, beta carotene in dark orange and dark green vegetables decreases the risk of developing cancer and enhances the immune system. In the future, vegetables naturally low in beta carotene, such as potatoes and corn, could be genetically altered to supply larger amounts of this vitaminlike substance.

Other health-promoting neutraceuticals include "flavonoids" in citrus fruits, "alliin" in garlic, "indoles" in broccoli, and "triterpenoids" in licorice root. Many foods could be genetically programmed to contain one or more of these and many more compounds, thereby increasing the total diet's content of food substances known to promote health. Designer foods are already available in Japan and other countries; however, it could be several more years before neutraceuticals enter the U.S. marketplace.

The Ten Worst Food Additives

Most additives in foods are safe. However, the following additives should be avoided because they have proven harmful or because there is insufficient evidence that they are harmless.

1. *Artificial colors.* Naturally derived coloring agents such as carotene and beet juice extract are presumed to be safe although they have been poorly tested. However, most processed foods are colored with combinations of synthetic dyes such as Green No. 3, Red No. 40, and Blue No. 2. Many of these colorants are suspected of causing cancer, and some have already been partially removed from the marketplace (such as Red No. 3, the coloring used in maraschino cherries and pistachio nuts, which causes tumors in laboratory animals).

2. *BHA and BHT.* These compounds retard rancidity in foods that contain oil. BHA is suspected of causing cancer in humans, yet it remains in hundreds of processed foods. Since other safe compounds could do the same job and many of the foods that contain these compounds do not need a preservative, there is no reason to use BHA and BHT.

3. *MSG.* Monosodium glutamate causes "Chinese Restaurant Syndrome" in some people, which includes headaches, tightness in the chest, and a burning sensation in the forearms, face, and back of the neck. MSG must be listed on the label; however, hydrolyzed vegetable protein, which contains small amounts of MSG, does not have to be listed and may appear only as "flavoring."

4. *Nitrites.* Sodium nitrite and sodium nitrate are used in processed meats such as bacon to preserve freshness, maintain color, and inhibit the growth of deadly botulism-causing bacteria. Although nitrites are harmless, they are converted to potent cancer-causing substances called nitrosamines when exposed to high heat or when ingested.

5. *Sulfites.* Sulfites prevent discoloration in dried fruits and freshly cut vegetables and inhibit bacterial growth and fermentation in commercial wines. Some people are allergic to sulfites, however, and develop breathing difficulties within minutes of consuming foods containing sulfites. These additives pose no harm to people who are not allergic to them.

6. *Saccharin.* This non-nutritive sweetener is linked to cancer in laboratory animals.

7. *Pesticides.* The pesticide level on fruits and vegetables varies according to the type of produce and the type of pesticide used during the growing season. Domestic vegetables and fruits are probably safer than imported ones, while cosmetically perfect produce could be an indication of higher exposure to pesticides. Washing with dishwashing soap and water, peeling, and purchasing unwaxed produce helps reduce exposure to pesticides in agricultural products.

8. *Bacteria.* Unintentional growth of bacteria such as aflatoxin in peanuts and peanut butter, listeria in vegetables and dairy products, and salmonella in eggs and other high-protein foods can cause food poisoning, disease, cancer, and even death. Proper food handling, avoiding spoiled or "old" food, and thorough cooking can help prevent exposure to these pathogens.

9. *Caffeine.* Excessive intake of caffeine causes nervousness, heart palpitations, nausea, headaches, and insomnia. Caffeine is also associ-

ated with hyperactivity in children and birth defects and infertility in adults.

10. *Salt.* Sodium chloride and other sodium-containing foods increase the risk of developing high blood pressure in salt-sensitive people. Americans consume as much as twenty-five times the recommended amount of salt, which for any other mineral would be considered a pharmacological dose.

Just because a compound is an additive does not mean it is necessarily harmful. Although their names may sound technical or foreign, many additives are considered safe, such as:

- thickening agents, such as propylene glycol alginate, sodium caseinate, and sodium carboxymethylcellulose
- emulsifiers, such as lecithin, sorbitan, monostearate, mono- or diglycerides, or naturally occurring gums (arabic, guar, karaya, locust bean, and tragacanth)
- preservatives, such as alpha tocopherol (vitamin E), ascorbic acid (vitamin C), calcium propionate, potassium sorbate, and sodium benzoate
- carrageenan, a carbohydrate derived from seaweed that is used in commercial milk shakes, meat extenders, ice cream, and other products.

Health Foods: The Good, the Bad, and the Glamorous

Labeling foods as "health foods" does not promise enhanced nutritional quality. Few states have a legal definition of "natural" or "organic" as it applies to food. Consequently, these descriptors can be used on a variety of products with no guarantee of quality. Even foods grown organically on soil fertilized with manure or compost could be contaminated by pesticides and artificial fertilizers used on neighboring fields.

There is no evidence that these foods are nutritionally superior to foods grown on soil fertilized with commercial fertilizers. Nutrient content varies more among varieties of a plant (that is, the vitamin C content of oranges varies depending on variety and growing location), the season, and the inherent mineral content of the soil (that is, the selenium content of a food is directly related to the selenium content of the soil in which it is grown).

"Health foods" also can be high in fat, cholesterol, salt, or sugar. For example, fertilized eggs, granola, coconut oil, and many snack items found in health food stores or in the health food section of a grocery store are similar in nutritional, fat, and salt content to conventional foods. Often the only difference is that the health food is more costly. However, some items in health food stores are nutritious bargains. Foods sold in bulk, such as grains, dried fruits, cereals, and beans, are less expensive than packaged items.

Peanuts in bulk, peanuts ground for peanut butter at the store, and small-brand peanut butters should be avoided, however, since they may be contaminated with the potent cancer-causing aflatoxin. Aflatoxin is a toxic substance produced by a mold that grows on peanuts. Although aflatoxin levels in the United States are relatively low, they are higher in regional and ground-in-store brands. Avoid peanuts that are moldy or have an off odor.

Some manufacturers are sincere in their attempts to provide quality organic foods. These products can be identified by asking the health food store manager for verification of a legal statement that the food has been grown or handled according to "organic" principles.

The best guidelines for selecting foods in health food stores are:

1. Read labels.
2. Avoid products not typically found in the diet, such as bee pollen, protein powders, and hormone extracts.
3. Avoid promotional claims that increase the price but not the nutritional quality of the diet.
4. Select foods that are minimally processed and fresh.

CHAPTER TWO

Preparing and Ordering the Healthy Woman's Diet

Knowing about nutrition, healthful shopping habits, and the nutrients important in preventing disease are helpful, but applying that knowledge to daily menu planning and food preparation, while keeping in mind that eating is still one of life's pleasures, is the true test.

Planning and Preparing Meals and Snacks

As with shopping, the most important rule for planning and preparing nutritious meals is to avoid fat. Fat is calorie-dense and nutrient-poor, so even small quantities can substantially increase the day's intake of calories and push fat calories above the recommended level of 30 percent or less. Adding fats for flavor, such as butter on a potato or cream cheese on a bagel, is one of the hardest dietary habits to give up, according to the Women's Health Trial, a Seattle study that investigated the effectiveness of a low-fat diet for the prevention of breast cancer. However, it is the best indicator of long-term success. The secret is to find tasty alternatives.

Limiting calorie-dense fats means you can reduce calories without reducing the quantity of food or make up the lost calories by eating a greater amount of low-fat foods. For example, a baked potato with sour cream and butter supplies approximately 400 calories, with 40 percent of those calories coming from fat. The same potato seasoned with chives, a no-calorie butter substitute, or nonfat sour cream contains half the calories, and only 1 percent of those are from fat. The only difference between a fried and a baked chicken breast is that the baked chicken has half the calories and considerably less fat.

Fat Consciousness

The first step in planning and preparing low-fat, nutrient-dense foods in the Healthy Woman's Diet is to become fat conscious. You must recognize what adds fat to recipes, menus, snacks, and meals. Visible fats are easy to spot and include the marbling in meat, oil in salad dressing, and cream bases of sauces and soups.

Hidden fats are trickier. They make a bran muffin look shiny, a potato chip leave a slick feeling in the mouth, and a cheese cube or a French fry leave a greasy feel on the fingertips. The hidden fats require fat-sleuthing skills.

The next step is to gradually reduce the amount of those fats or eliminate them entirely. Favorite recipes can be included in menu planning; just give them a low-fat face lift. When a recipe calls for ½ cup of butter or oil, reduce it to ¼ cup. If the quality, taste, and texture remain acceptable, try further reductions in fat the next time. Make pizza with more no-fat cheese, onions, green peppers, tomatoes, and other vegetables, and less fatty cheese or processed meats.

Preparation of convenience foods can also be fat-modified. Added butter and oils can be omitted when preparing preseasoned mixes such as noodle or rice mixes, with no change in taste or texture. When butter or stick margarine is required, use tub margarine made with canola oil instead and reduce the amount.

Fat-Free Cooking

Oils and fats can be eliminated from cooking methods with no loss of flavor or appearance.

- Simmer vegetables, chicken, fish, and other foods in a little wine, lemon juice, defatted chicken stock, or water and herbs.
- Select extra-lean cuts of meat (that is, less than 9 percent fat by weight) and trim all visible fat before cooking.
- Remove the skin from poultry.
- Bake, broil, grill, or stew extra-lean meats without added fat.
- Bake, broil, barbecue, braise, or stir-fry fish and poultry in lemon juice or chicken stock.
- Heat tortillas in a nonstick pan rather than frying them in oil.

The bottom line is to bake, steam, broil, microwave, grill, and barbecue to avoid using fat in food preparation.

Does microwaving food alter its nutritional content? During microwave cooking, most foods fare well and lose little nutrients, even those such as vitamin C and folic acid that are particularly susceptible to damage from other cooking methods. However, always cook in materials designed for microwaves. Plastic wraps and plastic cookware not specifically labeled microwavable can release "plasticizers" into the food during cooking, and these have been associated with an increased risk of liver damage.

Many foods can be basted with fat-free marinades made from numerous non-fat ingredients, including wine, tomato juice, fruit juice, nonfat milk, salsa, low-salt soy sauce, and spices. Lean cuts of meat, which might be tougher than fattier cuts, can be tenderized by cubing, grinding, pounding, or thinly slicing them; marinating in wine or beer; aging; or using commercial tenderizers (read labels for salt/sodium content). Some of the alcohol used in cooking does not evaporate during heating. A sauce made with wine retains approximately 5 percent of its alcohol after two and a half hours of cooking, while foods cooked for shorter amounts of time can contain 40 percent or more of the alcohol.

Since eggs are high in cholesterol, the weekly intake should be limited to three whole eggs or less. Better yet, one whole egg in recipes can be replaced by two egg whites. For example, three scrambled eggs for two people can be made with one whole egg and four egg whites. Or crumbled tofu can be mixed with the whole egg and egg whites. (See table 2-1.)

Planning Meals and Snacks with Vegetables, Fruits, and Grains in Mind

The second guideline for planning and preparing low-fat, nutrient-dense meals in the Healthy Woman's Diet is to plan the menu around foods of plant origin. Two-thirds to three-quarters should be vegetables, fruits, whole grain breads and noodles, and cooked dried beans and peas, with moderate servings of nonfat milk products. Extra-lean meats, poultry, or fish serve as condiments to the meal.

In fact, most of the day's protein should come from the combination of grains and cooked dried beans and peas rather than from fatty cuts of meat. For example, more kidney beans and less extra-lean meat can be added to chili. Spaghetti sauce can be made with less meat. Diced chicken adds protein to a vegetable stir-fry and deemphasizes the need for large servings of meat.

TABLE 2-1 Low-Fat Tricks of the Trade

The following tricks are only a few of the ways to reduce fat and increase the nutrient content of meals and snacks.

1. Eliminate egg yolks (use an egg substitute or use two egg whites for every whole egg), butter, cream, and salt. Substitute nonfat milk or evaporated nonfat milk, spices, and other seasonings.
2. Refrigerate stock and skim off the fat before preparing soup, stews, gravies, and sauces.
3. Baste with fat-free liquids and spices.
4. Mix either imitation or low-calorie mayonnaise with nonfat yogurt. Use for coleslaw, tuna salad, chicken salad, potato salad, and dressings.
5. Select low-calorie or nonfat salad dressings, lemon juice, nonfat yogurt–based salad dressings, and vinegar with a mixture of spices.
6. Simmer foods in defatted chicken stock. Use nonstick pans or nonstick sprays.
7. Use low-calorie jam, all-fruit preserves, or no-fat cottage cheese on toast.
8. Use nonfat milk with nonfat milk solids and flour or cornstarch to prepare cream sauces.
9. Use no-fat sour cream or nonfat yogurt with a dash of lemon for dips. Place nonfat yogurt in cheesecloth overnight, drain, and use yogurt curd as a substitue for sour cream.
10. In cooking, use no-fat sour cream or nonfat yogurt and blend with flour. Add the mixture after cooking and prior to serving.
11. Select plain nonfat yogurt and mix with fresh fruit.
12. Use nonfat milk with nonfat dry milk solids or evaporated nonfat milk instead of cream or whole milk. Partially frozen evaporated nonfat milk can be whipped into a foam for desserts or as a replacement for whipped cream.
13. Reduce the portion of cheese in sauces by one-third or one-half.
14. Prepare cream sauces with cornstarch and nonfat milk, water, or juice.
15. Prepare 2- to 3-ounce servings of meat and mix with whole grain rice or noodles and vegetables.
16. Roast garbanzo beans until crispy and season with garlic, chili, or cumin powder.
17. Prepare baked potatoes with chives or cut potatoes into strips and bake on an ungreased cookie sheet until brown and crispy.
18. Select whole wheat pita bread rather than hamburger buns.
19. Use a nonstick pan or nonstick spray to prepare grilled sandwiches.
20. Air-pop popcorn.

TABLE 2-1   Low-Fat Tricks of the Trade (continued)

---

21. Reduce sugar in recipes by one-third. Increase vanilla or cinnamon to give the impression of sweetness.

22. Prepare gelatin desserts with plain gelatin and unsweetened fruit juices.

23. Use herbs and spices, lemon juice, and low-sodium soy sauce.

Foods in the Right "Pro-Portion"

Even the best efforts at establishing good eating habits can be sabotaged unless you learn appropriate serving sizes. When you know how to assess portion sizes accurately, you can eat anything you want as long as *how much* and *how often* are considered. In contrast, even healthful snacks and meals can result in weight gain or imbalanced nutrition if consumed in excess amounts.

Women often assume that a diet that includes five servings of fruits and vegetables, six servings of grains, three servings of milk, and two servings of meat has more food than they can eat. However, this meal plan provides only 1,500 to 2,000 calories, depending on the choices made. It is serving size, not number of servings, that is misleading since most people underestimate how much they eat.

The recommended servings for various foods in the Healthy Woman's Diet are based on the following portion sizes.

Vegetables and fruits (five or more servings recommended):
- One serving of vegetables = one piece such as one carrot or one stick of celery; ½ cup cooked; 1 cup raw
- One serving of fruit = one piece such as one apple or one orange; ½ cup cooked such as applesauce; 1 cup raw; 6 ounces juice

Whole grain breads and cereals (six or more servings recommended):
- One serving = one slice of bread; ½ English muffin, bagel, or hot dog bun; ½ cup cooked grain such as rice, noodles, or oatmeal; ¾ cup ready-to-eat cereal

Cooked dried beans and peas (one or more servings recommended):
- One serving = 1 cup cooked lentils, beans, or split peas

Nonfat milk and milk products (three servings recommended):
- One serving = 1 cup nonfat milk, yogurt, or buttermilk; 2 cups nonfat cottage cheese; 1 ounce nonfat cheese

Extra-lean meat, chicken, and fish (no more than two servings recommended):
- One serving = 2 to 3 ounces without bones

It is easy to be fooled when estimating serving sizes, and a 1-cup serving can be mistaken for the recommended ½-cup serving unless carefully measured. Without portion control you are likely to consume too much of one food and not enough of another despite careful menu planning. You may also experience fluctuations in weight or not eat the recommended number of servings, assuming it is too much food.

The Five-Minute Meal

No matter how busy you are, there is always time to eat right. It takes no more time to eat a nutritious meal or a snack than it does to grab a candy bar from a vending machine or stop at a drive-up window for a hamburger and fries. Good food can be prepared in minutes, and it can be tasty and enjoyable if the following rules are followed:

1. Stock the kitchen with convenient, easy-to-prepare foods.
   - Fill the cupboards with low-fat crackers, cans of kidney or garbanzo beans, fruits canned in their own juices, canned clams, and tuna packed in water.
   - Fill the crisper with fresh fruits and vegetables and the freezer with frozen plain vegetables, fruit juices, and low-fat convenience entrées.
   - Store quick snacks in the refrigerator: nonfat yogurt, nonfat milk, no-fat and low-fat cheese, no-fat sour cream, and orange juice.
   - The bread box can contain other nutritious quick meals or snacks such as whole wheat bread, pita bread, and pumpernickel bagels.
2. Prepare foods in advance.
   - On the weekend, make a large pot of homemade soup, stew, or a casserole that will provide meals throughout the week.
   - Make basic, low-fat sauces such as tomato sauce or nonfat milk–based cream sauce, and freeze in individual portions. These sauces

can be thawed, mixed in a blender if needed, and seasoned in a variety of ways for quick meals during the week.

- Prepare a large pot of beans or rice that can be used for salads, pocket sandwiches, burritos, tacos, stews, mashed for refried (no-fat) beans, or used in casseroles.
- Make extra servings for dinner and use the leftovers the next day for lunch or snacks.
- Prepare and freeze sandwiches, bread products, and main dishes to thaw later in the week.

3. To avoid impulse snacking, carry low-fat foods such as apples, rice cakes, dried fruit, oranges, tomato juice, or a raisin bagel in your purse or briefcase, the glove compartment, or a work-desk drawer. These are nutritious alternatives to candy bars, doughnuts, and other temptations.

4. Develop a repertoire of low-fat, nutrient-dense meals that can be prepared in five to ten minutes. (See table 2-2.)

5. Snacks can be nutritious mini-meals as long as they contain one or two servings from the selection of low-fat, nutrient-dense foods. (See table 2-3.)

6. Use kitchen equipment that will save time—a microwave, Crock-Pot, food processor, blender, and electric mixer.

The Brown Bag Solution

Packing a nutritious lunch does not require hours of preparation if the following guidelines are followed.

- For sandwich fillings, use 2 ounces or less of extra-lean meats, chicken, fish, low-fat or no-fat cheeses, water-packed tuna, no-fat cream cheese, or homemade bean spreads.
- Generously garnish sandwiches with leaf lettuce, tomatoes, cucumbers, grated carrots or zucchini, sweet bell peppers, apple slices, sprouts, scallions, shredded cabbage, spinach, or mandarin oranges.
- Choose nonfat milk and plain yogurt.
- Take a thermos of homemade chili, stew, or soup (for example, bean soup or vegetable soup).

TABLE 2-2   Five-Minute Low-Fat, Nutrient-Dense Meals

- Breakfast: Top ½ whole wheat English muffin with 1 ounce no-fat cheese and broil until bubbly. Serve with a glass of orange juice.
- Breakfast: Add to 1 packet of instant plain oatmeal some nonfat milk, raisins, and a banana.
- Lunch: Fill whole wheat pocket bread with garbanzo beans, tomatoes, sprouts, grated low-fat cheese, and green onions.
- Lunch: Make a sandwich with whole wheat bread, 2 to 3 ounces of turkey, leaf lettuce, and a tomato slice. Serve with nonfat milk.
- Lunch: Stuff a large tomato with water-packed tuna mixed with low-calorie mayonaise and chopped celery. Serve with whole wheat crackers.
- Lunch: Fill a whole wheat tortilla with beans, low-fat cheese, tomatoes, and salsa. Serve with orange juice.
- Dinner: Reheat homemade soup. Serve with a whole grain roll, carrot sticks, and nonfat milk.
- Dinner: Slice fresh fruit onto no-fat cottage cheese and serve with a whole wheat roll, a baked potato (cooked in a microwave and seasoned with chives and Butter Buds), and a 3-ounce slice of lean beef or turkey.

- Choose whole grain pasta, cereals, breads, fresh fruits, and vegetables; for instance, potato salad with nonfat yogurt or sour cream dressing, whole wheat crackers, raw vegetables, a piece of fruit, or a fruit salad.
- Make pasta salads with no-fat or low-calorie dressing.
- Use spinach and leaf lettuce, which contains more vitamins and minerals than iceberg lettuce.
- Try new vegetables and vegetable combinations such as cherry tomatoes, Chinese pea pods, Jerusalem artichokes, jicama, mushrooms, radishes, spinach leaves, turnips, and zucchini. Dip in nonfat yogurt, fat-free cream cheese, or no-fat sour cream–based dressing.
- Beverages can include nonfat milk, nonfat buttermilk, fruit or vegetable juices, sparkling water or tap water, and iced herb tea.
- Leftover casseroles, chicken, turkey, fish, pasta dishes, soups, stews, and meatloaf are great brown bag lunches. Pack leftovers for tomorrow's lunch while cleaning up the kitchen at night.

TABLE 2-3 Healthy Snacks

- fresh blueberries
- fresh fruit and nonfat milk "milk shake"
- 3-bean salad prepared with no-oil marinade
- ½ papaya filled with nonfat yogurt
- ½ cantaloupe filled with chicken salad or cottage cheese
- toasted whole wheat pocket bread spread with spaghetti sauce, a sprinkle of Italian seasoning, and low-fat mozzarella cheese, and broiled
- air-popped popcorn
- "yogurt cheese" (nonfat yogurt placed in cheesecloth to drain excess liquid) can replace cream cheese on bagels, English muffins, or baked potatoes, and can be mixed with peanut butter, vanilla frosting, or mayonnaise to reduce fat and increase the nutritional content of these foods
- 2 rice cakes (toasted) with a thin slice of low-fat cheese
- crunchy vegetables
- crisp vegetables dunked in herbed nonfat yogurt dip
- peanut butter spread on a whole wheat bagel and topped with raisins or banana slices
- nonfat milk blended with fresh fruit and a tablespoon of frozen orange concentrate
- corn tortillas cut into triangles, baked until crispy, and served with salsa
- a glass of orange, pineapple, or tomato juice
- a slice of bread with apple slices and low-fat ricotta or no-fat cottage cheese
- fruit-filled shredded wheat, Cheerios, and other ready-to-eat cereals
- an English muffin topped with all-fruit jam
- tuna or chicken salad (made with a small amount of imitation mayonnaise) spread on whole wheat crackers

- Leftover pancakes can serve as tortillalike wrappers for ricotta cheese and fresh fruit snacks.

Forbidden Foods and Weekend Survival Skills

Any realistic lifelong nutrition plan must include a person's favorite foods, or it is likely to fail. Remember that nothing is forbidden but everything counts. You can include any food in your diet, but if it is high in fat, sugar, or cholesterol, plan it into your weekly nutrition program and consume it in moderation.

The Sugar Primer

Americans consume more than 125 pounds of sugar per person a year, or more than a quarter pound of sugar each day! We consume more than 450 servings per person per year of soft drinks; at 5 to 9 teaspoons of sugar per serving, that equates to 750 to 1,350 tablespoons of sugar from soft drinks alone.

It is difficult to avoid sugar since it is added to everything from ketchup, cereals, fruit drinks, granola bars, hot dogs, salad dressings, spaghetti sauce, and yogurt to desserts, pastries, and other typically sugary foods. Unfortunately, sugar supplies nothing besides calories and so can contribute to malnutrition in two ways. First, nutrient deficiencies can result if high-sugar foods replace low-fat, nutrient-dense foods. Second, excessive calories, mineral losses, and weight gain might result if sugary foods are added to an otherwise ample and nutritious diet. Weight problems, in turn, contribute to the development of heart disease, cancer, hypertension, diabetes, osteoporosis, and other degenerative disorders. Sugary foods, especially sticky foods or snacks between meals, also contribute to tooth decay and periodontal disease.

A direct link between sugar and disease is suspected but has not been proven, except as sugar relates to obesity and tooth decay. Sugar intakes common in the United States have been linked to the development of cancer, diabetes or hyperglycemia, gallstones, heart disease, kidney disease, ulcers, and nutrient deficiencies. Sugary soft drinks may result in drowsiness and mood swings. They also contain phosphorus, which reduces calcium absorption and can contribute to the development of osteoporosis if consumed in excess.

Naturally occurring sugars in fruits, vegetables, and milk do not produce the same effects as refined or added sugars. Small amounts of naturally occurring sugars are packaged with large amounts of fiber, vitamins, minerals, complex carbohydrates, and other nutrients and therefore are only a small part of low-fat, nutrient-dense foods.

The two exceptions to this rule are honey and the use of concentrated grape and pear juices as "natural" sweeteners in some convenience foods, such as mixed fruit juices. Both table sugar and honey are made up of the simple sugars glucose and fructose; the only difference is that honey contains a little more fructose. The minute amounts of a few vitamins and minerals contained in honey are insignificant to the total daily needs. Concentrated grape and pear juices are primarily sugar, not juice.

Sugar: Playing It Safe and Nutritious

Currently, sugar contributes more than 20 percent of the total calories in the typical American diet. Most national dietary recommendations suggest reducing this amount to no more than 10 percent of calories. Women who consume fewer than 2,000 calories a day must depend on low-fat, nutrient-dense foods from the Healthy Woman's Diet to guarantee adequate vitamin and mineral intakes, and so they should consume even less sugar.

To estimate sugar consumption, first identify your daily calorie intake. If it is above 2,000 calories, multiply the total calories by .10 to obtain the total day's calories that can be supplied by sugar. For example, a 2,500-calorie intake times .10 equals 250 acceptable sugar calories. This is the equivalent of the sugar in any one of the following:

- 5 tablespoons jam or jelly
- 3 bowls presweetened cereal
- 1 slice apple pie
- 1 cup sherbet
- 8 to 10 sweetened prunes
- 4 ounces fudge

A little sugar in the diet is safe and adds enjoyment and variety; however, your intake should be carefully planned and limited as all sugar is essentially calories with no redeemable nutrient qualities.

Weekend Nutrition Survival Skills

Weekends, vacations, and any other change in the daily routine can be a challenging time to stick with a nutrition plan. There are several options when approaching these "slip-prone" periods. You can eat more low-fat foods during the week and plan for impulse eating (in moderation) on weekends.

You might also plan weekends to include precisely determined amounts of higher fat foods, or anticipate slip-prone situations and decide ahead to stick with your nutrition plan. If you do splurge on weekends or vacations, include more exercise and exercise-related activities to offset the additional fat and calories. (See chapter 4 for more information on how to handle slips and relapses.)

Entertaining friends and family on the weekends while maintaining healthful eating habits can be simple and fun. As hostess you control the quantity and can offer foods that are enjoyable and low-fat. The secret to successful entertaining is not how rich the entrée is or how sweet the dessert but rather how creative and entertaining the presentation and how enjoyable the company.

Gourmet cooking from the Healthy Woman's Diet can be nutritious and tasty. Guests may not even suspect the food is low-fat! Plan the meal around favorite low-fat recipes or follow a light dinner with a "sinful" dessert served in small portions. Portion control can also be very resourceful. For example, cut a favorite cheesecake into twenty thin slices rather than eight thick pieces. A lavish serving of an all-fruit topping increases the serving size and nutritional content without adding fat.

Learn to enjoy socializing at friends' homes without compromising nutrition goals. The more you plan ahead, the easier it will be to stick with your low-fat eating plan. Plan to obtain the following information prior to the event:

- Will the meal be a sit-down meal or a buffet? (Buffets allow you more control over portion size and food selection.)
- Can guests bring anything? (If so, bring a low-fat, nutrient-dense food.)
- Will it be a formal or an informal event? (Informal events allow more flexibility for meal selection.)
- You also can ask for support depending on how well you know the host or hostess.

With this information in mind, decide to consume modest-sized servings of everything or to decline certain foods, such as sour cream on baked potatoes, sauces on meats, and salad dressing. Clearly define a modest serving so that the decision is made easily at the time of greatest temptation. Eat slowly to avoid an empty plate and the repeated offerings of more food. Remember that saying "no" to food is not a personal rejection of the host or hostess.

During the meal, refrain from taking seconds, avoid dressings, and leave sauces, gravy, meat fat, breading, and other fatty foods on your plate. Decline alcoholic or sugary beverages and ask for water or sparkling water with a twist of lemon or lime. Take large portions of low-fat foods and small servings of high-fat foods.

Dining Out Needn't Do You In

Since food labels, recipes, and other necessary decision-making tools are not available at most restaurants, it is difficult or impossible to know how much fat, salt, sugar, cholesterol, and calories are in a menu item. However, you can control the food preparation, portion size, and fat content of a meal if a few guidelines are followed in planning menu choices, ordering foods, and eating in restaurants.

Plan Ahead

Restaurants that prepare meals to order and accommodate special requests are usually small and privately owned. Cafeterias and restaurants that buy pre-prepared frozen entreés are less likely to accept special requests. Call the restaurant ahead of time and ask if food can be specially prepared. Be specific. Ask if the chicken can be dry broiled rather than sautéed, if sauces can be made with no oil, or if the food can be cooked without MSG.

The program of the American Heart Association (AHA), "Eating Away from Home," acknowledges restaurants that serve low-fat, low-cholesterol items. Ask if the restaurant serves food approved by the AHA. Beware of inexpensive restaurants; they often use more fat and sugar to compensate for the lack of more nutritious food.

Know your meal plan or carry a copy of your plan to the restaurant. Decide ahead of time what you will order based on that plan. Mentally rehearse ordering low-fat foods and prepare for possible stumbling blocks. If you plan to order a side of vegetables, remember to ask that it be served plain; otherwise it is likely to be served with butter. Request that salad dressing be served on the side and that butter and bread be removed from the table. Bring foods with you that are not offered at the restaurant, such as no-fat salad dressing, fruit or vegetable juices, or a favorite low-sodium seasoning.

How Much Will You Eat?

Practice with serving sizes to help recognize proper portions at the restaurant. Plan to leave at least one-half of the food on your plate or ask for a half-order.

Many restaurants serve more food or larger servings than designated by your meal plan. Split an entrée with a friend, give the extras to someone else, have the waiter/waitress remove the plate, or request a doggie bag.

Finally, if there is likely to be a wait at the restaurant, eat a low-fat snack or drink two glasses of water before leaving to avoid excessive hunger that can lower resistance to temptation.

Ordering in Restaurants

At the restaurant, do not hesitate to ask questions about how the food is prepared or ask for foods not listed on the menu. In addition,

- Park several blocks away and walk to the restaurant.
- Introduce yourself to the owner or waiter/waitress of a local restaurant. They are more likely to work with people who are frequent customers.
- Order without looking at the menu or order only from the à la carte section.
- Eat slowly and enjoy the company. Put the fork down between bites to allow time for the brain to catch up with the stomach and correctly register the level of fullness.
- Select soup *or* salad but not both unless that is the entire meal, or order a salad and share an entrée with a friend.
- Ask that foods be prepared without oils or fat; that salad dressings, gravies, or sauces be served on the side or not at all; that butter be removed from the table; and that the dessert menu not be brought to the table.
- Check foods when they are served to make sure your requests were fulfilled. For example, steamed vegetables that are served with droplets of oil in the juice probably were sautéed. The breading can be removed from chicken if an order for baked chicken arrives and it has been fried.
- Make special requests for whole wheat rolls, nonfat milk, vegetable platters (no cheese sauce or butter), fresh fruit for dessert, or plain oil and vinegar dressing (you can add mostly vinegar and little or no oil).
- Request low-fat milk for coffee or tea rather than nondairy creamers or whole cream.

TABLE 2-4   Ordering Low-Fat

APPETIZERS

Vegetable, bean, or tomato-based soups; vegetable juice; raw vegetable plates; fresh fruit cocktail; steamed seafood; shrimp cocktail; vegetables with dip on the side; low-fat dips such as salsa, yogurt-based spreads, or dips made from pureed vegetables

SALADS

All tossed salads and most salad bar items. Use lemon juice, low-calorie dressing, or plain oil and vinegar served on the side

ENTRÉES

2- to 3-ounce portions of extra-lean meat broiled; fish poached, broiled dry, grilled, baked, stewed, barbecued dry, or roasted; poultry without the skin; sauces on the side; vegetable and grain dishes; pasta with vegetable sauce (not cream sauce); and entrées served with wine sauces

SIDE ORDERS

Plain baked potato served with chives, cottage cheese, or nonfat yogurt; mashed or boiled potatoes; plain noodles or rice; beans, rice pilaf, or grain salads such as tabouli; steamed or raw vegetables such as artichokes, mixed vegetables, or sliced tomatoes; or mushrooms cooked in wine

DESSERTS

Gelatins, fruit ices, sorbet, fresh fruit, angel food cake, sherbet, frozen low-fat yogurt, or fruit juice

BEVERAGES

Nonfat milk, coffee, herbal teas, sparkling water, fruit juices, and vegetable juices

Avoid possibly high-fat menu items that may be described as:

refried	creamed
à la mode	au gratin
prime	au lait

(continues)

TABLE 2-4 Ordering Low-Fat *(continued)*

au fromage	in cheese sauce
Parmesan	basted
escalloped	Hollandaise
crispy	sautéed
béarnaise	

- Send back orders that are prepared incorrectly, and don't hesitate to leave a restaurant if there are no low-fat items on the menu and the establishment is unable to prepare a special order. (See table 2-4.)
- If you do overeat, eat less and exercise more the rest of the day and the next day.

Picnics, Cookouts, and Other Outings

Summer picnics and cookouts or camping trips can easily fit into a low-fat, nutrient-dense nutrition plan. From chili, corn-on-the-cob, and chicken at a picnic to instant oatmeal, raisins, and nonfat dry milk powder packed for a hiking trip, the choices for low-fat nutritious foods are endless. A picnic can be planned around a salad bar that includes a variety of textures, colors, and shapes. Salads for a picnic can be made with anything from fruit and vegetables to beans and pasta, and can be accompanied by a low-fat meat and no-fat cheese plate and a bowl of whole grain breads.

Safe Food

Since many of these foods will be exposed to air and high temperatures, the biggest concern when planning picnics and cookouts is to keep the food safe from contamination and spoilage. Refrigerate foods immediately after preparation. Wash hands before handling foods at home and at the outdoor event, and use a clean utensil to prepare and serve each dish. Avoid foods that spoil easily, such as egg dishes, cream desserts, chopped meats, and potato salads, or use special care to ensure that they are kept at cool temperatures (that is, at or below 40 degrees Farenheit). Blocks of ice, freezer packs, and dry ice are useful for maintaining low temperatures. Finally, store salad dressings in separate containers in the cooler and add to salads immediately before serving.

Fast Foods:
The Worst and the Best

Every ten seconds, one hundred people in the United States order hamburgers at a fast-food restaurant. The drive-up window has become a way of life. Despite increased concern about health and nutrition, Americans' favorite foods—hamburgers, hot dogs, whole milk, doughnuts, and French fries—and the sky-rocketing sales of soft drinks, pickles, and fried chicken reflect the fast-food phenomena more accurately than do the dietary guidelines.

The Worst

The two greatest nutritional concerns of the fast-food craze are calories and fat and their association with increased risk of developing numerous diseases and obesity. Fast foods are predominantly fat foods; approximately 40 percent to 60 percent of the calories in most of these meals comes from fat. For example,

- A sausage and egg croissant at Arby's contains 530 calories and 8 teaspoons of fat.
- A crescent sandwich with sausage at Roy Rogers contains 449 calories and 7 teaspoons of fat.
- Carl's Jr. Double Western Bacon Cheeseburger contains almost 900 calories, 63 grams of fat, 145 mg of cholesterol, and 1,810 mg of sodium.
- Two slices of Pizza Hut's Supreme Pan Pizza supply 30 grams of fat (14 of them from saturated fat) and 1,363 mg of sodium.
- Burger King's Whopper Double Beef with Cheese sandwich contains 946 calories and almost 15 teaspoons of fat.

- Taco Bell's Taco Light Platter contains 1,062 calories and 14 teaspoons of fat.

Even apparently harmless side dishes are fat-laden and calorie-dense:

- Wendy's Cheese Stuffed Potato contains 590 calories and 8 teaspoons of fat.
- Onion rings at White Castle contain 245 calories and 3 teaspoons of fat.
- A cherry danish at Roy Rogers contributes 271 calories and 3 teaspoons of fat.
- Carl's Jr. Zucchini contains 23 grams of fat and 1,040 mg of sodium.

A hamburger, French fries, and vanilla shake at a fast-food restaurant can supply 1,200 calories or more, which is more than 50 percent of the day's calories for the average woman. Unfortunately, the same meal does not supply equivalent proportions of essential vitamins, minerals, and fiber.

Even apparently "safe" foods can be deceptively high in fat. For example, one serving of McDonald's Chicken McNuggets contains the equivalent of five pats of butter in fat. A broccoli and cheese baked potato at Roy Rogers contains the equivalent of almost five pats of butter. Coleslaw may be 74 percent fat calories, and taco salads can be 60 percent fat calories.

The fat in fast foods is predominantly saturated fat. In addition, when polyunsaturated vegetable oils are used, they often are exposed to high temperatures in cooking, which raises the concentration of free radicals, highly reactive compounds that increase the risk of developing cancer, heart disease, and other disorders. Fast foods are also high in a type of cholesterol called cholesterol oxides, suspected to be highly atherogenic (causing atherosclerosis and heart disease). (See pages 240–44 for more information on free radicals and disease.)

The Best

The ten best bets at a fast food restaurant include the following:

1. plain baked potato
2. corn-on-the-cob

3. fresh fruit or fruit juice, salad bars, or individual salads (use low-calorie dressings such as McDonald's Lite Vinaigrette)
4. baked chicken or fish
5. McDonald's McLean
6. Hardee's Chicken Stix
7. Arby's Light Roast Beef or Light Roast Chicken Deluxe
8. Dairy Queen Fish Fillet sandwich
9. McDonald's milk shakes
10. low-fat milk

Wendy's also supplies low-calorie salad dressing and whole grain buns (although more than 80 percent of the flour in the bun is still enriched white flour).

Fast-Food Survival Skills

The goals when ordering at a fast-food restaurant are to limit the fat, salt, sugar, and cholesterol, and increase the complex carbohydrate, vegetable, and fruit content of the meal. To do this,

- Choose fast-food restaurants with a salad bar (avoid the potato or pasta salads and choose low-calorie dressing).
- Choose low-fat side dishes such as plain baked potato, corn-on-the-cob, orange juice, and shrimp salad.
- Select iced tea, low-fat milk, diet soft drinks, club soda, or water.
- Request no sauce on hamburgers, that the English muffin be served dry (it normally is served with a generous spread of butter), corn-on-the-cob without the butter, and salad dressings on the side. Removing the mayonnaise from a hamburger saves 150 calories. Hamburgers without cheese have 100 fewer calories.
- Avoid foods described as "double," "supreme," or "grande."
- Request more tomatoes and lettuce on sandwiches.
- Do not assume that chicken and fish are leaner choices than beef.
- Avoid anything that is deep-fat fried, including chicken, breaded items, French fries, and onion rings.
- Reduce the portion size. Order a "kiddie" plate (a Burger King Whopper Junior contains 300 fewer calories than the regular burger).

- Do not assume the calories are similar from one hamburger to another. A plain burger at Roy Rogers (456 calories) contains two times the calories of the McDonald's burger (263 calories).

An occasional fast-food meal is harmless. However, the vitamin, mineral, and fiber content of the weekly food intake might be low and the total fat intake high if more than three meals a week are chosen from fast-food fare.

CHAPTER THREE

Special Diets

Nutritional needs can be met in a variety of ways. The more restrictive the diet, however, the more difficult it becomes to ensure optimal intake of all nutrients. For example, people who avoid all dairy foods must be careful to include several daily servings of other foods high in calcium, vitamin B2, and vitamin D, since otherwise their diets will be inadequate. Avoiding meat, chicken, and fish could result in deficiencies of zinc, iron, and some B vitamins unless alternative sources of these nutrients are found. Restrictive rules about when foods should be consumed or in what order can also limit dietary intake and place demands on food selection.

Special diets can be developed that are nutritious and taste good. These diets simply require more nutrition know-how than diets based on a wide variety of foods from all the food groups.

Vegetarian Diets

Vegetarian diets have moved from the sidelines to the mainstream in the past two decades. A well-balanced vegetarian diet is safe, healthy, and can aid in the prevention of diseases such as arthritis, heart disease, cancer, and diabetes.

A well-balanced vegetarian diet easily meets the dietary recommendations for servings of fruits, vegetables, whole grains, and other foods of plant origin. By their nature, vegetarian diets are also higher in complex carbohydrates and fiber and lower in saturated fats and cholesterol than diets containing meat. Studies show that women vegetarians consume more fiber, vitamins, and minerals, and less fat and cholesterol than women who include meat in their diets.

There are several different types of vegetarian diets. A lacto-ovo vegetarian is someone who eats all fresh fruits and vegetables, whole grain breads and cereals, cooked dried beans and peas, nuts and seeds, dairy products, and eggs but avoids meat, chicken, and fish. A lacto vegetarian avoids meat, chicken, fish, and eggs. An ovo vegetarian avoids meat, chicken, fish, and milk products. Finally, a strict vegetarian, or vegan, consumes only foods of plant origin and avoids all animal-derived products, including meat, chicken, fish, eggs, and dairy products. People who avoid red meat but eat chicken and/or fish are not vegetarians.

Dispelling the Protein Myth

The biggest myth about vegetarian diets is that they do not supply enough protein. Except for the vegan diet, most vegetarian menus contain ample protein from dairy products and/or eggs, grains, beans, and nuts.

Protein is made up of building blocks called amino acids. More than twenty amino acids are needed to build tissues, red blood cells, and the hundreds of other protein-rich molecules that sustain life. The body can produce all but eight to ten of these amino acids, which must be obtained from the diet. This cluster of amino acids is called the "essential amino acids," not because they are any more important than the other amino acids but because it is essential that they be obtained from the diet.

Meat, chicken, fish, eggs, and milk products contain all the essential amino acids and are called "complete" or high-quality protein foods. Grains, dried beans and peas, nuts, seeds, and vegetables contain varying amounts of the essential amino acids and so are called "incomplete" proteins.

Complementary Proteins

Nature, in its infinite wisdom, balances the amino acids in grains and cooked dried beans and peas so that when the two are eaten together, the result is a complete or high-quality protein. For example, beans are low in the amino acid methionine and are high in the amino acid lysine, while grains are high in methionine and low in lysine. A bowl of baked beans served with brown bread, lentil and rice soup, or a peanut butter sandwich combines two incomplete proteins to make a high-quality protein. Combining a high-quality protein, such as cheese, with an incomplete protein, such as a bagel, also produces a complementary protein-rich meal.

All the essential amino acids are not required at the same meal. The body maintains an "amino acid pool," and normal protein metabolism is maintained, so as long as complementary proteins are consumed sometime during the day, normal protein metabolism is maintained. For example, an English muffin at breakfast and a bowl of lentil soup at lunch will still result in ample amounts of all the essential amino acids for normal body functions. Even vegetarian exercisers and athletes can consume enough protein to meet the extra demands of sports as long as three servings of milk products, two or more servings of cooked dried beans and peas, and at least 2,000 calories of nutrient-dense foods are consumed daily.

More Important Nutritional Considerations

For all vegetarians except vegans, complementing proteins is a minor issue since numerous combinations of protein-containing foods are included in the daily diet. Other nutrients are much more likely to be low unless care is taken to ensure the right proportion and amounts of nutrient-rich foods.

For example, red meat, chicken, and seafood are the best sources of iron and zinc. A vegetarian diet would not only exclude these choices but would interfere with iron and zinc absorption because of its high-fiber nature. In addition, the iron in plant foods is poorly absorbed compared to "heme" iron in meat. Consequently, some vegetarians consume too little of these minerals, and what is consumed is poorly absorbed. If a lacto-ovo or lacto vegetarian relies heavily on milk products for protein, the diet will almost certainly be inadequate in iron and zinc.

To ensure optimal dietary intake of these minerals, at least three servings of cooked dried beans and peas, nuts, and seeds should be included in the daily diet. Consider an iron supplement if intake is below 3,000 calories per day. (See table 3-1.)

A Closer Look at Vegans

The vegan is most susceptible to vitamin and mineral deficiencies, especially vitamins B2, B12, and D, calcium, iron, and zinc. Every day the vegan must consume foods rich in these nutrients or take a well-balanced vitamin-mineral supplement. (See chapter 6 for sources of these nutrients.)

TABLE 3-1   General Guidelines for the Lacto and Lacto-Ovo Vegetarian

The same low-fat, nutrient-dense dietary guidelines outlined in the Healthy Woman's Diet apply to lacto-ovo vegetarians except that more servings of cooked dried beans and peas replace the recommendations for meat. Ovo vegetarians also must consume more dark green vegetables, tofu, and calcium-fortified soy milk to meet their calcium and vitamin B2 needs, and they must find a supplemental source of vitamin D.

1. Limit empty-calorie foods high in sugar or fat, and choose a variety of fresh or frozen plain fruits and vegetables (5 servings or more).
2. Replace meat with eggs, cooked dried beans and peas, nuts and seeds (occasionally), and meat alternatives (4 servings or more).
3. Use low-fat or nonfat milk products such as yogurt, cheese, cottage cheese, kefir, and buttermilk (3 servings or more).
4. Select whole grains rather than refined or "enriched" grains (6 servings or more).
5. Include several servings daily of iron-rich and zinc-rich foods.

The only reliable plant sources of vitamin B12 are fermented soy products (for example, miso) and vitamin B12–fortified soy milk. Vitamin D is obtained from exposing the skin to sunlight, eating fortified foods, or taking supplements. (See table 3-2.)

In short, vegetarian diets can provide ample amounts of all nutrients if planned carefully. These diets should contain a variety of low-fat, nutrient-dense foods from each food category for optimal nutrition. A healthful diet with or without meat or milk should be easy to prepare and enjoyable to eat. (See table 3-3.)

Food Combining

Food combining, that is, restricting food intake based on certain combinations of foods, is a fad that dates back to the 1800s before people had a scientific understanding of digestion and food assimilation. In the past, food faddists have recommended not eating fruits and vegetables at the same meal, not combining citrus fruits with cereals, milk with coffee, or meats with fruit. The most recent version

---

TABLE 3-2 The Vegan Diet

The daily food guide for women on strict vegetarian diets includes the following:

VEGETABLES: 4 servings or more

At least 2 servings should be dark green leafy vegetables and 1 raw salad. One serving = 1 cup.

FRUITS: 3 servings or more

At least 1 iron-rich selection, such as strawberries or watermelon, and 1 vitamin C–rich selection, such as oranges or grapefruit. One serving = 1 piece of fruit or 6 ounces of juice.

GRAINS: 6 servings or more

Whole grain varieties only. One serving = 2 slices of bread, 4–6 crackers, 2 ounces ready-to-eat cereal, or 1 cup cooked brown rice, cereal, or noodles.

COOKED DRIED BEANS AND PEAS, INCLUDING SOY MILK: 3 servings

At least 2 cups calcium-fortified soy milk. Beans are preferable to nuts and seeds as a low-fat protein source. One serving = 1 cup cooked beans and peas, 2 cups soy milk, 6 ounces tofu, 4 tablespoons peanut butter, or 2 ounces nuts.

---

claims that carbohydrate-rich foods and protein-rich foods cannot be properly digested and absorbed when eaten at the same meal.

Proponents of this philosophy state that protein and carbohydrate cannot be mixed because they require different digestive enzymes that function at different pH (acid/alkaline) levels; pepsin digests protein in the stomach in a very acidic climate, while pancreatic amylase, sucrase, and other carbohydrate-digesting enzymes function best in the alkaline environment of the intestines.

There is no scientific or commonsense evidence for food combining. Protein- and carbohydrate-digesting enzymes do not destroy each other as the proponents of food combining state. Granted, all enzymes, including amylase and sucrase, are made from protein and are broken down and recycled by protein-digesting enzymes, but this has no effect on digestion and the absorption of food. These enzymes do not ferment or putrefy in the intestine, nor do they poison the

---

TABLE 3-3   Possible Nutrient Deficiencies for Adult Vegans

NUTRIENT	COMMON SOURCES	VEGAN SOURCES
Vitamin D	Fortified milk, fish oil	Sunshine, fortified foods, supplements
Vitamin B12	Meat, chicken, fish, milk, eggs	Fortified soy milk, miso, supplements
Calcium	Milk, cheese, canned salmon or sardines	Dark green leafy vegetables, supplements
Zinc	Meat, liver, eggs, seafood, chicken	Cooked dried beans and peas, wheat germ, whole grain breads and cereals
Iron	Meat, chicken, fish, leafy greens, "enriched" breads and cereals	Leafy greens, cooked dried beans and peas, dried fruit, iron cookware, supplements
Vitamin B2	Milk and milk products, meat, chicken, "enriched" breads and cereals, eggs	Leafy greens, Brewer's (nutritional) yeast, cooked dried beans, whole grain breads and cereals
Protein	Milk, milk products, meat, chicken, fish, eggs	Complementary vegetable proteins, soybean products

---

body or make a person fat as the proponents theorize. In fact, most foods, including grains, cooked dried beans and peas, and vegetables, contain a combination of protein and carbohydrate. Even breast milk, the perfect food for a newborn, contains protein, carbohydrate, and fat. A person must eat pure sugar or purified proteins to avoid consuming proteins and carbohydrates at the same time.

The truth is, the food eaten at one meal is broken down into its component nutrients, and these individual ingredients are mixed and churned until there is no distinguishing where an amino acid or a molecule of glucose originated. Some people might have unique differences in how their bodies handle foods, but often even these intolerances, when studied under controlled situations, are found to be

TABLE 3-4 Sample Menus for a Very Low-Fat Diet

EXAMPLE 1

Breakfast: 1 cup cooked oatmeal with 1 cup 1 percent low-fat milk and teaspoon of sugar, 1 slice whole wheat toast with 1 teaspoon butter, 1 cup of orange juice

Mid-morning snack: Apple, diet soda, and 2 glasses of water

Lunch: turkey sandwich on whole wheat bread with 1 teaspoon mayonnaise, 1 cup tossed salad with 2 teaspoons dressing, and iced tea with lemon

Mid-afternoon snacks: 1 cup low-fat yogurt, 6 ounces tomato juice, and water

Dinner: 3 ounces broiled salmon, baked potato with 2 tablespoons nonfat sour cream and chives, 1 cup Chinese pea pods and carrots, and 1 cup low-fat milk (1 percent)

Evening snack: 3 cups air-popped popcorn and water

Calories: 1,750
  Calories from protein: 22 percent
  Calories from carbohydrate: 58 percent
  Calories from fat: 20 percent

Fiber: 27 grams

EXAMPLE 2

Breakfast: 1 cup fresh fruit, 1 whole wheat bagel

Mid-morning snack: 1 cup 1 percent low-fat yogurt and water

Lunch: 2 slices pizza with lots of vegetables, 1 cup fruit juice

Mid-afternoon snack: 1 cup crunchy vegetables and water

Dinner: 4 ounces broiled chicken (2 pieces), pasta with vegetables (1 cup), 1 cup carrot sticks, 1 cup low-fat milk (1 percent)

Evening snack: 5 whole wheat low-fat crackers

Calories: 1,950
  Calories from protein: 26 percent
  Calories from carbohydrate: 57 percent
  Calories from fat: 17 percent

Fiber: 28 grams

more in their heads than in their stomachs. It is challenging enough to obtain consistently the recommended number of servings of low-fat, nutrient-dense foods in the daily menu without following unfounded diet claims that severely limit choices in planning a nutritious diet.

Beyond Low-Fat

In the 1970s, national dietary advice emerged recommending that Americans cut their fat consumption from the current 42 percent to 30 percent of total calories. More recently, the National Cholesterol Education Program and the American Heart Association have recommended that some people might need to cut fat even further, to 25 percent or less, in order to protect themselves adequately from heart disease and cancer. Additional research has also supported the health benefits of a diet that supplies as little as 20 percent fat calories. Although these recommendations might at first seem severe, in reality most people in the world consume diets similar to this. It is mostly in modern or industrialized cultures that fat intake is so high.

A diet that contains no more than 20 percent fat calories is based on the same foods as the Healthy Woman's Diet. However, the very low-fat diet contains more nonfat milk and milk products, little or no added fats or pre-prepared foods made with fat, and more grains, vegetables, and other plant-derived foods. (See table 3-4.)

CHAPTER FOUR

How to Stick with It: Ten Keys to Motivation and Habit Change

Each woman is born with a unique set of inherited genes that determines her range for health throughout life. Her habits decide where along that health continuum she will fall. Good food, regular exercise, strong social support, positive beliefs and attitudes, and effective stress-management skills swing the pendulum toward the optimally healthy end of her scale. Even the strongest genetic makeup, however, will succumb to unhealthy life-style habits.

Habits develop slowly. Day in and day out, year in and year out the same patterns and routines are repeated until they are well-worn habits. Therefore, changing these habits also takes time. Telling yourself to "eat right" or "exercise more" won't make lifelong habits go away. If you force yourself to do something, such as stop snacking or begin a strenuous exercise program after years of inactivity, you are likely to fail, and you'll believe that you don't have what it takes to make a healthful change. Nothing could be further from the truth!

The good news is that habits are developed, so they can be relearned or replaced with new habits. It is not a matter of willpower, it is a matter of following a few simple steps and practicing new behaviors until they become second nature. Identifying lifelong habits that need to be changed, setting realistic goals, practicing effective strategies for developing new habits and sticking with them are the foundations for success. Keep in mind that changes should be made gradually and that developing healthier habits becomes easier with each step.

Key Number One: Set Realistic Goals

Goals are the blueprint for developing a plan for health. If you set unrealistic goals, you will feel like a failure even when you have made tremendous progress. In fact, unrealistic goals, not lack of willpower, are often the cause of many failed attempts to change health behaviors. In contrast, if you set realistic goals, you will feel successful each step of the way.

Realistic Goals

Rather than choose some idealistic expectation for your eating habits, take time to reflect on what is reasonable for you based on your history, time demands, and health. Many people make the mistake of expecting perfection and wanting it "right now"! Goals must be realistic.

While the dietary guidelines in this book provide a benchmark for the ultimate healthful diet, it may be more reasonable to set your sights on making one or two changes now, such as eliminating the butter on your toast or using low-fat mayonnaise. Initial success gives you the motivation to stick with it and to try more challenging changes later on. Remember, the more realistic your expectations, the more successful you will be and the more motivated you will remain.

Specific and Measurable Goals

Goals should also be specific and precise. You should know exactly when you have reached your goal. "I will lose fifteen pounds in the next ten weeks by losing one to two pounds each week" is a measurable goal. "I will lose weight and start exercising" is not. The latter plan is so vague you won't know when you've reached the goal and won't notice the progress you have made along the way.

Mini-Goals

Long-range goals can be divided into mini-goals. Break down your long-range goal into weekly goals that are specific, precise, and realistic. For example, your long-range goal might be to eliminate oils and fats in cooking. Your first mini-goal might be to reduce the oil by half in all recipes. Once you have repeatedly practiced this mini-goal and are ready for the next step, you might experiment with other ways of cooking, such as simmering in chicken broth rather than butter or oil. Progressively, over the course of a year, with the help of mini-goals, you will slowly remove all oils from cooking and substantially reduce your fat intake.

A dietary goal to consume the recommended number of servings of fruits, vegetables, and whole grains specified in the Healthy Woman's Diet might start with a mini-goal to include one extra serving of fruit at lunch or to eat one extra serving of vegetables at dinner. Mini-goals are like stepping-stones to your long-range plans.

Evaluating Goals

You should routinely evaluate your progress toward your goals. Ask yourself each week, "Am I meeting my goals? Are my goals still realistic?" If you are not meeting your goals, that doesn't mean you are bad or lack willpower; it merely means you must adjust your goals or strategies to achieve success.

Key Number Two: Keep a Journal

Changing habits is possible only when you know what habits need to be modified. Since memory is biased and incomplete at best, a journal or written record of your actions is the only way to identify accurately what eating patterns are interfering with reaching your health goals. When you take the time to write down when, what, and why you eat, how you feel when eating, and how other people influence your behavior, you obtain accurate feedback that can be used to modify life-style habits and reach health goals.

You should keep detailed records for at least two weeks in order to detect habit patterns. The records should contain useful information related to eating, such as thoughts, events, and circumstances that trigger eating. Over time, behavior patterns should emerge. Some eating patterns will be useful or at least not harmful. Other patterns, such as snacking on candy bars at the mid-morning break, will interfere with health goals and might be targets for change. From the information you obtain from your records, you can develop strategies tailored to your individual needs, life-style, and time demands.

Write It Down While It's Fresh in Your Mind

Keeping records is not a test. There are no right or wrong answers, only feedback for making changes. The more honest and thorough you are in record-keeping, the more you will learn about your habits. Recording information immediately following or while you eat improves accuracy, while waiting until the end of the day or the next day to recall your food intake is likely to result in incomplete, inaccurate, or biased information.

Keep records whenever you need feedback on why you are eating inappropriately, gaining weight, or experiencing any problem that interferes with reaching your health goals. Although keeping records takes time and commitment, it is one of the most important life-style management skills you will learn! (See chart 4-1.)

Key Number Three: Analyze Your Records

After recording your eating behavior for two weeks, the next step is to analyze those records and look for patterns that might interfere with following the Healthy Woman's Diet.

Behavior doesn't just happen. You don't find yourself sitting on the couch eating a bag of cookies for no reason. Everything you do is always preceded or triggered by something else and is followed by a consequence or reward.

For example, you watch a TV show, have lunch with a friend, or go to a movie because of the enjoyment you gain. You might nibble on chips while reading the newspaper as a way to relax. Serving yourself extra dessert after an argument with a friend helps you cope with anxiety or anger. Eating a high-fat lunch at a fast-food restaurant might meet your need to socialize with friends.

Record-keeping helps you identify what triggers you to eat inappropriately. Sometimes the trigger is external; for example, you have an urge to eat after you smell food cooking, see or hear someone eating, watch a commercial on TV, notice the time of day, see an ice cream store, or attend a football game. Sometimes the trigger is internal. Thoughts such as "Everyone else eats this way, why can't I? One bite won't hurt" can trigger eating behavior that might be counterproductive to following the Healthy Woman's Diet. Other internal triggers include feeling relaxed, happy, angry, anxious, fatigued, or bored. Try to identify from your daily records what external and internal triggers interfere with your reaching your nutrition goals.

CHART 4-1   **The Daily Food Record**

DATE:

After each meal and snack, fill in the time and complete each column of the Food Record. Remember to be specific, honest, prompt, and thorough. Use the following scale for the *Hunger* category: 0 = not hungry, 5 = starving. Use this sheet to make additional copies.

Time	Food/ Beverage	Amount	Hunger	Where?	With Whom?	Doing What Else?	Feelings Before/After?

Consequences: The Whys of What You Do

If the consequences of your eating seem positive, you are likely to repeat those eating patterns. For example, if grabbing a Big Mac saves time during a busy workday, you are likely to pull up to the drive-up window again. If you are praised for your homemade cheesecake, you will probably make it again. The secret is to identify what happened before and what resulted from your inappropriate eating. Once you know this, you can develop new strategies for getting your emotional, social, or other needs met and still stick with your nutrition goals.

The following questions can help you get the most out of your records:

1. How do other people influence how, what, when, and where I eat?
2. Are specific thoughts, emotions, or attitudes associated with eating? Does loneliness, boredom, or unpleasant feelings influence my eating?
3. Does alcohol influence my food choices?
4. Am I likely to eat based on the time of day? the sight of food? the smell of food? after a glass of wine? at a party?
5. What prompts me to eat high-fat or high-calorie foods?
6. How much caffeine do I consume? Do caffeinated beverages influence my eating habits?
7. What times of day do I usually eat? Do I skip meals? How is my total day's food intake distributed throughout the day?
8. How hungry am I when I eat? How fast do I eat? What am I doing while I eat?
9. What excuses do I use to eat?
10. What precedes inappropriate eating or snacking?
11. What foods are difficult to resist?
12. What is the effect of exercise on my eating habits? Do I eat more, less, or differently?

Key Number Four: Develop a Plan

After setting realistic goals, identifying the behaviors you want to change, and recognizing what triggers these habits, the next step is to develop new habits that will lead you toward your nutrition goal.

There are basically three types of strategies for counteracting bad habits. First, you can avoid or eliminate whatever triggers the eating. If you can't resist the ice cream store on your way home from work, drive a different route.

Second, you can learn a new habit for an old situation. For example, if you snack on cookies or potato chips whenever you watch television, take this time to polish your nails, ride an exercise bicycle, or mend clothes. You also could replace fatty snacks with more healthful ones that fit into your eating plan.

Third, you can create a new situation for a new behavior. Place your walking shoes on top of the alarm clock, and when reaching over to shut off the clock, also reach for your shoes. This will remind you to set out for a quick morning walk instead of heading for the coffeepot to wake up. Developing friendships with fellow exercisers, taking a low-fat cooking class in the evening when you normally would be snacking on the couch, and bringing a nutritious lunch to work rather than going out to lunch are other examples of establishing new situations for developing new habits. (See table 4-1.)

Key Number Five: Manage Tough Situations

Tough situations are ones where you are most likely to revert to old habits. Without a plan it is difficult to stay on track. For example, your goal for the week is to avoid all fried foods, but here you are at a party nibbling on fried hors d'oeuvres. You can either stop as soon as you realize what is happening and find something else to do until a better choice comes to mind, or you can eat the hors d'oeuvres and take time later to plan how you will handle the situation in the future.

Your records are useful for identifying tough situations, where you are likely to overeat, eat high-fat foods, or engage in other unhealthy behaviors. Whether it is a party, a vacation, a person, or a mood, you can plan ahead and avoid succumbing to tough situations.

Key Number Six: Develop Support

The people who are most successful at making habit changes are those who have a strong social support network of family, friends, or co-workers. Those in your support system can help you through the slip-prone times, encourage you and

TABLE 4-1   Tips for Developing New Eating Habits

Shop from a list and do not shop when hungry.

Do not bring tempting food into the house.

Store food out of sight and immediately put away leftovers.

Enter the house through a door away from food.

Do not put bowls of food on the table.

Arrange business meetings at times other than lunch.

Eat slowly. Put the fork down between bites.

Monitor portion size.

Sit down to eat.

Leave food on the plate.

Include tempting foods in your food plan.

Redefine "problem" foods as "foods I eat occasionally."

Plan social events around exercise rather than eating.

Eat only at a designated eating spot.

Eat at regular intervals of 4 to 5 hours.

Plan ahead what and when you will eat before attending a party.

Replace negative thoughts with encouraging ones.

Ask for support, help, and encouragement from family and friends.

---

build your self-confidence, and even join in on the healthful changes you are making in your life. Most people will be supportive of your desires to eat more healthfully or exercise. However, any change in life can trigger changes in interpersonal relationships that can be beneficial or stressful.

Sometimes support does not just happen but must be nurtured and encouraged. The more you encourage support from others by openly and honestly asking for it and by modeling supportive behavior (that is, treating other people as you want to be treated), the more likely you will receive the type of support you need.

Key Number Seven: Practice Makes Habits

Realistic goals, accurate record-keeping, creative strategies, and a strong social support set the stage for changing habits. But the standing ovation comes only after practice. Including new habits in your routine every day is the way old behaviors are changed and new behaviors are developed, so practice, practice, practice.

Fortunately, the process gets easier with each step, and soon you automatically choose low-fat, nutrient-dense foods. You may even lose the taste for fattier foods. Many eating behaviors are only conditioned reflexes; if you eat just before going to bed every night, soon your body will crave a before-bed snack. By practicing a new habit, such as drinking a glass of water, riding your exercise bike for fifteen minutes, or giving yourself a facial just before bed, your body soon unlearns the food craving.

Slowly converting your diet to the low-fat, nutrient-dense Healthy Woman's Diet is much like learning to ride a bike: Practice, determination, patience, and encouragement are essential for success. Sometimes you fall off, and that's all right as long as you get back on and keep trying. Sometimes the process isn't fun, but you should attempt to remain motivated. The fun, health rewards, improved appearance, and feelings of well-being will come as long as you keep at it.

Key Number Eight: Reward Your Efforts

Motivation is the fuel that drives people toward their goals. It is the basis for all habits and especially habit change. Regardless of your health goals, motivation is the key to sticking with it.

Willpower is only a small fraction of what keeps you on track. Although many women feel that motivation is a gift—you either have what it takes to stick with it or you don't—nothing could be further from the truth. Anyone can stay motivated to reach her goals while enjoying the process; all it takes is a motivational plan.

What Is a Reward?

Rewards are anything that happens during or immediately following a new habit that increases the likelihood the behavior will occur again. Planning a trip to Mexico when you have lost twenty-five pounds is not likely to motivate you today. In contrast, going to a movie tonight if you follow your eating plan today is a more effective reinforcer.

An effective reward must increase the likelihood of sticking with a new habit. If putting a quarter in a jar toward the purchase of a new set of wineglasses every time you use low-fat cooking methods doesn't motivate you to follow your plan, then it is not a reward for you. When people say "Rewards don't work," what they are really saying is "I haven't found a reward that works for me."

Rewards are as numerous and individual as the people who use them. You can celebrate accomplishments with money, tally marks on a graph, or stars on a calendar that can be exchanged for other rewards such as going to a movie or buying a book. Rewards can be activities such as gardening and fishing. Rewards can be praise from friends and positive thoughts. However, never use food as a reward.

Reward Rules

There are a few "rules" to using rewards. First and foremost, plan daily how, when, and for what you will reward yourself. Second, a reward is effective only if you follow the "if . . . then" rule. In other words, *if* you eat a low-fat lunch, *then* (and only then) may you watch your favorite TV show. No low-fat lunch, no show.

Third, use more or multiple rewards at the start of a new behavior. For example, following the Healthy Woman's Diet might require using several rewards daily in the beginning. Later on, how you feel and the taste of the food might be rewards in themselves and few other rewards will be needed.

Finally, just as strategies must be updated frequently, a motivational plan must also be reviewed and updated. A reward that works today might not be effective once a health goal has been reached.

Key Number Nine: Handle Slips to Avoid Relapse

Everyone trying to change eating habits occasionally slips off the plan. The secret is not to allow the slip to progress into a relapse. An important characteristic of people who succeed in making lifelong habit changes is that they learn to identify a slip and handle it before it progresses to a relapse.

As mentioned above, everyone has tough situations where they are most likely to "fall off the wagon." The sooner you recognize that you are reverting to old habits and use that experience to learn more about yourself, the easier it is to prevent that slip from progressing and to avoid it in the future. (See table 4-2.)

Self-talk is also important in handling slips. Negative thoughts and attitudes

TABLE 4-2 Learning from Your Mistakes

If you are struggling with relapses, ask yourself the following questions:

1. What are the emotional states that challenge me the most? Am I likely to eat inappropriately when I am bored, happy, tense, relaxed?

2. How have I prevented relapses in the past?

3. How do worries about my willpower interfere with my health and fitness goals?

4. What type of positive thoughts help me to counteract self-defeating thoughts and keep me on track?

5. What is the most consistent and strongest reward for my efforts to change health-related behaviors?

6. What do I foresee as my biggest challenge to long-term health and fitness management? What can I do to minimize this challenge in the future?

that reinforce that you are a failure or lack willpower will encourage the slip to progress. Positive self-talk allows you to use mistakes to reevaluate and revise health and fitness plans and encourages long-term success. Monitor your self-talk. You can mentally set yourself up for relapse, so replace negative thoughts with positive ones.

When you realize that you have strayed from your eating or health plans, review your goals, records, strategies, and motivational plan. Identify troublesome situations and plan how you will cope with them in the future. Focus on the long-term benefits of feeling your best rather than the short-term payoffs of overeating or eating unhealthy foods. A piece of cake might taste good now, but the long-term effects of inappropriate eating might lower self-esteem, cause weight gain and frustration, interfere with optimal health, or prevent you from wearing well-fitting clothes.

Key Number Ten: Maintain It or Lose It

Learning to eat low-fat and nutrient-dense meals, losing weight, or beginning any new health habit is the first step. The biggest challenge is maintaining your new

TABLE 4-3   The Maintainer's Questionnaire

Ask yourself the following questions when analyzing your food records:

1. What do I want to improve in my maintenance habits?
2. What do I need to continue doing or thinking?
3. What do I need to do more frequently?
4. What characteristics of a healthy person do I currently exhibit?
5. What do I want to be doing or thinking 3, 6, or 12 months from now?
6. How much progress toward my goals do I want to have made in 3 months?

The answers to these questions provide you with information to update goals, develop mini-goals, and practice new strategies.

---

habits. The work is not complete when you reach your goals; however, maintaining those goals requires only that you continue to practice the same key steps that helped you get there.

First, never assume you've "made it." Overconfidence can be your worst enemy. Breaking an old habit, whether it be nail biting or eating high-fat foods, is a slow process. Eating a healthy diet is a lifetime process that requires careful attention, so don't be fooled into thinking that you have overcome your old habits forever!

Second, remember that no one is powerless, helpless, or hopeless when it comes to food. In fact, women who believe they can make a difference in their lives show increased power and ability to do so. Those who believe they can't make a difference are riddled with feelings of self-doubt, helplessness, and hopelessness, which interferes with success. Remind yourself that it is not the number or size of your obstacles but how you handle them and think about them that determines success or failure. You are limited only by your own expectations, aspirations, and beliefs. (See table 4-3.)

You have worked hard to reach your goals. You are healthier, more fit, and more confident than when you started. Focus on how to maintain your healthier condition and continue improving. Realistic goal-setting, record-keeping, effective strategy development, and your motivational system will continue to be essential for staying on track.

Surround yourself with people who also take their health seriously and who support your efforts. Strengthen your skills by repeating situations that you have handled successfully. Frequently monitor your thoughts and attitudes, and act immediately at the first sign of a slip. Finally, pay attention to your successes, be patient, and stick with it!

CHAPTER FIVE

Understanding Vitamin and Mineral Supplements

The best place to obtain daily requirements for vitamins and minerals is from the diet. However, not everyone is able to or wants to consistently consume a perfect diet; consequently, vitamin-mineral status might suffer unless an alternative source of these nutrients is found. During times of physical or emotional stress, such as surgery, depression, and competition in sports, nutrient needs might exceed the Recommended Dietary Allowances (RDAs), but food intake does not always increase to meet them.

The current questions are no longer concerned with minimal levels that prevent classic nutrient-deficiency diseases but ask "Are amounts known to prevent clinical deficiencies adequate to maintain optimal nutrition and health?" and "Does the 'balanced' diet supply not only adequate but optimal amounts of nutrients?" These questions lack definitive answers at this time; however, a well-balanced supplement that provides moderate doses of the vitamins and minerals is safe nutritional insurance. On the other hand, long-term use of larger doses of single or multiple nutrients is a form of self-medication and should be carefully monitored by a dietitian or physician trained in nutritional science.

The Rationale for Supplementation

Numerous national nutrition surveys conclude that the "balanced diet" is not well balanced and have reported deficiencies of vitamin A, vitamin C, the B vitamins, calcium, and iron. Nine out of every ten diets are marginal in chromium and contain only one-half of the RDA for magnesium. It is estimated that the average intake of folic acid is approximately one-half the adult RDA.

Life-style habits common to modern families are often a challenge to meeting daily recommendations for vitamins and minerals. People skip meals, snack on convenience foods, diet, and eat away from home. Family members often do not sit down for meals together, and the single-parent household has rearranged eating habits. Today, people consume fewer calories than their ancestors. A reduced food intake means that diets containing a large percentage of selections from highly processed or refined foods cannot guarantee daily recommended amounts of vitamins and minerals.

Who Is a Likely Candidate for Supplements?

Supplementation might be necessary for those who diet, have irregular eating habits, skip meals, or choose poorly from the wealth of food selections available. Women are at particular risk for nutrient deficiencies if they are menstruating, on low-calorie diets, pregnant, breast-feeding, or if they are seniors or are chronically ill.

Women who abuse alcohol, tobacco, or other drugs, those who are on long-term medications, are under stress, or who have poor eating habits are also included in this group. Strict vegetarians and food faddists are at particular risk for developing nutrient deficiencies unless a well-balanced supplement fills the nutritional gaps of the suboptimal diets.

Supplement Survival

The shelves of most grocery, drug, and health food stores are lined with vitamin and mineral supplements. It is easy to feel overwhelmed when facing this ocean of products, especially when little regulation has led to a mixture of quackery and quality.

The following steps are helpful in sifting fact from fallacy pertaining to supplements, food claims, and the media coverage of nutrition research:

1. Read or listen critically. Question everything. Ask for evidence of all claims and a written guarantee. If research is quoted, ask for

copies of all original research published in referenced, scientific, peer-reviewed journals.

2. Analyze the style. Is it written to appeal to emotions or intellect?

3. Critique the content. Are the claims exaggerated? Are the facts embellished? Is the content based on factual evidence or testimonials? Are references provided? Are the references current (within the last five years) and from scientific journals, or from popular books and magazines?

4. If the claim states a food or nutrient helps or cures a disease, ask how much is needed to see an effect and whom it helps. Is the amount realistic, or would it require dramatic deviations from a person's normal food intake? Are the effects seen in everyone or only in a specific subset of the population? A study on animals does not prove the same results could be obtained from humans.

5. Is the research on which the claim is based funded by an interest group? For example, a study funded by the Egg Board on egg consumption and blood cholesterol levels might draw different conclusions from one funded by the Soybean Growers of America.

6. Although consensus in the nutrition community is rare, do other trained nutrition experts also agree with these findings or claims? Judge each claim, article, study, and ad on its own merits.

7. Consider the source. The nutrition information published in popular magazines is more accurate now than it was a few years ago, but readers should still be aware that not all magazines offer sound nutrition advice. Check the nutrition credentials of the writer and the magazine's editor or editorial board.

8. Who is the author or speaker? What is his or her background in nutrition? What is the motive for writing or speaking? How does he or she interpret the facts? Is the product or program promoted by a celebrity who is not an expert on this topic?

9. Read other references on the topic. Double-check the information. Seek professional advice from well-respected nutrition groups such as the American Heart Association, state and local dietetic associations, nutritionists and dietitians at the public health department, or from the Food and Drug Administration, 5600 Fishers Lane, Rockville, Maryland 20857.

10. If the product was promoted through the mail, you can report suspicious advertising claims to the Federal Trade Commission, Bureau of Consumer Protection, Washington, D.C. 20850. Health fraud also can be reported to the state attorney general's office and the county prosecutor's office.

In truth, there are more useless products than worthwhile ones on the market. Supplement labels add insult to injury with words such as "organic," "therapeutic," "time-release," and "chelated." Confusion about optimal nutrient intake, the best type of nutrient, and the best ratio of nutrients can leave the shopper asking "How much of what is best?"

The Vitamin-Mineral Primer

The following are the most commonly misunderstood terms related to vitamin and mineral supplements.

Vitamin A and Beta Carotene: Vitamin A, or retinol, is the "active" form of the vitamin and is found in liver, eggs, and other foods of animal origin. It is potentially toxic if taken in large amounts (that is, 50,000 IU or more) for long periods of time.

Beta carotene is one of hundreds of carotenoids found in dark green and orange fruits and vegetables. It is converted to active vitamin A in the body (and therefore is called a "precursor" to vitamin A) or remains intact and functions independent of its vitamin A activity. Beta carotene is nontoxic even in high doses.

Vitamin A palmitate and vitamin A acetate are synthetic versions of vitamin A found in supplements and foods fortified with vitamin A. Tretinoin and isotretinoin are special forms of vitamin A used by prescription only in the treatment of acne; they are not true vitamins.

Vitamin E: Vitamin E is a family of compounds including the tocopherols. The most active natural form is d-alpha tocopherol. Synthetic vitamin E, or dl-alpha tocopherol, might not be quite as potent as its natural version. This fat-soluble vitamin is relatively nontoxic even in large doses taken for long periods of time.

B Vitamins: Although these water-soluble vitamins were thought to be nontoxic, recent research shows that temporary and even permanent damage can develop from overdosing with certain B vitamins, such as vitamin B6. More than likely, if the diet is low in one B vitamin, it is probably low in others, and since these vitamins work as a team, they are most effective if taken as a complex and in the proper ratio to one another (that is, 100 percent to 300 percent of the RDA for all B vitamins). Larger amounts of a single B vitamin are justified in special circumstances, such as vitamin B6 in carpal tunnel syndrome and folic acid in pregnancy. In most cases, a supplement manufacturer adds large amounts of the B vitamins because they are inexpensive, not because they are needed.

Vitamin C: Vitamin C, or ascorbic acid, is a relatively nontoxic, water-soluble vitamin that can be consumed by healthy adults in doses several times the RDA with no adverse side effects. However, people at risk for developing kidney stones should limit vitamin C intake to 500 mg or less.

The "vitamin C complex" is a nonregulated term that suggests other substances have been added to the supplement, such as any number of bioflavonoids. "Natural" vitamin C contains small amounts of naturally derived vitamin from rose hips or acerola berries mixed with a greater amount of synthetic vitamin C. Ascorbyl palmitate is added in small amounts to some mineral supplements as a preservative.

Calcium: Most calcium supplements are equally well absorbed. Choosing a supplement is therefore more a matter of convenience. Calcium carbonate and calcium citrate are 40 percent calcium, so fewer tablets are needed to reach the RDA than if calcium lactate (13 percent calcium) or calcium gluconate (9 percent calcium) are chosen.

Some antacids are inexpensive sources of calcium, providing the product does not contain aluminum, which might interfere with calcium absorption, or sodium, which adds to the total day's intake of salt. Bonemeal and dolomite are not recommended as regular sources of calcium since some brands contain toxic metals such as lead and cadmium. Calcium citrate is better absorbed in women with low stomach acid, a condition called achlorhydria. Calcium carbonate is best absorbed with food. In fact, most supplements should be consumed with food since the presence of other nutrients, such as vitamin D, magnesium, and lactose, aids in the absorption of calcium. Doses greater than 2,500 mg a day should be monitored by a physician.

Chromium: Not all chromium supplements are created equal. Brewer's yeast is an excellent form of well-used chromium, as are supplements containing chromium from yeast. In contrast, chromium chloride must first be converted by the body to the potent form of the mineral, and this conversion is incomplete in many people. Since there is no way to know if you are a good chromium converter, it is best to rely on yeast-based sources. Glucose tolerance factor (GTF) chromium sounds like an active form of the mineral, but few brands are good sources of chromium.

Magnesium: Most forms of magnesium are well absorbed when the mineral is consumed in small, divided doses of 100 mg per serving (that is, small-dose supplements several times a day rather than one high-dose supplement). Limited research shows that magnesium citrate might be slightly better absorbed than magnesium oxide, but if either the oxide or the acetate version of the mineral is consumed with food, this difference in absorption is likely to be small. Magnesium absorption decreases as calcium intake increases unless magnesium intake is increased at the same time, so keep the calcium-to-magnesium ratio at approximately 2 to 1. For example, 1,000 mg of calcium would require 500 mg of magnesium. Doses greater than 600 mg could produce a laxative effect.

Label Lingo

The following is a brief review of supplement terminology.

Therapeutic or super potency: The terms *super potency, megavitamins,* and *therapeutic* refer to doses in excess of ten times the RDA for one or more vitamins or minerals. The terms are deceiving since they imply more is better. In most cases, this is not the rule, and at best, the extra nutrient is excreted. At worst, as in the case of vitamins A, D, and B6, and several minerals, the nutrient can accumulate to toxic levels. Exceptions to the rule are vitamins E and C. These nutrients are safe in relatively large doses, although intakes should be limited to 400 IU and 1,000 mg, respectively.

A chelated mineral: A chelated mineral is one that is attached to another substance called a "chelator," such as an amino acid. Zinc gluconate is an example of a chelated mineral. Theoretically, chelated minerals are absorbed better than other minerals. However, chelation forms a weak bond between the mineral and the amino acid that is often easily broken once the supplement hits the stomach. The free-floating mineral is then absorbed at the same rate as a nonchelated mineral or dietary mineral. Nutrient absorption is affected more by the circumstances in which you take a supplement than by the supplement itself. For example, most minerals except iron are better absorbed with food.

Time-released vitamins: The theory supporting time-released supplements makes sense. Unfortunately, in reality, time-released vitamins and minerals are no better and even might be less effective than other supplements.

Time-released supplements are designed to dissolve and be absorbed slowly. This should prevent the rapid rise and subsequent loss of the nutrient through the urine and prolong the availability of the nutrient to the tissues; however, by the time most time-released tablets have dissolved, they have passed the portion of the intestine where they would be absorbed.

Organic and natural: "Organic" and "natural" vitamins and minerals are, in most cases, no better than synthetic ones. Often these terms only imply a higher cost. Exceptions to this rule might be chromium, selenium, and vitamin E. Yeasts grown on a selenium- or chromium-rich medium incorporate the minerals into their structure in an organic-like form that is better absorbed and used than are inorganic mineral salts, such as selenite and chromic chloride. The "natural" form of vitamin E, called d-alpha tocopherol, is more potent than the synthetic form, dl-alpha tocopherol.

Emulsified vitamins: The term "emulsified" is applied only to supplements that contain a fat-soluble vitamin such as A or E. An emulsifier separates the fat-soluble vitamin droplets into smaller droplets that are more readily absorbed from the digestive tract. They can be useful if you have celiac disease or other digestive tract problems that interfere with fat absorption.

Choosing a Supplement

A few simple guidelines take some of the mystique out of supplement shopping.

1. Choose a multiple vitamin-mineral preparation rather than several single supplements.
2. Select a supplement that provides approximately 100 percent to 300 percent of the U.S. RDA for the following vitamins and minerals: fat-soluble vitamins A (preferably beta carotene) and E; water-soluble vitamins C, B1, B2, niacin, B6, B12, folic acid, pantothenic acid, and biotin; calcium, copper, iron, magnesium, and zinc.

   Vitamin D can be particularly toxic, so total intake from fortified foods, such as milk and cereals, and supplements should be no more than 200 percent of the U.S. RDA. Most multiples do not contain adequate amounts of calcium or magnesium, and additional single supplements might be needed if the diet is low in these minerals. (See page 19 for more information on the U.S. RDAs.)

Choose a supplement that provides the following minerals in these approximate amounts: chromium (50 to 200 mcg), manganese (2.5 to 5.0 mg), and selenium (50 to 200 mcg).

3. Supplements that are taken in multiple doses allow you to take smaller doses several times a day, which helps maximize absorption. They also provide flexibility. The dose can be increased on days when the diet is not perfect and decreased on "good" days.

4. Avoid supplements that contain useless or potentially harmful substances, such as vitamin B15, hormone extracts, inositol, or nutrients in minute amounts. These ingredients falsely imply added benefits.

5. Consider taking extra vitamin C, vitamin E, and beta carotene.

Some amino acids, such as tryptophan and tyrosine, are building blocks for hormonelike substances in the body. Research is incomplete on the safety of these dietary factors, and large doses could trigger undesirable side effects. Consequently, amino acid supplements should be taken only under the supervision of a physician.

Designing Your Own Supplement Program

Review your answers to the questionnaire titled "Analyzing Your Diet" on pages 36–38. If you answered "no" to questions 2, 3, 5, 6, 7, 9, 11, and 13, your diet may not be adequate in certain vitamins and minerals. For example,

- A "no" answer to questions 5, 6, or 7 could mean your diet is low in vitamin C, beta carotene, vitamin E, folic acid, and magnesium.
- A "no" answer to question 9 could mean your diet is low in fiber, trace minerals, B vitamins, and vitamin E.

- A "no" answer to question 11 suggests inadequate intake of iron, zinc, protein, magnesium, and B vitamins.
- A "no" answer to question 13 could mean your diet is low in calcium, vitamin B2, magnesium, and vitamin D.
- Repeated dieting as indicated in question 2 suggests wide fluctuations in nutrient intake with suboptimal intakes often occurring.

Use of alcohol or medications, frequent or chronic stress, or restricted food intake could result in increased nutrient needs or limited nutrient intake. All vitamins and minerals could be suspect in these situations.

In addition, if you have a personal or family history of heart disease, hypertension, cancer, or diabetes; have allergies, food intolerances, or frequent colds and infections; engage in strenuous exercise; are pregnant or breast-feeding; use tobacco; or are recovering from illness or surgery, you might want to consider a broad-range vitamin-mineral supplement or specific single supplements in low doses to boost your nutritional status. (See individual diseases discussed in part III for a more detailed description of vitamin and mineral needs.) The table on page 35 also provides detailed information on the physical symptoms of various nutrient deficiencies, which is useful when designing a supplement program.

Table 5-1 provides a sample vitamin and mineral supplement program for the average healthy woman. If you have a family history of cancer or live in a metropolitan area with smog, you might use this supplement as a foundation and add additional antioxidant nutrients such as beta carotene, vitamin C, and vitamin E. If you are under considerable stress, add additional amounts of beta carotene, the B vitamins, magnesium, the trace minerals such as zinc, and vitamin C. If you are healthy and planning pregnancy, add additional folic acid and iron to this baseline formula.

Supplements: The Bottom Line

Supplements are no substitute for the low-fat, nutrient-dense eating plan outlined in the Healthy Woman's Diet. Many nutritive substances in foods, other than vitamins and minerals, protect against disease and improve health. For example, a substance in garlic called alliin is a natural antibiotic; compounds called indoles

TABLE 5-1 A Sample Vitamin and Mineral Supplement for the Healthy Woman

Two to four tablets taken daily with meals should supply the following nutrients:

	QUANTITY	PERCENTAGE OF U.S. RDA
Vitamin A (retinol)	2,500 IU	50
Beta carotene.	10 mg	*
Vitamin D	400 IU	100
Vitamin E (d-alpha tocopherol)	60 IU	200
Vitamin B1 (thiamin)	1.5 mg	100
Vitamin B2 (riboflavin)	1.7 mg	100
Niacin (niacinamide)	20 mg	100
Vitamin B6 (pyridoxine)	2 mg	100
Vitamin B12 (cobalamine)	6 mcg	100
Folic acid (folacin).	400 mcg	100
Biotin	300 mcg	100
Pantothenic acid (calcium pantothenate).	10 mg	100
Vitamin C (ascorbate)	150 mg	250
Calcium (calcium carbonate)	1,000 mg	100
Chromium (chromium from yeast)	200 mcg	*
Copper	2 mg	100
Iron (ferrous fumarate).	18 mg	100
Magnesium (magnesium citrate)	400 mg	100
Manganese	5 mg	*
Molybdenum	75–250 mcg	*
Selenium (selenomethionine)	200 mcg	*
Zinc (zinc gluconate)	15 mg	100

*No U.S. RDA has been established for these nutrients. The amounts listed are based on the Food and Nutrition Board's safe and adequate daily amounts.

in vegetables such as cabbage and broccoli protect against cancer; and saponins in cooked dried beans and peas help lower blood cholesterol levels. These non-nutrient substances are found only in a varied diet, not in supplements.

People often mistakenly believe that supplements protect them against disease, strengthen the immune system above normal levels, or prevent premature aging, even when other life-style habits remain unhealthy. This is not the case. However, supplements can be an inexpensive and practical means of ensuring adequate nutrition, especially for women at risk of developing nutrient deficiencies.

CHAPTER SIX

Nutrients and
Their Dietary Sources

Increase your intake of the antioxidants, such as vitamin C and beta carotene."

"You are likely to be iron deficient unless you consume several servings daily of iron-rich foods."

"If nursing, you must make sure you eat several calcium-rich foods daily."

These and other recommendations are easier said than done, unless you know what foods contain what nutrients. The following is a partial list of good food sources for most of the essential nutrients, including protein, vitamins, and minerals.

All Recommended Dietary Allowances (RDAs) listed are for nonpregnant women.

PROTEIN: *(RDA: 44–50 grams)*

Food	Quantity	Grams
Chicken, beef, pork	3 ounces	21
Fish	3 ounces	21
Dried beans and peas, cooked	1 cup	14
Nonfat milk	1 cup	8
Low-fat milk	1 cup	8
Egg	1 medium	7
Vegetables	½ cup	2
Bread	1 slice	2
Cereals	1 ounce	2
Fruit	1 serving	0

VITAMIN A/BETA CAROTENE *(RDA: 4,000 IU)*

Food	Quantity	IU
Beef liver	3 ounces	45,420 (A)
Carrot juice	1 cup	11,520 (BC)
Pumpkin	¾ cup	10,943 (BC)
Dandelion greens	½ cup	10,530 (BC)
Sweet potatoes	¼ cup	8,500 (BC)
Carrots	½ cup	7,610 (BC)
Spinach	½ cup	7,200 (BC)
Collard greens	½ cup	5,130 (BC)
Winter squash	½ cup	4,305 (BC)
Mustard greens	½ cup	4,060 (BC)
Cantaloupe	¼	3,270 (BC)
Broccoli	½ cup	2,363 (BC)
Romaine lettuce	3½ cups	1,900 (BC)
Dried apricots	4 halves	1,635 (BC)
Peach	1	1,320 (BC)
Tomato juice	½ cup	970 (BC)
Asparagus	½ cup	650 (BC)
Egg yolk	1	590 (A)
Oysters	15	555 (A)
Green peas	½ cup	430 (BC)
Summer squash	½ cup	410 (BC)
Brussels sprouts	½ cup	405 (BC)
Banana	1 medium	230 (BC)
Low-fat milk, fortified	1 cup	200 (A)

VITAMIN D *(RDA:* 400 IU)*

Food	Quantity	IU
Sardines	3½ ounces	1,150–1,570
Mackerel, fresh	3½ ounces	1,100
Cod liver oil	1 teaspoon	400
Herring, fresh	3½ ounces	315

*The previous recommendation of 400 IU for Vitamin D is used.

Food	Quantity	IU
Salmon, fresh	3½ ounces	154–550
Shrimp	3½ ounces	150
Milk, fortified	1 cup	100
Egg yolk	1 medium	25
Beef liver	3½ ounces	9–42
Cheese	1 ounce	3–4
Butter	1 pat	1.8

VITAMIN E *(RDA: 12 IU)*

Food	Quantity	IU
Wheat germ oil	¼ cup	63.6
Wheat germ	½ cup	27
Almonds	¼ cup	25
Safflower oil (preferably cold-pressed)	¼ cup	19.5
Cottonseed oil	¼ cup	13
Avocado	½	0.95–2.0
Broccoli	3 stalks	0.8–3.4
100% whole grain cereal	1 cup	0.4
100% whole wheat bread	1 slice	0.4

VITAMIN K *(RDA: 55–65 mcg)*

Food	Quantity	Mcg
Turnip greens	⅔ cup	650
Green peas	½ cup	225
Broccoli	⅔ cup	200
Lettuce	2 cups	129
Cabbage	⅔ cup	125
Liver, beef	3½ ounces	92
Spinach	⅔ cup	89
Asparagus	5–6 spears	57
Peach	1	16
Egg yolk	1 medium	11

Food	Quantity	Mcg
Tomato, raw	I medium	7
Potato, baked	I medium	6

VITAMIN B1 *(RDA: 1.0–1.1 mg)*

Food	Quantity	Mg
Wheat germ	¼ cup	.44
Ham	3 ounces	.40
Brewer's yeast	I tablespoon	.34
Oysters	¾ cup	.25
Beef liver	3 ounces	.23
Green peas	½ cup	.22
Lima beans	½ cup	.16
Collard greens	½ cup	.14
Orange	I	.13
Dried beans, cooked	½ cup	.13
Dandelion greens	½ cup	.12
Asparagus	½ cup	.12
Orange juice	½ cup	.11
Low-fat milk	I cup	.10
Noodles, enriched	½ cup	.10
Nonfat milk	I cup	.09
Potato	I small	.08
White bread	I slice	.06
Broccoli	½ cup	.06
Chicken, meat only	3 ounces	.05
Beef, lean	3 ounces	.05

VITAMIN B2 *(RDA: 1.2–1.3 mg)*

Food	Quantity	Mg
Beef liver	3 ounces	3.60
Low-fat milk	I cup	.52
Nonfat milk	I cup	.44

Food	Quantity	Mg
Yogurt, whole milk	1 cup	.39
Oysters	¾ cup	.30
Cottage cheese, creamed	½ cup	.30
Avocado	½	.22
Beef, lean	3 ounces	.19
Collard greens	½ cup	.19
Chicken, meat only	3 ounces	.16
Dandelion greens	½ cup	.15
Asparagus	½ cup	.13
Broccoli	½ cup	.12
Brussels sprouts	½ cup	.11
Spinach	½ cup	.11
Green peas	½ cup	.09
Strawberries	¾ cup	.08

NIACIN *(RDA: † 13–15 mg)*

Food	Quantity	Mg
Tuna, water-packed	½ can	13.0
Beef liver	3 ounces	12.3
Halibut, baked	3 ounces	6.06
Chicken	2 pieces	5.8
Salmon, baked	3 ounces	5.67
Beef, lean	3 ounces	5.1
Pork roast	3 ounces	4.27
Brewer's yeast	1 tablespoon	3.16
Avocado	½ medium	2.92
Tomato sauce	1 cup	2.82
Almonds	½ cup	2.39
Miso (soybean product)	1 cup	2.37
Pinto beans	½ cup	2.1

† The niacin in food tables is only a fraction of the total niacin available to the body. It does not include the amount that is converted from the amino acid tryptophan. Sixty milligrams of tryptophan are considered equivalent to 1 milligram of niacin.

Food	Quantity	Mg
Lentils, homemade	1 cup	2.1
Tortilla, flour	one 10-inch	1.93
Wheat germ	¼ cup	1.70
Brown rice, cooked	½ cup	1.50
Nectarine	1 medium	1.37
Kidney beans, canned	1 cup	1.29
Green peas	½ cup	1.18
Whole wheat bread	1 slice	1.09
Whole milk	1 cup	.2+
Banana	1 medium	.8
Orange	1 medium	.5
Carrot, raw	1 medium	.4
Egg	1	.03+

VITAMIN B6 *(RDA: .5–1.6 mg)*

Food	Quantity	Mg
Beef liver	3 ounces	.569
Banana	1 medium	.480
Avocado	½ medium	.420
Chicken	3 ounces	.340
Corn, cooked	½ cup	.246
Wheat germ	¼ cup	.220
Collard greens, cooked	½ cup	.170
Spinach, cooked	½ cup	.161
Tomato	1 medium	.148
Brown rice, cooked	½ cup	.127
Green peas	½ cup	.110
Broccoli, cooked	½ cup	.107
Nonfat milk	1 cup	.098
Orange	1 medium	.098
Peanut butter	1 tablespoon	.046
Apple	1 medium	.045
Whole wheat bread	1 slice	.041

Food	Quantity	Mg
White rice, cooked	½ cup	.030
White bread	1 slice	.009

FOLIC ACID *(RDA: ‡ 400 mcg)*

Food	Quantity	Mcg
Brewer's yeast	1 tablespoon	313
Black-eyed peas, cooked	1 cup	240
Beef liver	3 ounces	123
Kidney beans, canned	1 cup	126
Baked beans, homemade	1 cup	122
Spinach, freshly chopped	1 cup	109
Spinach, raw	1 cup	106
Orange juice	6 ounces	102
Lettuce, Romaine	1 cup	98
Spinach, cooked	½ cup	82
Avocado	½ medium	81
Wheat germ	¼ cup	80
Asparagus, fresh	½ cup	70
Beets, cooked	½ cup	66
Collard greens, cooked	½ cup	65
Grapefruit juice	1 cup	52
Honeydew melon	1 cup	51
Papaya	1 medium	48
Broccoli, cooked	½ cup	44
Brussels sprouts, cooked	½ cup	28
Strawberries, fresh	1 cup	28
Bread, whole wheat	1 slice	16
Bread, white	1 slice	10
Lettuce, iceberg	1 cup	0–20

‡Because of controversy over the accuracy of the reduced RDAs (180 mcg for folic acid and 15 mg for iron) established in 1989, the previous recommendations of 400 mcg and 18 mg, respectively, are used.

VITAMIN B12 *(RDA: 2 mcg)*

Food	Quantity	Mcg
Beef liver	3 ounces	68
Clams	½ cup	19.1
Oysters	3½ ounces	18
Salmon, baked	3 ounces	4.93
Trout, baked	3 ounces	2.40
Snapper, baked	3 ounces	1.60
Tempeh (soybean product)	1 cup	1.39
Tuna, canned	2 ounces	1.32
Yogurt, low-fat plain	1 cup	1.28
Nonfat milk	1 cup	0.95
Cottage cheese, creamed	½ cup	0.70
Miso (soybean product)	1 cup	0.57
Chicken	3 ounces	0.36
Cheese, cheddar	1 ounce	0.23

BIOTIN *(RDA: 30–100 mcg)*

Food	Quantity	Mcg
Beef liver	3 ounces	82
Oatmeal, cooked	1 cup	58
Soybeans, cooked	½ cup	22
Clams	½ cup	20
Salmon, baked	3 ounces	10
Brown rice	½ cup	9
Shrimp	3 ounces	9
Low-fat milk	1 cup	7
Avocado	½ medium	6
Banana	1 medium	6
Peanut butter	1 tablespoon	6
Cantaloupe	¼	3
Orange	1 medium	3

PANTOTHENIC ACID *(4,000–7,000 mcg)*

Food	Quantity	Mcg
Beef liver	3 ounces	6,035
Egg	1 medium	1,100
Avocado	½ medium	1,100
Chicken, meat only	3 ounces	826
Nonfat milk	1 cup	806
Low-fat milk	1 cup	788
Chicken	3 ounces	765
Tomato sauce	1 cup	757
Soybeans, cooked	½ cup	525
Sole, baked	3 ounces	500
Cottage cheese, low-fat	1 cup	486
Orange juice	1 cup	476
Banana	1 medium	450
Orange	1 medium	450
Collard greens	½ cup	425
Potato, baked	1 medium	400
Almonds	½ cup	335
Broccoli, cooked	½ cup	315
Cantaloupe	¼	300
Brown rice, cooked	½ cup	300
Apricots, fresh	3	254
Peanut butter	1 tablespoon	238
Oatmeal, cooked	½ cup	234

VITAMIN C *(RDA: 60 mg)*

Food	Quantity	Mg
Green pepper	1 large	128
Red bell pepper	½ cup	95
Orange juice	6 ounces	90
Grapefruit	1 medium	76
Kiwi	1	74

Food	Quantity	Mg
Brussels sprouts	½ cup	68
Orange	1 medium	66
Strawberries	½ cup	66
Broccoli	½ cup	52
Collard greens	½ cup	44
Grapefruit juice	6 ounces	38
Cantaloupe	¼	32
Blackberries	1 cup	30
Beet greens	½ cup	30
Tomato juice	6 ounces	30
Cabbage	½ cup	24
Baked potato, flesh only	1 medium	20
Asparagus	½ cup	19
Green peas	½ cup	17

CALCIUM *(RDA: 800–1,200 mg)*

Food	Quantity	Mg
Nonfat milk	1 cup	296
Nonfat dry milk	⅓ cup	293
Yogurt	1 cup	272
Oysters	¾ cup	170
Canned salmon with bones	3 ounces	167
Collard greens, cooked	½ cup	145
Dandelion greens, cooked	½ cup	126
Cottage cheese	1 cup	116
Spinach, cooked	½ cup	106
Mustard greens, cooked	½ cup	97
Orange	1 medium	54
Broccoli, cooked	½ cup	49
Dried beans, cooked	½ cup	45
Lima beans, cooked	½ cup	40
Tangerine	1 medium	34
Cabbage	½ cup	32
Green beans	½ cup	32

Food	Quantity	Mg
Winter squash	½ cup	29
Summer squash	½ cup	26
Whole wheat bread	1 slice	25
Brussels sprouts	½ cup	25
White bread	1 slice	21
Rye bread	1 slice	19
Asparagus, cooked	½ cup	15

CHROMIUM *(RDA: 50–200 mcg)*

Food	Quantity	Mcg
Brewer's yeast	1 ounce	168
Scallops	6	90
Clams	6	46
Baked beans	1 cup	24
Romaine lettuce	2 cups	22
Oysters	6 medium	20
All-bran cereal	1 cup	14
Wheat germ	½ cup	12
Mozzarella cheese	1-inch cube	11
Spinach, raw	1 cup	11
Corn flakes	1 cup	11
Lentils, cooked	½ cup	11
Puffed rice	1 cup	10
Orange juice	1 cup	9.6
Turkey, meat only	3 ounces	9
Peach	1 medium	8
Peanut butter	1 tablespoon	5
Strawberries	1 cup	4.5
Molasses	2 tablespoons	4.4
Cheese	1 ounce	4.4
Walnuts	1 tablespoon	4
Whole wheat cereal	1 cup	3
Sunflower seeds	1 tablespoon	3
Green beans	½ cup	2

COPPER *(RDA: 1.5–3.0 mg)*

Food	Quantity	Mg
Oysters	6 medium	8.92
Sesame seeds	½ cup	4.90
Sunflower seeds	½ cup	1.26
Clams, canned, drained	1 cup	1.10
Soybeans, cooked	1 cup	.70
Almonds	½ cup	.67
Garbanzo beans, cooked	1 cup	.58
Tofu	½ cup	.48
Tomato sauce	1 cup	.48
Baked beans	1 cup	.40
Wheat germ	½ cup	.35
Spinach noodles, cooked	1 cup	.29
Salmon, baked	3 ounces	.26
Brewer's yeast	1 tablespoon	.26
Whole wheat spaghetti, cooked	1 cup	.23
Brown rice, cooked	1 cup	.20
Whole wheat cereal	1 cup	.20
Peanut butter	1 tablespoon	.18
English muffin	1	.18
Beet greens, cooked	½ cup	.18
Chard, cooked	1 cup	.17
Green beans	1 cup	.13
Oatmeal, cooked	1 cup	.13
White rice, cooked	1 cup	.13
Banana	1 medium	.12
Whole wheat bread	1 slice	.10
Low-fat yogurt, plain	1 cup	.09
Apricots, fresh	3	.09
Low-fat ricotta cheese	1 cup	.08
Cantaloupe	1 cup	.07
Beef, extra lean	3 ounces	.07
Low-fat cottage cheese	1 cup	.06
Low-fat milk	1 cup	.06
Nonfat milk	1 cup	.05

Food	Quantity	Mg
White bread	1 slice	.04
Chicken, meat only	3 ounces	.04

IRON *(RDA: ‡ 18 mg)*

Food	Quantity	Mg
Oysters	¾ cup	10
Beef liver	3 ounces	8
Dried beans, cooked	1 cup	5
Beef, lean	3 ounces	3
Hamburger, lean	3 ounces	2.7
Prune juice	¼ cup	2.6
Spinach, cooked	½ cup	2.4
Lima beans	½ cup	2.2
Tuna, water-packed	3 ounces	1.6
Dandelion greens, cooked	½ cup	1.6
Green peas	½ cup	1.5
Chicken, meat only	3 ounces	1.4
Mustard greens, cooked	½ cup	1.3
Strawberries	¾ cup	1.1
Tomato juice	½ cup	1.1
Brussels sprouts	½ cup	.9
Dried apricots	4 halves	.8
Whole wheat bread	1 slice	.8
Blackberries	½ cup	.7
Noodles, enriched	½ cup	.7
Broccoli, cooked	½ cup	.7
Peanut butter	1 tablespoon	.6
White bread	1 slice	.6

‡Because of controversy over the accuracy of the reduced RDAs (180 mcg for folic acid and 15 mg for iron) established in 1989, the previous recommendations of 400 mcg and 18 mg, respectively, are used.

MAGNESIUM *(RDA: 280–300 mg)*

Food	Quantity	Mg
Almonds	½ cup	210
Cashews	½ cup	178
Chard, cooked	1 cup	150
Soybeans, cooked	1 cup	148
Peanuts	½ cup	131
Baked beans	1 cup	110
Refried beans	1 cup	99
Halibut, baked	3 ounces	87
Spinach noodles, cooked	1 cup	87
Black-eyed peas, cooked	1 cup	86
Brown rice, cooked	1 cup	84
Kidney beans, canned	1 cup	79
Garbanzo beans, cooked	1 cup	78
Artichoke, steamed	1	72
Oatmeal, cooked	1 cup	56
Malted milk	1 cup	52
Succotash	½ cup	51
Nonfat yogurt	1 cup	43
Whole wheat spaghetti, cooked	1 cup	42
Cod, baked	3 ounces	42
Avocado	½	35
Red snapper, baked	3 ounces	34
Bran muffin	1	34
Papaya	1	34
Nonfat milk	1 cup	28
Orange juice	1 cup	28
White rice, cooked	1 cup	27
Whole wheat bread	1 slice	26
Grapefruit juice	1 cup	26
Chicken, meat only	3 ounces	25
Peanut butter	1 tablespoon	25
Pineapple, fresh	1 cup	21
Beef, lean	3 ounces	20

Food	Quantity	Mg
Low-fat cottage cheese	1 cup	14
White bread	1 slice	6

MANGANESE *(RDA: 2–5 mg)*

Food	Quantity	Mg
Raisins	1 small box	.201
Spinach, cooked	½ cup	.128
Carrots, cooked	½ cup	.120
Broccoli, cooked	½ cup	.119
Orange	1 medium	.052
Green peas, cooked	½ cup	.051
Apple	1 medium	.046
Low-fat milk	1 cup	.046
Wheat bran	½ cup	.024
Chicken, meat only	3 ounces	.019

MOLYBDENUM *(RDA: 75–250 mcg)*

Food	Quantity	Mcg
Beef kidney	3½ ounces	2,140
Pork, lean	3½ ounces	368
Tomato sauce	½ cup	280
Wheat germ	¼ cup	144
Yam, cooked	1 cup	118
All-Bran, Kellogg's	½ cup	77
Green beans	1 cup	66
Egg noodles, cooked	1 cup	34
Quaker Puffed Rice	1 cup	26
Strawberries	1 cup	20
Winter squash, cooked	1 cup	18
Spinach, raw	1 cup	14
White bread	1 slice	7

Food	Quantity	Mcg
Beef, lean	3 ounces	6
Brussels sprouts	10 medium	4

SELENIUM *(RDA:§ 50–55 mcg)*

Food	Quantity	Mcg
Organ meats	4 ounces	149.6
Seafood	4 ounces	37.9
Lean meat	4 ounces	22.7
Chicken, meat only	4 ounces	22.7
Refried beans	1 cup	14
Low-fat cottage cheese	1 cup	14
Egg	1 medium	12
100% whole wheat bread	1 slice	12
100% whole grain cereal	½ cup cooked	12
Baked beans	1 cup	12
Nonfat milk	1 cup	7
Vegetables	1 serving	.7–316 (1.6 average)
Fruits	1 serving	.9 (average)

ZINC *(RDA: 12 mg)*

Food	Quantity	Mg
Oysters	6 medium	124.9
Lobster	3½ ounces	7.9
Crab	1 cup	6.7
Pork roast	3 ounces	5.1
Beef, extra-lean	3 ounces	4.6
Liver, beef	3 ounces	4.6
Turkey, dark meat only	3 ounces	3.7

§The selenium content of plants depends on the selenium content of the soil in which they are grown.

Food	Quantity	Mg
Liver, cooked	3 ounces	3.3
Wheat germ	¼ cup	3.1
Lima beans, cooked	½ cup	2.7
Lentils, cooked	1 cup	2.0
Almonds	½ cup	2.0
Split peas, cooked	1 cup	2.0
Turkey, light meat only	3 ounces	1.8
Parmesan cheese	1 ounce	1.5
Spinach, cooked	1 cup	1.3
Yogurt, plain	1 cup	1.3
Tuna, water-packed	1 can	1.3
Brown rice, cooked	1 cup	1.2
Almonds	¼ cup	1.2
Oatmeal, cooked	1 cup	1.0

CHOLINE *(estimated adequate intake: 700–1,000 mg)*

Food	Quantity	Mg
Soybeans, uncooked	3½ ounces	340
Brown rice, cooked	1 cup	218
Egg yolk	1 medium	170
Wheat germ	¼ cup	112
Beef, lean	3½ ounces	68
White rice, cooked	1 cup	58
Wheat bran	¼ cup	52
Whole milk	1 cup	49
Cashews	1 ounce	37
Brewer's yeast	1 tablespoon	24
Green beans	1 cup	1.8
Molasses	1 tablespoon	17
Cabbage	1 cup	16
Avocado	½ small	14
Carrot, raw	1 medium	11
Mustard greens, raw	1 cup	7

CHOLESTEROL *(consume less than 300 mg a day)*

Food	Quantity	Mg
Calf's liver	3½ ounces	300
Egg	1 medium	225
Lemon chiffon pie	1 serving	181
Custard, homemade	⅗ cup	165
Custard pie	1 piece	155
French toast	1 slice	111
Ice cream (16% fat)	1 cup	84
Macaroni salad with mayonnaise	1 cup	84
Clams, cooked	½ cup	80
Potato salad with mayonnaise	1 cup	65
Waffles, homemade	1	64
Ice cream (10% fat)	1 cup	53
Egg noodles, cooked	1 cup	50
Ricotta, part skim	½ cup	40
Pumpkin pie, homemade	1 piece	40
Cinnamon roll	1 medium	39
Salmon, cooked	3½ ounces	35
Creamed cottage cheese	1 cup	34
Cream	2 tablespoons	34
Whole milk	1 cup	34
Cornbread	1 piece	31
Cheddar cheese	1 ounce	30
Whole-milk yogurt	1 cup	30
Bologna	1 slice	28
American cheese	1 ounce	27
Doughnut	1	27
Cake, vanilla with icing	1 piece	22
Mozzarella cheese	1 ounce	22
2% fat milk	1 cup	20
Whipping cream	1 tablespoon	20
2% fat cottage cheese	1 cup	18
Potatoes, scalloped with cheese	½ cup	18
Mozzarella cheese, part skim	1 ounce	15

Food	Quantity	Mg
Low-fat yogurt, plain	1 cup	14
Ice milk	1 cup	13
Butter	1 teaspoon	11
1% fat milk	1 cup	10
Mayonnaise	1 tablespoon	10
Salad dressing, Russian	1 tablespoon	10
Salad dressing, Thousand Island	1 tablespoon	9
Chocolate chip cookie	1	9
1% fat cottage cheese	1 cup	9
Pork and beans	1 cup	8
Cupcakes	1	5–10
Nonfat milk	1 cup	5
Nonfat yogurt, plain	1 cup	4
Eggbeaters	¼ cup	0

PART TWO

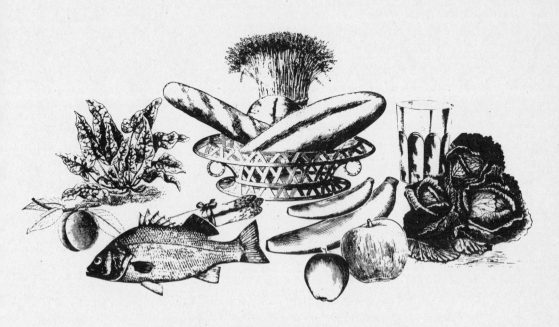

Nutrition and
Specific Life Events

CHAPTER SEVEN

Managing Your Weight

Years ago, body weight was thought to be a simple matter of calories in versus calories out (that is, what you ate and how much you exercised). Researchers now recognize the weight-management issue is much more complicated than previously thought. Weight is a result of genetics combined with physical, psychological, and even social factors. Women have a slower metabolic rate and more body fat than men, so they gain weight more easily on lower calorie intakes. More important, the type of calories and the frequency of dieting determine a woman's weight.

A calorie is not the same for two different people. Compared to lean women, overweight women have higher amounts of an enzyme called lipoprotein lipase that converts fats in the blood into fatty acids that are stored in fat tissue; consequently, an overweight body is more efficient at storing body fat. Willpower is only a small factor in a complex interplay among genetics, environment, and lifelong habits in determining body weight.

Why Lose Weight?

Regardless of the cause, excessive body fat is a health risk. Women who are 20 percent or more above their desirable body weight are at increased risk of diabetes, hypertension, certain cancers, elevated blood fats and heart disease, skin problems, and bone and joint disorders. The obese woman also has an increased risk of early-onset menstruation, abnormal or discontinued menstrual flow, irregular periods, and reduced fertility.

In an effort to attain America's dream-girl figure, millions of women (approximately half the adult female population) diet regularly. Fad diets come, go, and are resurrected, while diet soft drink sales have never been higher. Yet Americans continue to get fatter. More than 98 million people are overweight despite repeated attempts to diet. Even traditional treatments, from very low calorie diets to drug therapy and surgery, do not produce consistent weight loss or long-term success for most people.

Women can and do lose weight and keep it off if they have the knowledge and skills necessary to make life-style changes. Although it is beyond the scope of this book to discuss all the aspects of weight management, the following pages provide a brief overview of what to look for when choosing a weight-loss plan. (For more information on how to make habit changes, refer to chapter 4.)

The Only Way to Lose Weight and Keep It Off

The truth is there is no quick fix when it comes to weight management. No pill, potion, powder, or food combination will miraculously and effortlessly melt body fat. Losing weight and, more important, keeping it off require time, effort, and a lifelong commitment to nutrition, physical activity, and habit change.

Weight Management: The First Step

Before starting a weight-management program, there are a few very important considerations and steps that should be taken. First, make sure this is the best time to lose weight. Do you have the time and energy to devote to learning the skills and making the changes necessary to keep the weight off? If not, it is better to wait until the time is right. Second, plan for success rather than setting yourself up for failure.

The Chronic Dieting Syndrome and Yo-Yo Dieting

The chronic dieting syndrome addresses the common problem many women face of constantly dieting or being overconcerned with their weight. These women feel frustrated because their dieting attempts never work and they always gain back any lost weight.

In an attempt to lose weight fast, women often jump on the diet bandwagon with little preplanning. Consequently, even if weight is lost, it is regained. These repeated bouts of weight loss and weight gain are called "yo-yo" dieting or weight cycling, and they might be more harmful than not dieting and remaining slightly overweight.

Controversies rage over whether yo-yo dieting teaches the body to be fat. One theory states that the body loses both fat and lean tissue during the weight-loss phase but gains back more fat during the weight-gain phase. Therefore, the body becomes more fuel efficient since fat is less metabolically active than muscle tissue. Metabolism slows, and it becomes increasingly more difficult to lose the unwanted pounds. For example, a woman may drop from 145 pounds to 125 pounds and lose 15 pounds of fat and 5 pounds of muscle. When she regains the weight, however, she may gain 18 pounds of fat and only 2 pounds of muscle, becoming fatter as a result of dieting.

In contrast, other researchers believe weight cycling or yo-yo dieting has no effect on body fat but does significantly increase the risk of developing heart disease and premature death.

Are You an Apple or a Pear?

As body fat is gained, a greater proportion of fat accumulates in the abdominal and chest areas, creating a more apple-shaped body. This body shape is associated with an increased risk of heart disease, diabetes, and high blood pressure. Men are more likely to accumulate fat above the waist, while women usually gain upper body fat only when they have reached a higher level of obesity.

However, as a woman gains more upper body fat and becomes more apple-shaped, the risk of heart disease increases to match that of men. Dr. David Schapira, a professor of medicine at South Florida College of Medicine, reports that "apples" are fifteen times more likely to develop endometrial cancer. Apples also are five times as likely to develop breast cancer than women who store their excess body fat in the thighs and hips (called pear-shaped or gynoid body fat distribution).

This does not mean a woman should give up trying to lose weight. Women who already have an apple-shaped body and are 20 percent or more above a desirable body weight should seriously consider making changes to lose weight. However, those who are more pear-shaped are at a lower risk for developing disease, so their desire to lose weight is based more on vanity than health. These women

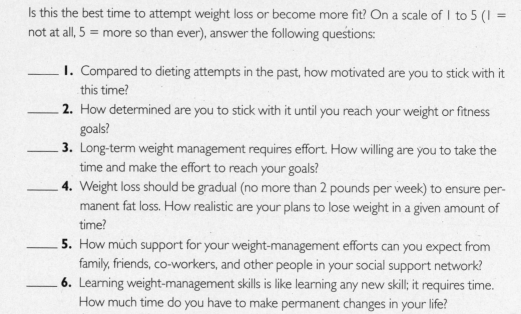

TABLE 7-1   Am I Ready to Make a Change?

Is this the best time to attempt weight loss or become more fit? On a scale of 1 to 5 (1 = not at all, 5 = more so than ever), answer the following questions:

_____ **1.** Compared to dieting attempts in the past, how motivated are you to stick with it this time?

_____ **2.** How determined are you to stick with it until you reach your weight or fitness goals?

_____ **3.** Long-term weight management requires effort. How willing are you to take the time and make the effort to reach your goals?

_____ **4.** Weight loss should be gradual (no more than 2 pounds per week) to ensure permanent fat loss. How realistic are your plans to lose weight in a given amount of time?

_____ **5.** How much support for your weight-management efforts can you expect from family, friends, co-workers, and other people in your social support network?

_____ **6.** Learning weight-management skills is like learning any new skill; it requires time. How much time do you have to make permanent changes in your life?

Add up your scores. A score of 6 to 16 reflects a low commitment to weight management and a high likelihood of failure in losing weight or keeping it off. Wait and try another time. A score of 17 to 23 reflects a moderate commitment to weight management, but you still need to work on motivation. A score of 24 or higher reflects high motivation. This may be the best time to begin losing weight.

could have more to lose than just weight. An unsuccessful weight-loss attempt will increase their body fat and their risk for disease. Pear-shaped women should approach dieting cautiously and should attempt weight loss only if they are committed to making it work. (See table 7-1.)

Establishing Realistic Goals

The best way to ensure that body fat is lost and the new weight is maintained is to lose weight slowly, that is, no more than 2 pounds per week. Gradual weight loss ensures that most of the lost weight is fat, avoids the metabolic slowdown experienced with rapid weight loss, and reflects a slow change in eating and exercise habits to keep the lost weight off.

Body Fat Is Where It's At

Weight is not the entire issue—fat is the issue. Jumping on a scale won't tell you how fat you are. You can be within your desirable body weight range and still be fat.

The combination of healthful eating and physical activity will result in a loss of body fat and a gain in lean tissue, which weighs more than fat tissue. Consequently, a woman might show little change in total body weight, but her body is slimmer and her clothing size drops.

Body fat can be measured by a trained health professional using calipers, by underwater weighing, by bioelectric measurements, or by other methods. The number received reflects the percentage of body fat. A recommended desirable body fat for a trim woman is 18 percent to 22 percent but no more than 30 percent of total body weight. Body fat should not drop below 16 percent, because the body needs some fat to cushion internal organs, regulate body temperature, and maintain health. Take time to set realistic expectations and goals. You may feel fine and look great at a weight above the recommendations on a height-weight chart. What you weighed in high school is probably not an ideal weight at age forty-five. At what weight would you feel most comfortable? Why? Remember, you should be more concerned about body fat, not total body weight. How long will it take to lose that weight based on a loss of two pounds per week (divide the number of pounds to be lost by two to reach the total weeks necessary to reach the goal)? Losing weight faster than this could be setting yourself up for failure. (See chart 7-1.)

What to Look for When Choosing a Weight-Loss Plan

Any program that promises quick and easy weight loss is lying. It took you months, years, sometimes a lifetime of habits to develop the body you have today. It will take some time to develop a new body. Keep in mind that how you look and feel reflects how you live. The only way to permanently lose excess fat or

CHART 7-1　Charting Your Weight-Management Course

Current Weight: _____ pounds　　Current Body Fat: _____ %

Desirable Weight: _____ pounds　　Desirable Body Fat: _____ %

Pounds to Lose: _____ pounds　　Body Fat to Lose: _____ %

Based on the 2-pounds-per-week rule, how long will it take to lose the weight? _____ weeks or _____ months

Use the following chart to record your weight loss. Daily fluctuations are deceiving, so weigh yourself only once a week. Fill in the date at the top and your weights in the left-hand column of the chart, beginning with your starting weight. Each square represents two pounds. Record your weekly weights and connect the marks to create a graph.

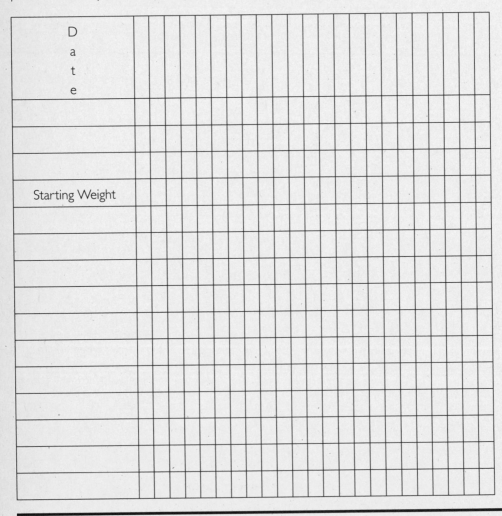

become more fit is to permanently replace the habits that put on the weight in the first place.

Diets don't change habits. Anything short of taking a strong look at your life, exercise and eating habits, stress, social support, self-esteem, or body image, and other key weight-management factors is a Band-Aid approach to a much more complex issue. In essence, in order to change your body, you must change your life.

Fad diets come in a variety of shapes and disguises, but they all have one thing in common: They promise miracles with little effort. In addition, since they do nothing to change the eating patterns that cause weight problems, it is no wonder that 90 percent of the people who follow these diets regain the weight and often gain more weight. Seldom do these diets supply optimal amounts of all nutrients, thereby increasing risk of developing marginal deficiencies. In addition, most fad diets result in one or more health complications. (See table 7-2.)

Ketogenic Diets

The most popular fad diet is the high-protein or ketogenic diet. This diet has entered the market under a variety of names. In the 1960s it was called the Air Force Diet; in 1964, the Drinking Man's Diet; in the late 1960s, The Stillman Diet; and in the 1970s, The Atkins' Diet. In recent years this diet has become more sophisticated, with exact measurements of ketones (intermediate by-products of fat breakdown) in the blood and urine that monitor how well the diet is "working." Without carbohydrates in the body, fat cannot be efficiently burned and fat fragments or ketones accumulate in the blood. Excreting ketones is supposed to waste calories and help a person lose weight; however, only about 100 calories are lost in a twenty-four-hour period when ketones are excreted.

Reports that a low-carbohydrate diet stimulates fat-mobilizing enzymes have not been substantiated by well-designed research studies. Weight loss occurs, not because of the protein, but because one can eat only so much of the limited selection of foods and, thus, consumes fewer calories. The initial loss of weight on these diets is mostly due to water loss as tissue carbohydrate stores are depleted and bound water is released. Little fat weight is lost.

In addition, high-protein diets are harmful to a person's health. Common complications include nausea, vomiting, diarrhea, constipation, faintness, muscle cramps, fatigue, irritability, weakness, cold intolerance, hair loss, and dry skin. More serious complications include cardiac arrhythmia, gout, dehydration, and low blood potassium levels. Any diet that is high in protein is also high in fat and

---

TABLE 7-2 Judging the Diets

The following red flags should alert you to questionable weight-loss diets:

1. The diet is restrictive and does not include a variety of low-fat foods, including whole grain breads and cereals, fresh fruits and vegetables, cooked dried beans and peas, extra-lean meat or chicken, fish, and nonfat or low-fat milk products.
2. You are required to purchase special foods, devices, or books.
3. The program or plan is not supervised by a dietitian, physician, or qualified medical personnel, or the staff was not trained by one of these health professionals.
4. The program reports weight losses greater than 2 pounds per week.
5. The advertising makes sensational claims such as "eat all you want," "lose weight in your sleep," "spot reduction," or "burn off cellulite."
6. The plan recommends appetite-suppressant pills.
7. The literature is based on testimonials and anecdotal stories from successful clients rather than on scientifically documented evidence of how to lose weight.
8. The diet does not include sound nutrition information, exercise, and behavior modification.
9. The total calorie intake is lower than 1,000 calories.
10. The program or plan focuses on "ideal weights," predetermined meals, or specific food combinations rather than providing flexibility for your individual body, life-style, and preferences.

---

cholesterol, thus increasing the risk for developing atherosclerosis and heart disease.

Ketogenic Clones

Variations on the high-protein theme include the Woman Doctor's Diet for Women and the Scarsdale Diet, both of which contain slightly more carbohydrates. However, these diets contain excessive amounts of protein, and in all cases, weight loss occurs because fewer calories are consumed, not because of a special proportion of protein or a certain combination of foods.

According to Dr. Judith Wurtman at the Massachusetts Institute of Technology, consuming a low-carbohydrate diet is counterproductive to long-term weight loss because it alters brain chemical levels, increases the desire for snacks high in sugar and starch, and is likely to cause episodes of binge eating and depression.

Special Weight-Loss Foods

Specific foods are sometimes touted as miracle weight-loss aids, hence the Grapefruit Diet, the Cottage Cheese Diet, the Potato Diet, and the Skim Milk and Banana Diet. Again, weight loss is due to a lower caloric intake, not to any magical quality of these specific foods. Most of the weight loss is water and lean tissue, with only small amounts of body fat. The weight is almost inevitably regained, often with increasing amounts of body fat.

Cellulite

Other fad diets promise to shed specific types of body fat. It has been incorrectly claimed that combinations of grapefruit and toast will burn off fat from the hips and that fish and green beans will melt away a type of fat called cellulite.

Spot reduction is a myth; the only way to lose inches off the waist and hips, for example, is to lose total body weight and firm the underlying muscles in these areas through exercise. The rippling type of fat touted as cellulite is only subcutaneous fat that is caught in a webbing of fibrous tissue connected from the skin to deeper tissue layers. When the fat cells increase in size, the compartments of fat bulge and produce a waffled appearance on the skin. The only treatment that removes "cellulite" or any body fat is a low-fat, nutrient-dense diet plus exercise.

Food Combining and Other Myths

Other fad diets propose that certain food ingredients are weight-loss aids. These diets take portions of accurate information and distort it or make up new information to sell a product. Some diets report that fruits supply powerful digestive enzymes to help increase food assimilation. There is no truth to this theory because the enzymes in fruit are weak in comparison to the digestive juices and enzymes in a person's stomach and intestines.

Another diet takes current research on how certain amino acids (the building blocks of protein) might affect mood and distorts it by categorizing foods into "happy" foods and "sad" foods. This leap from scientific inquiry is meant to sell books, not provide accurate information. In all cases, weight loss on these diets can be attributed to lower caloric intake.

Liquid Diets, Shakes, and Supplemental Fasts

The 1990s is the decade for meal-replacement shakes, a resurrection of the breakfast drinks popular back in the 1960s. The nutrient content has improved since the "liquid diets" of the late 1970s that resulted in at least sixty deaths, mostly from arrhythmias. Today's drinks contain high-quality protein and carbohydrates plus a smattering of vitamins and minerals. When used as a total replacement for food, the diet plan is called "supplemented fasting" and should be monitored by a physician if energy intake falls below 800 calories.

Supplemented fasting results in rapid weight loss for the very obese person; however, without concurrent physical activity and intense habit change skills, the person is likely to gain back the weight. The shake temporarily replaces food rather than teaching new eating habits. Consequently, you either must remain on the shake for life or resume old eating habits and regain the weight. Most people do not stick with a supplemented fasting program long enough to reach their goals, or if they do reach their goals, they are three times more likely to regain weight than those who lose it slowly.

Supplemented fasting products are useful for truly obese patients under the supervision of a physician. However, any very low calorie diet is dangerous for non-obese people who are at risk of losing lean tissue and are most likely to self-monitor their weight-loss plans. Over-the-counter drinks used for crash dieting by marginally overweight women encourage yo-yo dieting and increase body fat and health risks, including heart arrhythmias and gallbladder disease. Using over-the-counter drinks as a replacement for one meal a day is probably no better or worse than eating the equivalent in protein- and carbohydrate-rich foods. However, it doesn't teach a person how to eat right, so it is only a small piece in the weight-management process.

The Bottom Line

Approach any new fad diet with a wary eye. If the program or plan promises quick or easy weight loss, is based on a special combination of foods or excludes entire food categories, or stands alone without also providing exercise and habit change skills, then it is bound to fail and is not worth risking your health to try.

Physical Activity and Eating:
The Balancing Act

Despite the individual uniqueness of body fat regulation and the complexity of skills necessary to manage body weight, the bottom line for losing weight remains the same: Calories consumed must be less than calories expended in physical activity.

There are no shortcuts to fitness. Physical activity is an essential component of weight management and becomes increasingly more important as a woman ages. Both aerobic exercise and strength training increase calorie expenditure, burn body fat, increase lean body tissue such as muscle, and help prevent the metabolic slowdown associated with dieting.

Exercise, in fact, is a critical factor in whether or not weight lost from dieting is maintained. Without exercise, the weight inevitably is regained. More important, once started, exercise must be continued for life. Studies show that animals who discontinue exercise revert back to previous body fat levels and disease risk. In short, exercise is not a quick fix but a permanent one.

The common belief that exercise increases food intake is not true. Researchers at Washington University School of Medicine monitored food intake in men and women exercisers and nonexercisers, and found that exercise does not increase calorie intake and, in fact, places you in negative calorie balance (that is, calories in are less than calories out so you lose weight).

Another misconception about exercise is that you must exercise vigorously in order to see results. Research shows that increased physical activity, including moderate recreational and leisure activities, improves energy output and helps maintain a desirable body weight. Since women struggling with their weight often exercise less than leaner women, even small increases in activity can improve health and weight status.

How Much of What and for How Long?

For safe and effective weight loss, exercise must use up or burn fat fragments called fatty acids from fat stores while protecting against muscle loss. Losing weight too fast, even with exercise, results in loss of muscle and other lean tissue. In contrast, the proper balance between calories in and calories out in the form of exercise guarantees maximum fat loss and minimum muscle loss.

This is accomplished best with slow, continual movement for long periods of time. Fast stop-and-start exercises, such as tennis and volleyball, burn mostly body sugars and have less of an effect on weight loss. Therefore, a single session of long duration (that is, a long walk or a jog) is more beneficial in terms of burning fatty acids than the same duration of exercise divided into several short sessions. (However, when beginning an exercise program, start slowly and work up to longer sessions.)

Recent research has shown that strength training exercises also increase muscle mass and improve weight management. How much exercise affects weight loss is specific to each individual. In general, the length and quantity of exercise is equated with the quantity of weight lost and maintained; only long-sustained physical activity, not just for a few days or weeks but for months and years, will have a significant effect on lifelong weight management. The basic formula for exercise is as follows:

Frequency: five times a week

Duration: a minimum of thirty minutes, preferably forty-five minutes to one hour

Intensity: exercise hard enough that you perspire but can still talk while exercising.

The Nutritional Plan

The best diet is one you can stick with for the rest of your life. The dietary guidelines for weight loss, therefore, are the same low-fat, nutrient-dense dietary guidelines outlined in the Healthy Woman's Diet.

To lose weight simply experiment with the amount of calories until you find the balance between calories in and calories out during daily activity and exercise. If you are gaining weight, your calorie intake is too high or your exercise level is too low. If you are maintaining weight, the calorie intake is balanced with the calorie output. Weight loss reflects a negative balance between calories in and calories out.

A daily intake of less than 2,000 calories, even of nutrient-dense foods such as fruits and vegetables, whole grain breads, nonfat milk, and extra-lean meats, cannot ensure optimal intake of all the essential vitamins and minerals. Consequently, a moderate-dose multiple vitamin-mineral supplement should accompany lower calorie diets.

Fat Is Fattening

Not all calories are the same. Calories from fats and fatty foods and from alcohol are more likely to end up in the body's fat stores than are calories from carbohydrates and protein. According to a study at the University of Tennessee, the most consistent predictor of body weight in women is the amount of fat in the diet. Granted, ounce for ounce fat has more than twice as many calories as carbohydrates and protein; however, why dietary fat is particularly good at making fat bodies goes beyond just calories.

First, it is easier for the body to convert dietary fat into body fat than it is to turn carbohydrates or protein into fat. According to researchers at the University of Massachusetts Medical School in Worcester, the body uses 3 percent of the calories in fat to convert it to body fat, while 23 percent of the ingested calories in carbohydrates are used when converting them to fat.

Second, the body resists converting dietary carbohydrates into fat. In fact, some studies show that you would have to eat large amounts of carbohydrates before your body began storing them as fat. (That is not a license to overeat sugars and starches, especially since many overweight women have difficulty handling carbohydrates and are prone to diabetes.)

Third, while you burn more carbohydrates for energy when eating starchy foods, the more fat you consume the more fat you will store. Dr. Eric Ravussin at the National Institute of Diabetes in Phoenix states, "The body is able to cope with excess protein and carbohydrate, but not excess fat." This is supported by studies showing that women lose weight on low-fat diets even when their calorie intake increases.

Women with weight problems might have a "fat" tooth rather than a "sweet" tooth. Some overweight women report eating the same amount of calories as do lean women but with more of the calories coming from fat. Another study showed that, given the choice between a low-fat and high-fat version of the same food, overweight people will choose the high-fat selection. These and other findings suggest that whatever makes people fat also contributes to a craving for fatty foods. (See the section following on food cravings.)

The issue is more complicated than just fat: Many people eat a typically fatty American diet, yet only one-third of them become overweight. Studies on animals reflect this discrepancy as well. Mice fed low-fat diets stay slim; however, body shape begins to change as fat is added to their diets. Some mice grow fat, others are slightly overweight, and others remain slim—just like people. Obviously, genetics and other factors contribute to obesity and weight problems, but reducing calories and dietary fat is one factor you can control.

THE NIBBLER'S DIET

In addition to the amount and type of food eaten, the frequent of meals may be an important factor in weight management. Consuming the total day's calories in three or fewer large meals triggers the body to store more of those calories as fat. In contrast, eating frequent small meals and snacks, even when the total calorie intake is the same, reduces fat storage and improves weight management.

Other Weight-Management Tools: Chromium, Fiber, and Water

Several other dietary factors have been implicated in weight management. Recent scientific findings report that a supplemental form of chromium called chromium picolinate might improve body composition and cause weight loss regardless of physical activity. This evidence is preliminary, however, and further studies are necessary before recommendations for chromium picolinate can be made. A high-fiber diet lowers hunger and helps manage weight, while diluting dietary intake by drinking several glasses of water each day reduces calorie intake and helps facilitate weight loss.

Food Cravings

Some women can't "just say no" to some foods. They battle cravings for sweets, chocolate, or pasta. A craving for a specific food is one of the most common and intense food experiences, and although many scientists would argue that food cravings are based on taste alone, cravings may be the body's way of satisfying a nutritional deficiency or counteracting mild depression.

Women report food cravings more frequently than men do, possibly because of hormonal and taste fluctuations caused by menstruation and pregnancy. Food cravings have been documented in women with Seasonal Affective Disorder (SAD)—a condition characterized by mild depression in the fall and winter; during pregnancy and Premenstrual syndrome (PMS); and in dieters. Women with SAD often lose their food cravings when they are exposed to bright artificial light for one to two hours in the morning.

Both women with PMS and women who crave carbohydrates while dieting sometimes are able to control their cravings more easily if they consume mini-meals and snacks throughout the day, including some complex carbohydrate foods, such as whole grain breads, and some protein-rich foods, such as a slice of cheese or a broiled chicken leg. In addition, planning a carbohydrate-rich snack during the time of day when cravings are at a peak sometimes alleviates binge eating later.

Carbohydrate craving might result from low brain levels of a nerve chemical called serotonin. This chemical regulates mood, sleep, and other psychological functions, and a low serotonin level is associated with depression, irritability, and feeling agitated. According to Richard Wurtman, Ph.D., at Massachusetts Institute of Technology, these metabolic imbalances can be induced by fad diet-ing. Serotonin is manufactured in response to dietary intake of its building block, an amino acid called tryptophan. Brain levels of serotonin also rise when carbohydrate-rich foods are consumed, because these foods contain few other amino acids that compete with tryptophan for entry into the brain. If this theory is correct, then the high-protein fad diets would lower brain serotonin levels and result in carbohydrate cravings in some people.

Drs. Richard and Judith Wurtman have conducted research showing that mood improves in carbohydrate-sensitive individuals when they consume starchy snacks. Carbohydrate cravers report feeling more energetic and less depressed after a sugary or starchy snack, while noncravers feel drowsy and fatigued. Although interesting, this theory remains controversial. (See pages 349–56 for more information on sugar, food cravings, and mood.)

Other research indicates that certain types of compulsive behaviors are associated with alterations in brain chemicals. For example, ex-smokers who counter-act nicotine withdrawal by eating more usually choose sweet foods. Some evidence shows that a high-carbohydrate, high-tryptophan diet might help ex-smokers stay off cigarettes and refrain from bingeing on sweets.

Chocolate cravings pose a more confusing problem. Dr. Judith Wurtman, of the Department of Brain and Cognitive Sciences at Massachusetts Institute of Technology, speculates that "people crave chocolate because it satisfies their need to eat a high-carbohydrate food, which then affects serotonin levels in the brain, which will in turn calm them down." However, chocolate is higher in fat than it is in carbohydrate. Chocolate also is a source of caffeine, which would give a lift to a dropping energy level and temporarily soothe a mild depression, and a compound in chocolate called phenylethylamine is suspected of improving mood and feelings of well-being.

Suggestions for controlling chocolate cravings include the following:

1. Keep portions small by eating chocolate with or soon after a meal.
2. Buy chocolate in small serving sizes rather than large bars or boxes.
3. Regularly include small servings of chocolate to avoid binge eating associated with abstinence.
4. Use cocoa powder, which has only 30 percent of its calories from fat, when making homemade desserts.
5. Try chocolate-flavored syrup with only 3 percent fat calories as an alternative to fudge or candy. Use it as a dip for fresh strawberries or other fruits.

Although poorly understood, cravings for foods other than sweets and starches might indicate a nutritional need for something in that food. People who are protein-deficient choose high-protein foods, while people who are adequately nourished in protein choose only approximately 15 percent of their food intake as protein. Sometimes cravings for salty or spicy foods indicate changes in taste. For example, elderly people, especially if they are zinc deficient, have lowered taste sensations and will add sugar or excessive amounts of salt to foods in order to taste them.

Cravings for coffee, cola drinks, or tea are likely to be a mild addiction to the caffeine in these beverages rather than a craving. Caffeine is the most widely used drug in the United States that provides several reinforcing effects, such as contentedness, improved mental clarity, and improved feelings of well-being and euphoria. These effects linger for three to four hours after ingestion. It is unlikely that one to two cups of coffee daily pose a health threat; however, reports of withdrawal symptoms, including tightness in the neck, insomnia, headache, nervousness, and mild depression, have been noted in heavy coffee drinkers when they discontinue their daily intake.

Many food cravings are merely habits. The body becomes accustomed to a mid-morning doughnut or learns to anticipate an evening snack. If a food craving interferes with weight loss,

1. Learn a new response to the situation such as taking a walk.
2. Substitute a lower-fat food or beverage such as mineral water or air-popped popcorn.
3. Go "cold turkey" and stop eating the food until cravings subside (usually a week or more).
4. Avoid food craving situations, such as the lull in the afternoon or television in the evening.
5. Brush your teeth as a signal that eating is finished.

Often, cravings for sweets slowly subside when all sugar is removed from the diet.

Sugar Highs, Sugar Lows

The pick-me-up effect of sugar results from the rapid rise in blood sugar levels following ingestion of a sugary food. That temporary quick energy might be an antidote to the mid-morning, mid-afternoon, or early evening doldrums, but the effect doesn't last. Elevated blood sugar levels trigger the pancreas to secrete extra doses of a hormone called insulin that removes sugar from the blood. Excess blood sugar means excess insulin, which can result in too much sugar being removed from the blood and subsequent low blood sugar.

One study at Kansas State University measured mood changes in college women one hour after the ingestion of a 12-ounce glass of either water or Kool-Aid sweetened with sugar or with a sugar substitute. Within thirty minutes, the women who had ingested the sugary Kool-Aid were the sleepiest. Limited evidence also suggests that coffee with sugar might lower energy levels even more than sugar or coffee alone in some sugar-sensitive individuals.

Sugar also stimulates other brain chemicals called endorphins, which are naturally occurring morphinelike compounds that produce feelings of well-being and euphoria. The sugar-endorphin theory has not been tested in adults, but it does provide an interesting link between the consumption of sweets during Premenstrual syndrome (PMS), alcohol or tobacco withdrawal, bulimia, and an almost immediate relief from depression, tension, or fatigue. In these cases, a sugary snack provides a temporary "quick fix."

Sugar Substitutes

Sugar substitutes such as aspartame (NutraSweet) might supply sweetness without calories, but they probably won't help you lose weight. Studies repeatedly show that beverages sweetened with aspartame have no effect on curbing appetite. In fact, in some cases appetite increases and more weight is gained in women who drink diet sodas compared to those who drink water or sugared sodas.

Although controversial, some researchers speculate that artificial sweeteners trigger hunger, especially cravings for carbohydrates. A few studies reported harmful effects, including seizures and depression, with aspartame consumption; however, recent reports show no health risks when aspartame is consumed in moderate amounts. Other artificial sweeteners such as cyclamates and saccharine are potentially cancer-causing and should be avoided.

Beyond Desirable: When Thin Isn't Enough

Negative body image and obsession with weight control have become the norm rather than the exception in the United States. More than 80 percent of college women are concerned about their weight, while only 8 percent actually are overweight. As many as 25 percent of women who have negative attitudes about their weight or body image have used some severe method of weight control, including the use of diuretics and laxatives, vomiting, or other forms of purging.

Severe body distortion such as anorexia nervosa, once thought to be peculiar to adolescent and young women, is now observed in older women as well. Anorexia, bulimia, obesity, and emotional eating problems are all related eating disorders that vary in their health consequences from minor inconveniences to death.

Anorexia Nervosa

Anorexia is characterized by a vigorous pursuit of a thin body and a fear of weight gain. The hallmarks of anorexia are a resistance to eating and an obsession with weight loss. In addition, the anorexic may vomit, exercise excessively, or abuse laxatives and diuretics to lose weight.

Women are ten times more likely to develop anorexia than are men. This progressive disorder often results in fatigue, loss of menstruation, constipation, severe loss of weight (that is, more than 15 percent of average body weight), and in severe cases heart arrhythmias and death.

The causes of anorexia are complex and poorly understood. Initially, a desire for thinness motivates the prospective anorexic. Vigorous dieting becomes a compulsion, however, and is associated with dramatic alterations, such as in the brain chemicals that regulate female hormones and the thyroid hormones. Higher-than-normal growth hormone and cortisol also are noted in anorexic patients. It is likely these hormonal changes are a result rather than a cause of anorexia.

Several studies show a correlation between zinc status and anorexia. Poor appetite is common in zinc deficiency, and in the early 1980s researchers at the University of Reading reported that anorexics with zinc deficiency who subsequently were given 15 mg of zinc three times daily showed improvements in appetite and mood within two weeks. The researchers concluded that the onset of anorexia might be related to social and psychological factors; however, its progression might relate to altered taste perception and sense of smell, which is associated with zinc deficiency.

Researchers at the University of Göteborg in Sweden and at the University of Kentucky Medical Center in Lexington have since confirmed these findings and recommend zinc supplementation as adjunct therapy in the treatment of anorexia. Severe calorie restriction also results in numerous deficiencies, which also have been documented in anorexics, and might contribute to the progression of the disorder and its symptoms, such as depression and mood swings.

Bulimia

Bulimia is an eating disorder characterized by excessive binge eating (as much as 5,000 calories consumed in one episode), often followed by purging in an attempt to lose weight. Purging behaviors include self-induced vomiting and the abuse of laxatives and diuretics. As many as one in every twenty young women maintains her weight by compulsive vomiting. Complications from this disorder include dehydration, imbalance in body salts, loss of tooth enamel and dental decay, rupturing of the esophagus and stomach, enlargement of the throat muscles, mood swings and other personality problems, heartbeat irregularities, and low blood sugar. Death occurs in severe cases.

Mineral deficiencies are common in bulimics. Researchers at the University of Kentucky state that zinc deficiency is common in bulimics and might contribute to the progression of the disorder, while zinc supplementation in addition to primary therapy might be useful for rehabilitation. Low blood levels of magnesium and potassium are also found in bulimic patients, which might contribute to muscle weakness, heartbeat irregularities, restlessness, reduced concentration, muscle cramps, and poor memory.

The treatment for both anorexia and bulimia focuses on changing behaviors, not curing symptoms. With the help of trained health professionals, a recovering patient learns to manage food without fear or compulsiveness, and to reassess expectations about her body, her appearance, and herself. Structured, regular meals and an understanding of nutrition and meal planning are included in the rehabilitation. Serious cases may require hospitalization to stop the binge-purge syndrome and to ensure adequate nutritional intakes.

CHAPTER EIGHT

Nutrition Through Pregnancy and Breast-feeding

Nutrition is more important prior to, during, and immediately following pregnancy than at any other time in life. The mother's nutrient intake has an effect on the development and the lifelong health of the growing infant. In fact, part of what is now regarded as a genetic contribution to heart disease and other disorders may be the effect of nutrition during pregnancy and in early childhood.

A normal-weight woman who consumes a well-balanced, nutritious diet prior to and during pregnancy has a much better chance of experiencing a pregnancy and delivery free from serious complications and of having a healthy, normal-weight baby than does a woman who is malnourished prior to pregnancy or who consumes a poor diet throughout pregnancy. For example, poor nutrition can result in low-birth-weight infants (5½ pounds or less) who are at increased risk for complications during delivery and impaired intelligence or early disease and death later in life.

Gearing Up for Pregnancy

In the past, people believed that regardless of the mother's nutritional status prior to conception or her dietary habits during pregnancy, the baby would draw all necessary nutrients from the mother's nutrient stores. It was thought that if a mother's diet was iron depleted, the baby still would obtain ample iron by draining iron reserves from the mother's body. This myth perpetuated a generally careless attitude toward the diet and weight gain of pregnant women.

It is now recognized that every choice you make, from cereal and supplements to caffeine consumption, will directly affect your baby. Every gram of protein, every microgram of folic acid, every drop of water, every trace of copper that the growing baby receives will come from your diet.

Some essential nutrients come from the limited tissue stores stockpiled prior to pregnancy if your diet is optimal. Other nutrients are not stored in the body or are stored in such limited amounts that the diet is virtually the only place the baby can obtain them. Consequently, nourishing a baby begins before conception. If you wish to get pregnant and give birth to a healthy, robust infant, follow the dietary guidelines of the Healthy Woman's Diet for several months prior to conception. This is not a time to try severe diets or lose weight. However, since obesity is associated with several complications of pregnancy, if you are very overweight, you might wish to lose weight prior to considering pregnancy.

Optimal nutrition is essential as soon as a woman begins trying to get pregnant, because nutritional deficiencies seriously affect fetal development, especially in the initial few weeks following conception.

Smoking or exposure to other people's cigarette smoke is harmful to the mother and baby, so tobacco smoke should be avoided. If caffeine produces birth defects, it is most likely to have its effect before pregnancy is detected. Limit caffeine-containing beverages (including soda pop, tea, and coffee) to no more than two servings daily and avoid medications that contain caffeine when trying to conceive.

Pregnancy: Nourishing the "We" of Me

The daily intake of protein, calories, vitamins, and minerals during the first few months of development provides necessary ingredients for diverse and specialized changes in cell types, while the size of the developing infant (at this stage called an embryo) remains tiny.

A new organ called the placenta develops inside the uterus to supply nutrients and oxygen to the growing infant. The muscles supporting the growing uterus increase in size, as does the blood volume and the volume of other body fluids. Breast tissue increases in preparation for lactation, and there is also an increase in the fat or energy stores. The overall gain in weight from increased maternal body tissues and the child is dependent on a constant supply of nutrients and calories.

This increased demand for nutrients is represented in the differences between the RDAs for nonpregnant and pregnant women. For example, greater amounts of calcium, magnesium, and protein are required to supply the building blocks for developing bones in the infant and to increase maternal stores in preparation for lactation. Folic acid needs increase because of this vitamin's role in cell growth in the infant and for the increased blood volume and expanding tissues in the mother. Iron needs increase to supply the increased oxygen demands of the tissues. The Healthy Woman's Diet provides ample amounts of all nutrients to ensure optimal stockpiling in preparation for and during pregnancy, except perhaps for folic acid and iron. (See chart 8-1.)

CHART 8-1   The RDAs for Vitamins and Minerals for Pregnant and Nonpregnant Women

	PREGNANT	NONPREGNANT	INCREASE (%)
Vitamin A	4,000 IU	4,000 IU	0
Vitamin D	400 IU	200 IU	50
Vitamin E	10 mg	8 mg	25
Vitamin B1	1.5 mg	1.1 mg	36
Vitamin B2	1.6 mg	1.3 mg	23
Niacin	17 mg	15 mg	13
Vitamin B6	2.2 mg	1.6 mg	38
Folic Acid*	800 mcg	400 mcg	100
Vitamin B12	2.2 mcg	2.0 mcg	10
Vitamin C	70 mg	60 mg	17
Calcium	1,200 mg	800–1,200 mg	0–50
Iodine	175 mcg	150 mcg	17
Iron*	48–78 mg	18 mg	167–333
Magnesium	320 mg	280 mg	15
Zinc	15 mg	12 mg	25

*The current RDAs (1989) are substantially reduced levels for these nutrients and have been met with considerable controversy. Previous RDA levels (1980) are used here.

Weight Gain During Pregnancy

Weight gain during pregnancy is directly related to the birth weight and survival of the infant; a weight gain between 25 and 35 pounds is optimal, whereas a weight gain of less than 20 pounds is associated with low birth weight and an increased infant death rate. Underweight women entering pregnancy should gain slightly more, or between 28 and 40 pounds, while weight gain should be slightly less (that is, 15 to 25 pounds) for pregnant women who begin pregnancy over-weight.

The rate of weight gain also is important. During the first three months of pregnancy, weight gain should be 2 to 4 pounds. An average weight gain during the last six months of pregnancy should be approximately three-quarters to 1 pound each week.

Dieting during pregnancy is dangerous. Calorie and food restriction can cause a toxic condition called ketosis that deprives the growing infant's brain of needed sugar and can result in congenital deformity. On the other hand, women who gain too much weight during pregnancy do not necessarily give birth to bigger babies. Excessive food intake increases the mother's fat stores rather than promoting the growth of the baby, thus making weight loss more difficult after pregnancy.

Protein, Calories, Fat, and Carbohydrates

Optimal protein intake is important during pregnancy. Adequate intake of protein and calories prior to and during pregnancy results in few pregnancy-related complications and the likelihood of healthy, moderate to big babies who are at low risk for illness and death.

Protein powders are not necessary, and supplementing the diet with individual amino acids (the building blocks of protein) might interfere with the growth of the baby and weight gain in the mother. Protein needs are easily met by consuming a few additional servings of nonfat milk products, extra-lean meat, chicken, fish, and/or cooked dried beans and peas.

At least 1 to 2 tablespoons daily of safflower oil should be consumed to ensure optimal intake of linoleic acid, the essential fatty acid. In addition, several servings each week of fish, which contains fish oils, might be "an easy and cheap intervention to avoid preterm delivery," according to researchers at the University of Aarhus in Denmark. Fatty acids in fish oils, called the omega-3 fatty acids, are also suspected to be essential for the normal development of eye function and vision in the growing fetus, further strengthening the argument to include fish in the diet during pregnancy.

The fatigue associated with labor might be partially relieved by consuming a high-carbohydrate diet (that is, several servings daily of pasta, breads, starchy vegetables, and cooked dried beans and peas) during the last few weeks before delivery. Researchers at St. Louis University Medical School speculate that carbohydrate loading, the same dietary practice used by athletes prior to an endurance event such as a marathon, might increase tissue glycogen stores (the storage form of carbohydrate) and help supply extra energy for labor and delivery.

Salt

Mild water retention is common in pregnancy and should not be treated with salt restriction unless prescribed and monitored by a physician. No less than 2 to 3 grams of sodium, the equivalent of 1 teaspoon of salt, should be consumed each day in the total diet. This amount is easily obtained by consuming a varied diet of wholesome, minimally processed foods with no salt added during cooking or at the table or in processed or fast foods.

Vitamin A

Vitamin A needs during pregnancy are a matter of balance. A severe deficiency of vitamin A can cause birth defects, while excessive intake might result in abnormal development of the infant's nervous system. For this reason daily vitamin A intake should be limited to no more than 8,000 IU. In contrast, beta carotene, even in large doses, is not associated with vitamin A toxicity or birth defects, although there is no reason to consume beyond recommended amounts.

Vitamin D

A severe vitamin D deficiency might produce rickets in the developing infant, which is responsive to vitamin D supplementation. Premature infants and their mothers often show low levels of vitamin D in their blood, and supplementation raises blood levels of the vitamin, improves maternal weight gain, and reduces the risk of low blood calcium levels in infants. These low levels are most likely to develop in a newborn during the winter when the mother has limited exposure to sunlight (the body makes vitamin D when the skin is exposed to sunlight) or avoids vitamin D–fortified milk.

Vitamins E and K

The requirement for vitamin E might increase during pregnancy, but there is no evidence of damage to the newborn when vitamin E intake is marginal.

There currently are no recommendations for vitamin K other than normal adult intake. Although vitamin K status appears to be maintained in the mother from diet and from bacterial manufacture of the vitamin in the digestive tract, little is known about how much of this vitamin is transferred to the developing baby. Infants are born vitamin K deficient, so medical staff are required to administer a dose of the vitamin soon after delivery.

Folic Acid

By far the B vitamin most closely related to pregnancy outcome is folic acid. The MRC Vitamin Study at the Medical College of St. Bartholomew's Hospital in London provided landmark evidence of a direct link between folic acid and neural tube defects (NTDs). This study found that folic acid supplementation in high-risk women around the time of conception and during pregnancy reduces the risk of NTDs, a condition where the embryonic neural tube that forms the future brain and spinal column fails to close properly.

NTDs are the second leading cause of death from birth defects in this country. Even mild folic acid deficiency during pregnancy increases the risk of spontaneous abortion, low birth weight, and poor growth, whereas folic acid supplementation improves pregnancy outcome and increases birth weight, while lowering the risk of fetal growth retardation.

Low blood levels of folic acid are found in approximately one-fifth of women who show no obvious signs of folic acid deficiency. No toxicity symptoms from excess intake of folic acid have been reported. Supplements of folic acid (400 mcg to 800 mcg) are necessary before and during pregnancy for women who do not consume several servings each day of folic acid–rich vegetables or for women with conditions that increase daily requirements, such as multiple pregnancies, long-term use of oral contraceptives, or anemia.

Other B Vitamins

Vitamin B12 works with folic acid in cell growth and is essential to the normal development of the infant. Anemia from chronic vitamin B12 deficiency is rare in women who consume milk products, meat, chicken, or fish. However, women who follow a strict vegetarian diet for years without vitamin B12 supplementation are at risk of deficiencies. When a deficiency does occur, it is accompanied by infertility or increased risk of having a child who is stillborn.

Inadequate vitamin B6 might jeopardize a mother's health, the development of her baby, and the bonding between mother and child. Mothers with low intakes of vitamin B6 have low blood and milk levels of the vitamin and give birth to infants with lower Apgar scores than mothers with normal to high intakes of vitamin B6. (The Apgar score reflects a baby's condition sixty minutes after delivery, based on heart rate, respiratory effort, muscle tone, reflexes, and color.) In addition, low vitamin B6 intake during pregnancy might harm the infant's nervous system and increase irritability.

The diets of pregnant women are consistently low in vitamin B6, according to a study conducted by the U.S. Department of Agriculture. Only 6 percent of the women studied met or exceeded the RDA for vitamin B6 before and after pregnancy.

Vitamin B6 supplements might reduce poor appetite, depression, and the morning sickness associated with the first few months of pregnancy. One study from the University of Iowa College of Medicine in Iowa City reported that nausea and vomiting were significantly reduced in pregnant women when supplemental doses of vitamin B6 were added to the diet.

Choline, a vitamin B-like substance, also might be necessary for normal brain development in the growing baby. Eggs are the primary dietary source of choline, but with egg consumption on the decline, some pregnant women might not consume adequate amounts of this compound and should include alternative choline sources in the diet, such as Brewer's yeast, wheat germ, soybeans, peanuts, and green peas.

Vitamin C

Poor intake of vitamin C lowers blood levels of the vitamin and might increase the risk for pre-eclampsia and premature births. Pre-eclampsia, a type of toxemia that occurs during pregnancy, is characterized by water retention, headache, the presence of a type of protein called albumin in the urine, and increased blood pressure.

On the other hand, excessive intake of vitamin C during pregnancy might produce "rebound scurvy" in the newborn. Some researchers speculate that a newborn's body exposed to large doses of vitamin C becomes conditioned to breaking down and excreting more of the vitamin, and when vitamin C intake decreases following birth, the baby develops scurvy in the presence of otherwise adequate amounts of the vitamin. Although this theory remains controversial, there is no benefit to taking large doses of any vitamin, including vitamin C, during pregnancy.

Calcium

More than 30,000 mg of calcium accumulates during pregnancy, primarily in the developing infant's skeleton, with the greatest accumulation occurring during the last three months of pregnancy. Increased calcium intake improves bone strength and density in both mother and infant.

Calcium deficiency is associated with toxemia or eclampsia. One study at Brown University in Providence, Rhode Island, reported that low calcium intake (as well as low magnesium and potassium intake) during pregnancy increased the risk of elevated blood pressure in the newborn, while calcium intake of 1,000 mg to 2,000 mg each day lowered blood pressure and reduced the risk of eclampsia in pregnant women.

Fluoride

Children whose mothers consume adequate amounts of fluoride during pregnancy have fewer cavities than children whose mothers' diets were lacking in fluoride during pregnancy. The infant's primary teeth begin forming during the first few months of gestation, and the adult teeth begin to form during the last three months. Fluoride intake has a significant effect on the strength and later susceptibility to tooth decay of the developing infant. On the other hand, an excessive intake of fluoride, that is, more than 12 ppm (parts per million) in drinking water, during pregnancy might produce mottled teeth in the offspring.

Iron

Iron needs increase considerably during pregnancy because of the increase in the mother's blood volume and the demands of the developing infant. The number of red blood cells in the mother's blood increases 20 percent to 30 percent, depending on the available supply of iron. The increased daily food intake during pregnancy usually provides only 1 mg to 2 mg. This inadequate consumption, coupled with low iron stores and inadequate dietary intake of iron prior to conception, makes iron deficiency a common occurrence in pregnant women. Daily supplementation of 30 mg to 60 mg of elemental iron is usually recommended to prevent anemia or marginal iron deficiency.

The consequences of iron deficiency are greater than anemia alone. The iron-deficient woman is less able to tolerate blood loss during delivery and is more susceptible to infection following delivery. Iron deficiency increases the risk of spontaneous abortion, premature delivery, low-birth-weight infants, stillbirth, and infant death. Infants born of anemic mothers are at greater risk of developing anemia during the first year of life. All of these complications are avoided if iron intake is optimal prior to and during pregnancy.

Zinc

Zinc deficiency results in congenital birth defects, low birth weight, spontaneous abortion, premature delivery, mental retardation, and behavior problems in the offspring. Maternal zinc status also might be associated with the ease of pregnancy and delivery, infant weight, and head circumference. Complications during pregnancy and frequency of infections might increase in women with low blood levels and low dietary intake of zinc. In animals, marginal zinc deficiency in the mother produces offspring with reduced resistance to infection and disease, while optimal zinc intake strengthens the immune system.

Adequate dietary intake of zinc is required during pregnancy since maternal stores of the mineral might not be available to the developing infant. Evidence shows, however, that pregnant women frequently do not consume even the RDA for zinc, and either supplementation or increased consumption of foods high in zinc is necessary to maintain adequate blood levels of this trace mineral. In one study, only women who took supplements consumed adequate amounts of zinc and copper and maintained normal blood levels of these minerals.

Putting It All Together: Dietary Recommendations

Pregnancy is not the time to diet or restrict calories and other nutrients. In fact, caloric intake should increase by 300 calories a day during the last six months of pregnancy in order to gain the recommended weight.

The dietary guidelines for pregnant women are simple. If a woman consumes the Healthy Woman's Diet prior to pregnancy, then moderate increases in whole-some foods, such as nonfat milk products, fresh fruits and vegetables, whole grain breads and cereals, cooked dried beans and peas, fish, chicken, or extra-lean meat will meet the increased nutrient demands of pregnancy. If the diet was poor prior to pregnancy, then more dramatic changes must be made to compensate for the prepregnancy diet and to meet the added nutritional needs of pregnancy.

Regardless, calorie needs increase less during pregnancy than vitamin and mineral needs, and food choices should be made from nutrient-dense foods that supply few calories in relation to nutrients. See the detailed guidelines of the Healthy Woman's Diet.

The daily menu: The daily diet should include three to four servings of low-fat or nonfat milk, cheese, or yogurt. Calcium-rich dairy foods can be added to soups, custards, puddings, and flavored beverages. Foods from this group contain calcium, vitamin D (from fortified milk), magnesium, vitamin B2, and protein. For women with a lactose intolerance who cannot drink milk, small amounts of cheese, yogurt, or milk can sometimes be consumed with a meal. If not, then calcium supplements might be required. (See table 8-1.)

Include three 3-ounce servings of chicken (skinned), very lean red meat, or cooked dried beans or peas daily and two to three servings of fish weekly. Selections should be baked, steamed, or broiled rather than sautéed or fried in oils and fats. Foods from this group provide iron, protein, zinc, B vitamins, and selenium. Cooked dried beans and peas also contain fiber.

Vegetarian diets that include several servings daily of cooked dried beans and peas and low-fat dairy products are safe during pregnancy. Strict vegetarians who avoid all foods of animal origin should consult a dietitian for dietary advice since their diets might be low in several nutrients, including protein, calcium, vitamin B2, vitamin D, and zinc.

Two or more servings of dark green leafy vegetables, two or more servings of other vegetables, and one or more servings of a vitamin C–rich fruit should be consumed each day. Folic acid and iron-rich selections are particularly important.

TABLE 8-1   A Sample Menu for Pregnancy*

Breakfast: Cooked oatmeal with raisins and nuts (½ cup)
Nonfat milk (½ cup)
Whole wheat toast (2 slices)
Orange juice (6 ounces)
Herb tea

Snack: Cold chicken (½ breast)
Mineral water (8 ounces)

Lunch: Split pea soup (½ cup)
Cornbread (1 piece)
Cheese slices (1½ ounces)
Fresh fruit salad (1 cup)
Yogurt dressing (½ cup)
Herb tea

Snack: Broccoli spears (4)
Carrot sticks (½ cup)
Celery sticks (4)
Yogurt curry dressing (½ cup)
Water

Dinner: Salmon, baked (3 ounces)
Brown rice (½ cup)
Spinach salad (1 cup)
Salad dressing (1 tablespoon)
Summer squash (½ cup cooked)
Nonfat milk (1 cup)
Strawberries (½ cup)

*This day's menu provides 100% or more of all vitamins and minerals (iron supplements would be needed to raise iron intake to 30 mg or more); 24% of calories are from protein, 52% from carbohydrate, and 23% from fat.

Dark green leafy vegetables are excellent sources of folic acid and iron. Other nutrients supplied by these foods include vitamin A, fiber, some protein, trace minerals, vitamin E, and vitamin C.

Six or more servings of whole grain breads and cereals, such as brown rice and oatmeal, 100 percent whole wheat bread, and whole wheat noodles, will provide trace minerals, vitamin E, fiber, some protein, and B vitamins in the daily menu. In addition, include one to two tablespoons of safflower oil in salad dressings or cooking.

There is little room in the diet for "empty" calories supplied by sugar and fat, so candy, potato chips, other commercial snack foods, pastries, desserts, and soft drinks should be chosen only after all other nutrient-dense foods have been consumed. These "junk" foods provide little or none of the vitamins, minerals, and fiber necessary for the development and growth of the infant and health of the mother, and contribute to excessive fat accumulation in the mother. Artificial sweeteners, such as saccharin, should be avoided since they have been shown to cause cancer in the offspring of pregnant animals.

Fluid intake: Fluid intake should increase during pregnancy to six or more glasses of water each day. Alcohol can slow the growth of the developing infant and result in irreversible problems that appear at birth or become apparent months to years later. So-called moderate alcohol intake, such as one to two drinks a day, is not advisable, and the safest recommendation is to avoid alcohol prior to and during pregnancy.

Coffee consumption during pregnancy is controversial. Some evidence shows caffeine from soft drinks, nonprescription medications, tea, and especially coffee increases the risk of spontaneous abortion, birth defects, small head circumference, and low-birth-weight babies. In addition, coffee consumption increases the amount of magnesium and calcium lost in the urine. To be safe, avoid caffeinated beverages throughout pregnancy or limit them to no more than two 5-ounce cups a day.

Eating and life-style habits: When, where, and how often nutritious foods are consumed is flexible. Foods can be consumed in three square meals a day or in several snacks throughout the day as long as the recommended number and types of foods are chosen. Foods can be seasoned to taste or left bland, depending on personal preference; however, moderate use of iodized salt will ensure that iodine intake is sufficient to prevent deficiency. In addition, a prenatal multiple vitamin-mineral supplement that supplies approximately 100 percent of the Recommended Daily Allowance (U.S. RDA) for all vitamins and minerals with extra iron and folic acid should be considered.

Other life-style factors have a strong influence on the course of pregnancy. Healthy behaviors include regular exercise; avoidance of drugs, tobacco, second-hand smoke, and caffeine; effective coping skills for stress; adequate weight gain; and an active support team of family and friends. Working during pregnancy has no adverse effects on pregnancy outcome. However, strenuous work or long work hours should be avoided.

Complications of Pregnancy Related to Nutrition

Morning sickness or nausea is common in the first three months of pregnancy, and excessive vomiting might result in vitamin and mineral deficiencies. Frequent small meals, saltine crackers prior to rising in the morning, and vitamin B6 supplements are successful in some cases. Drink fluids between meals rather than with them. Learning to recognize what foods trigger nausea (and avoiding them) and what foods appear and smell palatable are more important than any hard rules about what to eat during nausea.

Heartburn is common during the latter months of pregnancy and is caused by the pressure of the baby and the enlarged uterus on the stomach. The symptoms of heartburn are reduced if frequent, small, low-fat meals are consumed rather than large meals. Also, eat slowly, wear loose-fitting clothes, remain in a sitting position after eating, and consult your physician about the use of antacids.

To alleviate constipation during pregnancy, drink at least 2 to 3 quarts of water every day, eat plenty of fresh fruits and vegetables and whole grains, and increase physical activity. Avoid laxatives unless recommended by your physician.

Food cravings are common during pregnancy and usually pose no harm to the mother or infant. Enjoy the foods that taste good, but remember to consume the recommended number of servings of other foods as well. Food aversions also are common and usually subside after pregnancy. Try substituting other foods within the same food group to ensure optimal nutrition.

Toxemia sometimes develops during the last three months of pregnancy in young women and teenagers, in women who are pregnant for the first time, or those who consume a nutrient-poor diet. The causes of toxemia or eclampsia are unknown; however, the syndrome is associated with poor diet and inadequate vitamin and mineral intake. In addition, altered blood levels of polyunsaturated fats are noted in women with toxemia and pre-eclampsia, while increased intake of linoleic acid in safflower oil or fish oils might help prevent or slow the development of the condition and pregnancy-induced high blood pressure. The correction of dietary inadequacies and vitamin-mineral supplementation might help reduce the risk of toxemia.

Breast-feeding: Staying Nourished

The caloric requirements of the mother are greater during lactation than during pregnancy, and the quality and composition of the mother's diet can affect the composition of the breast milk. However, a poor diet is more likely to cause decreased quantity rather than a decrease in the nutrient quality of the milk. When the mother's diet is deficient in these important nutrients, maternal body stores rather than the infant's needs will suffer.

Vitamins

There is an increased requirement for vitamin A or beta carotene during lactation; the adult RDA of 4,000 IU is increased to 6,000 IU. The concentration of vitamin A can be increased fourfold in breast milk by an increase in the mother's diet of beta carotene–rich foods, such as dark green or orange vegetables.

The level of vitamin D is low to moderate in breast milk and directly reflects maternal stores and dietary intake, so the mother's diet should provide approximately 400 IU daily in order to prevent rickets in breast-fed infants. Vitamin D–fortified milk is the only reliable source of this fat-soluble vitamin, and women who avoid fortified milk might require a supplement. (Yogurt and other dairy products are not fortified with vitamin D.)

In adults, vitamin K is normally produced by bacteria in the large intestine; however, this may be a problem in the newborn who has a sterile intestine with no bacteria for several days after birth. Since levels of vitamin K may be low in breast milk, a physician sometimes recommends supplementation for an infant to protect against any problems with bleeding.

Recommended dietary intakes for the B vitamins and vitamin C are in general slightly higher than recommendations during pregnancy. Concentrations of these water-soluble vitamins in breast milk are very responsive to the mother's food intake and show immediate improvement when the dietary intake is increased or supplements are added to the diet.

Minerals

The lower mineral content of breast milk as compared to cow's milk probably protects against stress on the newborn's immature kidney. The minerals in human breast milk are also better absorbed than the minerals in cow's milk.

Calcium and protein are the most important of all the nutrients consumed by lactating women. When maternal intake is inadequate, the needs of the infant are still met at the expense of the mother's long-term health. Calcium requirements increase by 50 percent during lactation to 1,200 mg for women more than twenty-four years old and are even higher for young women below the age of twenty-four.

Iron is very important for the lactating woman, especially if still recovering from blood loss during delivery or depletion of body stores during pregnancy. Continued supplementation of the mother for two to three months, and often up to one year, after the baby is born may be advisable in women with low blood "ferritin" levels or high "total iron binding capacity" (more sensitive blood tests than hemoglobin or hematocrit tests for iron status).

Recommended magnesium intake increases above both normal and pregnancy levels during lactation. Pregnancy, delivery, and lactation are stressful periods for both mother and infant, causing losses of magnesium that should be replaced through good dietary intake. (See table 8-2.)

TABLE 8-2 The RDAs for Vitamins and Minerals: Lactating Women

NUTRIENT	FIRST 6 MONTHS	SECOND 6 MONTHS
Vitamin A	6,500 IU	76,000 IU
Vitamin D	400 IU	400 IU
Vitamin E	12 mg	11 mg
Vitamin C	95 mg	90 mg
Vitamin B1	1.6 mg	1.6 mg
Vitamin B2	1.8 mg	1.7 mg
Niacin	20 mg	20 mg
Vitamin B6	2.1 mg	2.1 mg
Folic Acid*	500 mcg	500 mcg
Vitamin B12	2.6 mcg	2.6 mcg
Calcium	1,200 mg	1,200 mg
Phosphorus	1,200 mg	1,200 mg
Magnesium	355 mg	340 mg
Iodine	200 mcg	200 mcg
Iron*	30–60 mg	30–60 mg
Zinc	19 mg	16 mg

*The current RDAs (1989) are substantially reduced levels for these nutrients and have been met with considerable controversy. Previous RDA levels (1980) are used here.

Putting It All Together: Dietary Recommendations

The breast-feeding mother is a milk factory and her body requires foods that resemble the nutrient composition of breast milk for this production to continue. An excellent source of these additional nutrients, such as protein, calcium, vitamin B2, and magnesium, is cow's milk. Other foods similar in nutrient composition, such as cheese, soy milk, dark green vegetables, and yogurt, must be consumed by those who cannot tolerate milk. At least three to four servings of calcium-rich foods should be consumed each day. Nutritious foods selected from whole grains, fruits and vegetables, and lean meat or cooked dried beans and peas provide the additional calories and nutrients necessary to maintain optimal health for the breast-feeding mother and newborn.

Large amounts of fluids are lost in breast milk and the nursing mother should consume at least eight glasses of water and other fluids each day to replenish these losses. Other than the increased calcium, protein, and calorie needs that can be met by increases in low-fat dairy products, water, and nutritious foods, the dietary guidelines for the breast-feeding mother are similar to those described in detail on pages 168–70.

Severe or restrictive weight loss diets should be avoided during lactation. However, selecting nutritious foods and food preparation methods that are low in calories can supply all the necessary vitamins and minerals for optimal milk production while allowing a slow and steady loss of weight (no more than 2 pounds per week).

Substances consumed by the mother other than nutrients are also found in breast milk. Compounds such as nicotine in tobacco, caffeine in coffee and cola drinks, aspirin, marijuana, morphine, oral contraceptives, alcohol, and hormones are excreted from the body through breast milk and affect the nursing infant. The breast-feeding mother should avoid these substances and all medications not specifically prescribed by a physician.

A breast-feeding woman will retain some extra weight in the breasts and fat stores, but this weight drops off quickly when breast-feeding is stopped. In fact, studies on animals show that increased fat stores are used up by the end of the nursing period, while animals that do not breast-feed retain the extra body fat and are likely to gain increasingly more body fat with the next pregnancy. In short, women who do not breast-feed remain fatter for a longer period of time than women who nurse.

The Post-Pregnancy Diet

The number-one agenda of many women after pregnancy and breast-feeding is to return to their prepregnancy weight. Many women become needlessly discouraged when they don't achieve their weight loss goals overnight. However, the best and most successful way to lose the pregnancy weight is to do it slowly—no more than 2 pounds per week. Remember, it took nine or more months to gain the weight, and it is likely to take at least that long to lose it.

Between 10 and 30 pounds are lost within the first week or two following delivery. (The higher weight loss reflects greater water retention during pregnancy.) To lose the remaining extra pounds, a non-breast-feeding woman should follow the Healthy Woman's Diet and exercise daily. Include several glasses of water daily and avoid alcohol, low-nutrient "junk" foods high in sugar or fat, and smoking.

Some women find it useful to add a period of "abstinence" to the diet; that is, they stop eating all sugar (or whatever food is contributing to keeping the weight gained) for one to two weeks before beginning a moderate weight loss program.

If you do not breast-feed, you still have special dietary needs after pregnancy. Good nutrition will speed recovery and will provide the energy required to care for a new baby. The same dietary principles outlined in the Healthy Woman's Diet apply to the post-pregnancy period.

Your food intake no longer directly affects your growing child, so moderate amounts of caffeine and/or alcohol or an occasional sugary dessert can now be included in the diet. Iron supplementation is sometimes recommended for the first few months to one year following delivery to replenish depleted tissue stores. Since hemoglobin and hematocrit tests are insensitive indicators of tissue iron stores, you should specifically ask for "serum ferritin" and "total iron binding capacity" tests, which reflect iron levels in the tissues.

Your food intake may indirectly affect your child since the example you set is a strong influence on the eating patterns he or she will develop. Healthful eating habits are much easier to establish when a child is young than they are later in life.

Eating for the Next Baby

It is never too early to start nourishing a new baby. Since some babies are planned and others are surprises, maintaining optimal nutritional status during the childbearing years is an essential part of being a mother. The Healthy Woman's Diet provides an opportunity to build nutritional reserves before a baby starts tapping them, to alleviate nutritional deficiencies, and to adapt dietary habits while there is time and less pressure to change. The best time to make dietary changes that will benefit both the mother and the future new baby is prior to morning sickness, heartburn, and other pregnancy-related problems that interfere with good nutrition.

Pregnancy and breast-feeding are two of life's most nutritionally stressful experiences. Having several babies or having them in quick succession can seriously tax the body's nutritional status. Ideally, waiting two to three years between pregnancies while following a nutritious diet and exercising regularly is the best plan for maintaining optimal health for the mother and the baby.

In contrast, severe dieting between pregnancies might result in nutrient deficiencies and increased risk of complications during the next pregnancy. Even a nutrient-dense diet can be low in one or more nutrients if the energy level is below 2,000 calories, in which case a moderate-dose multiple supplement that supplies 100 percent of all the vitamins and minerals might add a safe level of nutritional insurance to an already good diet.

CHAPTER NINE

Women Athletes: Does Exercise Increase Nutritional Needs?

Fitness has become a way of life for many women. Some include moderate physical activity in their weekly routines for health or weight reasons. For others, the love of exercise has grown beyond recreational or weekend sports and has resulted in a new class of exercisers who work out intensely for personal enjoyment and occasional competition. Finally, the female athlete is someone who trains every day for a specific event and whose life revolves around training and competition.

The study of physical activity is broad, ranging from the health benefits of moderate exercise for the average person to optimal performance for the competition athlete. Although the issues pertinent to these two ends of the spectrum might appear unrelated, in reality many physiological and nutritional factors are common for all women engaged in physical activity.

Why Exercise?

Women who exercise regularly are healthier than those who are sedentary or who consider themselves busy but never engage in planned, regular exercise. Exercisers are less likely to develop hypertension, heart disease, or diabetes, and are less likely to die from these diseases. They also live longer than their inactive counterparts. More important, exercisers feel better and younger throughout life and maintain their independence longer than sedentary women. It does not matter whether you are a recreational walker or an Olympic athlete; both activities offer similar health benefits. In short, exercise keeps you feeling younger and helps reduce the effects of aging and age-related disease.

Nutrition for the Athlete and the Recreational Exerciser

Exercise ability is reflected in more than just a runner's race time, a dancer's performance, or a swimmer's endurance. Underlying an athlete's performance is a symphony of complex metabolic and physiological adaptations to the stress of exercise training. This response to exercise results from progressive increases in how long, how hard, and how often you exercise. In addition, optimal athletic performance occurs only if all the nutrient requirements for the growth, maintenance, and repair of body tissues are present during training, competition, and recovery from exertion.

Women athletes continually search for the perfect diet or the right combination of protein, carbohydrate, vitamins, and minerals to maximize exercise performance. Even recreational exercisers want to enhance their health and exercise program by eating the right foods in the right combinations. Ironically, several studies report that women athletes do not always eat right. For example, the diets of recreational exercisers and athletes are often low in several nutrients, including vitamin C, vitamin B1, vitamin B6, calcium, iron, magnesium, and zinc. (See table 9-1.)

The common belief that exercise increases food intake is incorrect; exercise often does not increase calorie intake and in fact might place you in negative calorie balance, eating fewer calories than are needed to maintain weight. Poor diet combined with increased requirements for vitamins, minerals, and other nutrients might jeopardize athletic performance and general health.

Exercise and Body Composition

In general, women who exercise have more muscle and less body fat than those who do not. In addition, the more intense and frequent the exercise, the more the ratio shifts toward muscle and away from body fat, regardless of age. Compared to men, women are more flexible and have the same muscular strength, unit for unit. However, women have approximately 10 percent more body fat than men of the same age.

Because body fat does not contribute to muscle contraction and athletic performance, many female athletes believe they should lower their percentage of body

---

TABLE 9–I   Nutrition and Athletics: Facts and Fallacies

Fact: Complex carbohydrates such as breads and cereals are the best form of fuel for endurance sports.

Fallacy: Sugar is the perfect fuel for sports.

Fact: The athlete needs little or no more protein than is provided in the typical American diet.

Fallacy: Athletes require more protein than is provided in the diet, and protein powders are necessary to meet this daily need.

Fact: Vitamin and mineral requirements for competition athletes are similar to or only slightly greater than the RDAs.

Fallacy: Everyone who exercises needs amounts of additional vitamins and minerals beyond the recommendations established by the RDAs.

Fact: Water should be consumed every 15 to 20 minutes during exercise.

Fallacy: It is best to restrict fluids during training.

Fact: Salt tablets and electrolyte replacements are usually not necessary unless more than 4 quarts of water have been lost during training or an endurance event. Water should always be replaced before salt tablets are taken.

Fallacy: Salt tablets are beneficial for replacing sodium lost in sweat, and commercial "activity" drinks are better fluid replacements than water.

Fact: Physically active people should follow the same low-fat, high-fiber dietary guidelines outlined in the Healthy Woman's Diet.

Fallacy: Physically active people can eat anything they want because exercise "burns" excess cholesterol.

---

fat. There is no general agreement on optimal body fat for athletes in any sport, and body fat percentages range from 6 percent to 20 percent in elite women athletes. Researchers do agree, however, that reducing body fat below a critical percentage (12 percent to 15 percent) can jeopardize health. In addition, the dietary practices used to severely reduce body fat, such as bulimia and restrictive calorie intake, are harmful to health and exercise performance. Athletes who wish to achieve a safe body fat percentage should follow the general weight-management guidelines in chapter 7.

Protein

Protein is necessary for the growth, repair, and maintenance of muscle and other lean tissues. Many athletes and exercisers believe that protein will increase muscle mass and strength. Intakes greater than normal requirements have no effect on building muscle, however; only training increases muscle mass and strength. The typical American diet supplies two to three times the recommended amount of protein and is more than adequate to meet all protein needs of athletes and exercisers. The only exception to this rule might be protein needs for women bodybuilders.

Certain amino acids, the building blocks for protein, might enhance athletic performance. During endurance exercises, muscles use the branched-chain amino acids (BCAA)—isoleucine, leucine, and valine—for fuel. When glycogen stores are low, more BCAAs are used for energy, suggesting that intense exercise breaks down muscle tissue when glycogen is depleted. In one study, athletes who supplemented their diets with BCAA prevented exercise-induced muscle loss and actually gained muscle mass despite heavy training. More information is needed on the long-term health and exercise effects of BCAA before recommendations can be made.

Carbohydrates: When, What, and How Much?

Carbohydrates are the primary fuel used by athletes engaged in anaerobic sports such as tennis, volleyball, and sprinting, and are the kindling fuel necessary for optimal fat "burning" for endurance-sport athletes such as race walkers, runners, swimmers, cross-country skiers, and cyclists. Daily high-intensity training and/or endurance events lasting more than one hour deplete these stores and jeopardize performance, while ample glycogen storage determines the athlete's tolerance to repeated days of heavy training and to prolonged exertion. This is the underlying reason for the diet practice of "carbohydrate loading" and consuming carbohydrate-fortified drinks during heavy endurance training and competition events.

Women engaged in moderate to vigorous physical activity should consume at least 60 percent of their calories in the form of carbohydrates, such as fruits, vegetables, whole grain breads and cereals, and cooked dried beans and peas. However, athletes typically consume only 45 percent to 55 percent of their energy from carbohydrate-rich foods. The amount of carbohydrates in the diet is directly related to glycogen storage and athletic performance.

Consumption of a high-carbohydrate diet results in a greater buildup of muscle glycogen and power output during training than a moderate-carbohydrate diet (45 percent to 55 percent of total calories). A low-carbohydrate diet (less than 45 percent of total calories) lowers glycogen stores, reduces athletic performance, and affects several mood and behavioral factors in athletes, including increased tension, depression, fatigue, anger, mental confusion, and reduced vigor.

Drinking or eating easily digested forms of carbohydrates such as fruit juices or carbohydrate-rich sports drinks during lengthy aerobic exercise (that is, one hour or more of running, brisk walking, cycling, swimming, or aerobic dance sessions) helps slow the rate of muscle glycogen depletion, helps maintain blood sugar concentrations, and helps prevent subsequent fatigue. However, the best proportion of glucose to water remains somewhat controversial.

Sports drinks that contain too much carbohydrate slow the rate of emptying from the stomach and limit the delivery of fluids to the body during exercise. Beverages containing "glucose polymers," such as maltodextrin, help maintain a high blood sugar level when consumed during endurance events and do not affect fluid replacement any more than water ingestion does. Isotonic beverages are the best. This form of carbohydrate can provide as much as 40 percent of the carbohydrate calories expended during the latter stages of moderately intense, long-term exercise.

How the body uses carbohydrate before, during, and after exercise is also influenced by the amount of carbohydrate consumed on the days prior to and the hours after exercise. A high-carbohydrate diet consumed during the week prior to an endurance event will have a greater impact on stocking the body's glycogen stores than will a big "pre-event meal" the night before.

An overnight fast (eating nothing since dinner the night before a morning athletic event) improves blood sugar levels during the early stage of exercise; however, consuming a carbohydrate-rich snack prior to exercise might or might not improve performance. Some studies show that ingestion of a carbohydrate-rich meal thirty to sixty minutes before the event might lower blood sugar levels and interfere with athletic performance, while other studies show a mixed-nutrient snack (one that contains some protein and some carbohydrate) has no effect on performance but does help speed recovery after exercise. It is clear that eating a high-carbohydrate snack after exercise increases muscle glycogen stores by 100 percent.

Fluids and Electrolytes

Dehydration resulting from inadequate fluid replacement is the most common contributor to reduced athletic performance. Some athletes avoid eating or drinking before a performance. A dancer might lose 2 to 3 pounds of water during a practice, while a runner can lose 5 pounds or more of water during a race. Gradual dehydration develops unless the entire fluid loss is replaced.

While a runner is savvy to these needs and often uses water or sports drinks to replenish water loss, other athletes such as dancers often choose soda pop or coffee, which further dehydrate the body by acting as diuretics. A common symptom of dehydration is reduced exercise performance and fatigue, accompanied by increased risk of injuries.

Since thirst is a poor indicator of fluid needs, a general rule is to drink twice as much water as is needed to quench thirst. Athletes and exercisers should drink water prior to, during, and following all training and sports events as well as regularly throughout the day.

The importance of fluid loss during exercise is well documented, but electrolyte losses—potassium, sodium, and chloride—and their effects on performance remain controversial. In general, fluid losses exceed sodium, potassium, and chloride losses during exercise. This is especially true in the well-trained, acclimatized athlete who perspires more but loses fewer electrolytes than the untrained exerciser. Replacing electrolytes prior to fluid replacement could be detrimental to health since this would super-concentrate electrolyte levels in the blood and aggravate the dehydrated state. That is one reason it is important to drink water first.

Consumption of potassium-containing beverages rather than water during intense exercise has no additional effect on minimizing exercise-induced disturbances in blood electrolytes or blood volume. Athletes who consume electrolyte-replacement drinks show no differences in body temperature, blood volume, or blood levels of potassium, chloride, calcium, or sodium compared to athletes who consume nonelectrolyte-containing drinks. In addition, any potassium lost during exercise can be replaced by eating a few high-potassium foods, such as bananas, potatoes, and other fruits and vegetables.

B Vitamins

Theoretically, requirements for many of the B vitamins, including vitamins B1, B2, B6, niacin, pantothenic acid, and biotin, should increase when calorie and carbohydrate intake increase since these nutrients are essential for the conversion of carbohydrate to energy. As long as nutrient-dense carbohydrate-rich foods are consumed, such as whole grain breads and cereals, then the intake of B vitamins also will increase.

However, selection of highly refined carbohydrates, such as white bread, egg noodles, and sugary foods, would increase carbohydrate intake without providing ample B vitamins to convert those foods to energy. Consequently, health and athletic performance suffers. There is little evidence, however, that intakes of any of the B vitamins (except possibly vitamin B2 and pantothenic acid) or the "B complex" in amounts greater than RDA levels improve athletic performance.

One study reported that active women might need slightly higher amounts of vitamin B2 than more sedentary women. Whereas the RDA is 1.2 mg to 1.3 mg, exercisers and athletes might require as much as 1.6 mg per 1,000 calories. Another study of older women showed that at least 4.4 mg of vitamin B2 per 2,000 calories was needed to meet the increased nutrient demands of exercise. Subsequent studies have reported contradictory results, however; some confirmed the increased need for vitamin B2 while others showed that normal dietary intake was sufficient to maintain optimal vitamin B2 status.

Exercise alters vitamin B6 metabolism. Blood levels of vitamin B6 increase during the exercise session, possibly because vitamin B6–dependent enzymes are released from muscle storage or the vitamin is transferred from the liver to the muscles. There is no evidence, however, that increased dietary or supplemental intake improves vitamin B6 status or athletic performance.

One study reported that supplementation with pantothenic acid (a B vitamin) might improve aerobic performance in distance runners. For two weeks the runners took either a 2-gram daily supplement of pantothenic acid (the RDA is 4 mg to 7 mg) or a placebo and then were tested to determine changes in aerobic capacity and exercise performance. The results of this study showed that supplemental doses of pantothenic acid might improve aerobic capacity and endurance performance in runners; however, more research is needed before recommendations can be made.

Antioxidants

Athletes and recreational exercisers breathe in more oxygen than sedentary women do. They therefore are exposed to greater quantities of oxygen fragments or free radicals. (See pages 240–44 for more information on free radicals.) Recent evidence shows that repeated or long-term exposure to free radicals impairs athletic performance, while daily administration of the antioxidant nutrients might help prevent free radical–induced tissue damage, decrease muscle fatigue, and improve endurance performance and high-altitude training. Research shows that normal ranges for the antioxidant nutrients might not be adequate to ensure a balance between free radical and antioxidant systems during intense exercise.

The antioxidants might also help protect athletes from the damaging effects of air pollution. Ozone is a component of air pollution that reacts with polyunsaturated fats in cell membranes to form free radicals. Ozone also impairs immune function. Vitamin E and other antioxidants protect immune and respiratory tissues from this damage, thus potentially increasing resistance to infectious diseases and cancer.

In contrast, inadequate levels of vitamin E are associated with increased tissue damage from ozone. Numerous studies show that supplementation with vitamin E above the recommended dietary requirements might be necessary to provide a strong defense against ozone exposure, especially in athletes who inhale greater amounts of this damaging compound.

Minerals

Female athletes are much less likely to supplement minerals, possibly because they express less concern for mineral status. However, exercise might deplete the body of certain minerals, including iron, magnesium, and some trace minerals, which could affect exercise performance and general health unless these marginal deficiencies are prevented or corrected.

MAGNESIUM

Magnesium serves numerous roles in the development and maintenance of muscle tissue. For example, magnesium helps convert glycogen to energy, regulates muscle building and relaxation, helps muscles and nerves communicate, and regulates the heartbeat and blood pressure. One study reports improved muscle strength when magnesium intake was increased to 8 mg per kilogram of body weight, or approximately 490 mg daily for a 135-pound woman.

Strenuous exercise alters magnesium concentrations in muscle and blood, which might affect performance and general health. Blood levels of magnesium are low after endurance exercise such as marathon running and cross-country skiing, and they remain below pre-exercise values for as long as several months after the strenuous training session or competition event. Levels of hormones, such as norepinephrine and epinephrine (adrenaline), rise in response to strenuous exercise, and these hormones also increase urinary loss of magnesium. In addition, muscle concentrations of magnesium can be low despite normal blood concentrations of the mineral. Thus, low blood levels reflect potentially serious tissue depletion of magnesium as a result of frequent and intense exercise.

Stressful conditions such as intense physical training and competition events increase the need for magnesium. Furthermore, dietary surveys show that self-selected diets often contain 200 mg to 250 mg of magnesium per day, which is below the RDAs of 280 mg to 350 mg for adults. The best dietary sources of magnesium—nuts, legumes, whole grain breads and cereals, soybeans, and seafood—are typically low in the athlete's diet.

In addition, controversy exists over the adequacy of the RDAs, especially for athletes and other people engaged in physically stressful activities. For example, the RDAs for magnesium are based on 4.5 mg to 5 mg per 2.2 pounds of body weight each day. However, magnesium-balance studies show that some people require 6 mg or more per 2.2 pounds of body weight each day to maintain optimal magnesium status. Although RDA levels might be adequate for the recreational exerciser, higher amounts are possibly necessary for women engaged in strenuous activity.

CALCIUM

Female athletes who do not consume adequate amounts of calcium are at increased risk for stress fractures, shin splints, weakened or porous bones, strains, poor ability of bone fractures to heal, and ultimately osteoporosis. Increased loss of calcium also occurs during periods of inactivity, such as during recovery from injury, stress, low vitamin D intake or low exposure to sunshine, high protein or fiber intakes, or abuse of antacids or diuretics.

As many as 50 percent of competition runners and approximately 45 percent of ballet dancers are amenorrheic (that is, have stopped menstruating). In the past, amenorrhea was considered a harmless side effect of intense athletic training. The condition is now recognized as very harmful to long-term health and athletic performance because of its effects on the bones. These athletes often have the bone density of women ten years older, and many women with long-standing amenorrhea have the bones of women twice their age. The reduction in bone mass can result in exercise-related bone fractures that are resistant to healing and increase the risk for later development of osteoporosis. A primary treatment is reduction in exercise training and increased weight gain and/or calorie consumption. Early management to prevent this rapid bone loss also might include increasing calcium intake to 1,000 to 1,500 mg per day.

IRON

Distance runners are most likely to develop iron-deficiency anemia, although any athlete is at risk. Keep in mind that anemia is one of the final stages of iron deficiency. Long before the red blood cell or hemoglobin counts drop, the tissue stores of iron have slowly drained, which has compromised aerobic performance and health.

Symptoms of iron deficiency include reduction in total exercise time, increased heart rate, decreased oxygen consumption, increased blood lactic acid concentrations, decreased exercise tolerance, and compromised exercise performance. Other symptoms of iron deficiency include lethargy, irritability, poor concentration, and headache. Iron deficiency in athletes can result from poor dietary intake, increased metabolic requirements, increased breakdown of red blood cells caused by training (called footstrike hemolysis), and/or increased iron losses in sweat.

The term "sports anemia" is used to describe lower than normal blood values for hemoglobin or red blood cells because of an exercise-induced increase in blood volume, which dilutes otherwise normal blood values. The increased fluid in the blood in the presence of normal amounts of iron-containing blood constituents might be an adaptive response to increase oxygen transport to the tissues and is not associated with iron deficiency. In contrast, iron deficiency has similar low blood counts for red blood cells and hemoglobin but reflects poor iron status, not increased blood volume.

As many as 80 percent of exercising women consume inadequate amounts of iron, and the increased metabolic demands of even moderate exercise aggravate an otherwise borderline condition. Whether a woman has symptoms of poor iron status, sports anemia, or iron-deficiency anemia, it is best to have additional blood tests done beyond just the hemoglobin and hematocrit test, including serum ferritin, total iron binding capacity (TIBC), and transferrin, to ensure that iron status is optimal.

OTHER TRACE MINERALS

Athletic performance affects the utilization, excretion, and metabolism of several other trace minerals. As a result of exercise, blood levels of chromium, zinc, and copper often decrease, while urinary excretion of these trace minerals can increase. Optimal dietary intake helps prevent exercise-induced depletion of mineral stores.

Zinc status might be altered in athletes, especially runners, possibly because of increased urinary and perspiration losses combined with redistribution of zinc in the body and marginal dietary intakes. Zinc loss is apparently associated with training intensity, with high-intensity exercise causing increased urinary excretion of zinc released from damaged muscle. Poor zinc status could affect energy production, tissue repair, and an athlete's resistance to colds and infections.

Caffeine and Athletic Performance

Caffeinated beverages might improve endurance capability by increasing the availability of fat for muscle use. In endurance exercise, the primary cause of fatigue is glycogen depletion. Increased circulating levels of special fats called free fatty acids are associated with glycogen sparing and improved performance. Caffeine increases the mobilization of free fatty acids and inhibits the production of lactic acid. Consequently, the athlete is able to perform more work or to exercise at a greater intensity.

However, researchers at the University of Cape Town Medical School report that well-stocked glycogen stores and a high-carbohydrate diet negate the free fatty acid response to caffeine. Other studies have also reported no benefits to fuel utilization or athletic performance when caffeine is consumed prior to an aerobic exercise session. Consequently, caffeine's effect on athletic performance remains controversial.

Should an Athlete or Exerciser Supplement?

Many athletes take vitamin and/or mineral supplements, sometimes in dosages greater than fifty to one hundred times the RDAs, in an attempt to improve performance and gain the "competitive edge." However, scientific studies have not found a consistent benefit in supplementation for athletes who already consume good diets. Supplementation should be considered for those female athletes and exercisers who don't eat a perfect diet every day.

Although both marginal deficiencies and/or supplementation might not overtly affect athletic performance, more sensitive tests of nutritional status show that blood, tissue, and urinary levels of many nutrients are affected by both moderate-intensity and strenuous exercise. In addition, other environmental factors, such as air pollution, and other health parameters, such as the immune system and an athlete's susceptibility to colds and disease, influence nutritional status and might increase requirements for certain vitamins or minerals.

For example, iron supplementation might be necessary for some athletes, especially women engaged in endurance sports. Iron supplementation in the "ferrous" form is absorbed best, especially if consumed on an empty stomach or with a vitamin C–rich food. High-dose iron therapy produces nausea, diarrhea, or constipation in some women. However, even moderate increases in iron intake, that is, 18 mg to 20 mg, improve tissue and blood levels of the mineral without causing stomach upsets. In addition, frequent consumption of iron-rich foods, such as lean meat and dark green leafy vegetables, and cooking foods in cast-iron cookware can improve iron status.

Calcium supplementation can interfere with iron absorption, reducing its absorption by as much as 50 percent. Consequently, if the two minerals are supplemented in the diet, they should be consumed at different times during the day, or an enteric-coated iron supplement should be taken that delays the release of iron into the small intestine, thus preventing nutrient interactions. In addition, the ratio of calcium to magnesium is important. Increased calcium intake should always be accompanied by increased magnesium intake in a ratio of 1.5 to 2 parts calcium for every 1 part magnesium—for example, 800 to 1,000 mg of calcium and 500 mg magnesium.

The Healthy Woman's Diet provides RDA levels of most of the antioxidant nutrients such as vitamin C and beta carotene, but it is difficult to obtain from dietary sources alone the 200 IU or more of vitamin E recommended to combat free radical exposure. Consequently, moderate-dose supplementation combined with a vitamin E–rich diet might be considered for this vitamin.

The recreational exerciser who follows the Healthy Woman's Diet is likely to consume ample amounts of all other nutrients, including magnesium, zinc, chromium, the B vitamins, vitamin C, beta carotene, and copper. Moderate-dose supplementation (that is, 100 percent of U.S. RDA) for the exerciser would provide nutritional insurance only when dietary habits are not optimal or consistent.

The athlete engaged in frequent strenuous training and competition would benefit from both a nutritious diet and a moderate-dose vitamin-mineral supplement to ensure adequate intake of all nutrients. There is no reason, however, to take megadose levels (that is, more than ten times the RDA) of any nutrient at any time, and there is no need for protein powders or other fabricated nutritional products. (See pages 109–16 for additional guidelines on choosing a supplement.)

Putting It All Together: Dietary Recommendations

The Healthy Woman's Diet is the foundation for diet planning for the "weekend warrior" or the recreational exerciser who engages in moderate activity two to three times a week. The female athlete who exercises five or more hours a week, competes in athletic events, or places stress on the body with increased exercise intensity should adapt the Healthy Woman's Diet so that at least 60 percent of total calories come from minimally processed carbohydrate-rich foods. The diet should revolve around pasta, fruits, vegetables, and cooked dried beans and peas, with small amounts of lean meat, chicken, and fish (that is, no more than 6 ounces per day). This means eating twelve or more servings of grains, four or more servings of fruit, one to two servings of cooked dried beans and peas, and five or more servings of vegetables daily. A sample diet could contain:

Breakfast: whole grain cereals, fruit, and nonfat milk

Lunch: salads, sandwiches, fruit, nonfat milk or juice

Dinner: pasta dishes (beware of fatty sauces), bread, vegetables, and beans

Snacks: more of the same, plus six to eight glasses of water (See table 9-2.)

Both the athlete and the recreational but avid exerciser should divide food intake into several small meals and snacks throughout the day, that is, eat every three to four hours. Always eat breakfast, and combine protein and carbohydrate during the midday meal to avoid fatigue in the afternoon.

Preparing for Endurance Events

The endurance athlete who eats a high-carbohydrate diet does not need to change dietary habits prior to a training session or competition event that lasts less than two hours. However, when preparing for a marathon, triathlon, or other strenuous endurance event, consume an even higher carbohydrate diet (70 percent to

---

TABLE 9–2　A Sample Diet for the Endurance Athlete (3,000 calories)

This diet meets or exceeds the RDA for all vitamins and minerals.

Breakfast:
Cheerios, 2 cups
Whole wheat toast, 1 slice
Margarine, 1 teaspoon
Peach, 1 medium
Nonfat milk, 1 cup

Snack:
Whole wheat bagel, 1
Peanut butter, 2 tablespoons
Raisins, ½ cup

Lunch:
Cheese sandwich:
　Cheese, 2 ounces
　Whole wheat bread, 2 slices
　Lettuce
　Mustard
　Mayonnaise, 1 teaspoon
Tossed green salad, 1 cup
Dressing, 2 tablespoons
Orange, 1 medium

Snack:
Apple juice, 1 cup
Mixed dried fruit, 3 ounces

Calories: 3,000
Protein: 125 grams
Carbohydrate: 508 grams
Protein: 16%
Carbohydrate: 65%
Fat: 19%

Dinner:
Linguini with clam sauce:
　Clams, 3 ounces
　Low-fat milk, ½ cup
　Onions, celery, garlic
　Cornstarch, 1 tablespoon
　Pasta, 3 cups
Broccoli, 3 spears
Three-bean salad, ⅔ cup

Snack:
Nonfat milk, ½ cup

---

75 percent) the week prior to the event, and drink extra water to ensure optimal hydration.

The night before the event, consume a moderate-size carbohydrate-rich meal that is easily digested. The pre-event meal or snack (within one to three hours before the event) should consist of easily digested carbohydrates, such as cereal, toast, and fruit. Avoid sugary foods that might lower blood sugar levels. This snack should be light—less than 500 calories of low-fat foods.

During the event, consume plenty of water and/or diluted sports drinks that contain glucose polyesters (maltodextrin) or a combination of glucose polyesters and fructose that help maintain blood sugar levels and prevent glycogen depletion. For exercise sessions that last more than ninety minutes, consuming approximately 100 calories of carbohydrate every thirty minutes during the exercise helps maintain blood sugar levels and allows the athlete to continue exercising longer without "hitting the wall" or tiring. After the event or training session, begin restocking glycogen stores by consuming a carbohydrate-rich snack such as a bagel with fruit or a bag of Cheerios.

Strength Training and Bodybuilders

Realistic and healthful dietary guidelines for women who strength-train or body-build depend on several factors, including how often, how hard, and how long they work out; body size (the bigger the body, the greater the calorie and protein demands); and metabolic differences based on genetic makeup. Most dietary needs are met by a diet similar to that consumed by other athletes, with the exception of protein.

Carbohydrates

Glucose derived from starchy vegetables and whole grain breads and cereals is the only fuel needed to power muscles during anaerobic exercises, such as weight lifting, that involve short, intense bursts of energy. In contrast, muscles obtain between 85 percent and 90 percent of their energy from fat and only 10 percent from glucose when resting. Thus, consuming a high-carbohydrate, low-fat diet helps the body maximize glycogen storage while burning unwanted body fat. In addition, consuming a high-carbohydrate snack following a workout helps the body rebuild glycogen stores for the next exercise session. In all cases, complex carbohydrates rather than sugary foods are best.

Protein

The typical "reference" person (the 5-feet 4-inch woman weighing 138 pounds with approximately 20 percent body fat) needs 0.8 grams of protein for every 2.2 pounds of body weight, or 50 grams of protein. The bodybuilder is not the typical woman, however. She may weigh more than 170 pounds with as little as 10 percent body fat. Research shows that bodybuilders might need as much as 1.5 grams to 2.0 grams for every 2.2 pounds of body weight, so that the same 138-pound

TABLE 9–3   A Sample Diet for the Bodybuilder (3,500 calories)

This diet meets or exceeds the RDA for all vitamins and minerals.

Breakfast:
Whole wheat toast, 2 slices
Peanut butter, 1 tablespoon
Whole wheat cereal, 1 cup
Low-fat milk, 1 cup
Orange juice, 1 cup

Snack:
Mixed fruit salad, 1 cup
Low-fat cottage cheese, 1 cup
Graham crackers, 6
Apple juice, 1 cup

Lunch:
Tuna sandwich
    Tuna, 2 ounces
    Bread, 2 slices
    Lettuce
Pasta Salad
    Macaroni, ½ cup
    Peas and carrots, ½ cup
    Mayonnaise, 2 teaspoons
Tomato juice, 1 cup
Broccoli, raw, 2 cups
Nonfat yogurt dip, 1 cup

Snack:
Blueberries, 1¼ cups
Mixed dried fruit, 3 ounces

Calories: 3,500
Protein: 161 grams
Carbohydrate: 581 grams
Protein: 18%
Carbohydrate: 63%
Fat: 19%

Dinner:
Beef stroganoff
    Lean beef, 3 ounces
    Noodles, 1 cup
    Peppers, 2 tablespoons
    Tomato sauce, ⅔ cup
    Sour cream, ¼ cup
Corn-on-the-cob, 1

Snack:
Sherbet, ⅓ cup
Carrots, raw, 2 cups

woman who is bodybuilding might need 126 grams of protein, or more than double the recommended protein intake for the average woman.

On the other hand, excessive protein intake interferes with strength-training and health. Any protein consumed in excess of body needs is broken down for energy or stored as fat. The waste products of this process are toxic to the liver and can damage the kidneys. In the kidneys' attempt to eliminate protein fragments from the body, extra water is lost, resulting in dehydration and potential mineral deficiencies.

To avoid excessive intake while ensuring adequate protein consumption during bodybuilding or weight lifting, follow the dietary guidelines outlined in the Healthy Woman's Diet and consume 1 ounce or 2 ounces more of protein-rich meat, chicken, or fish. (See table 9-3.)

L-carnitine and Amino Acids

L-carnitine is a compound made in the body from two dietary amino acids: lysine and methionine. L-carnitine transports fats into the cells' powerhouse centers, called the mitochondria, for conversion to energy. Thus, L-carnitine helps burn body fat and spare muscle glycogen. L-carnitine also helps regulate energy use during exercise since it monitors when, how much, and how fast the exercising muscles burn fat and glucose.

Despite depletion of carnitine stores during intense workouts, a carnitine deficiency is unlikely in women who consume a moderate amount. The Healthy Woman's Diet provides ample amounts of the amino acids necessary to restore carnitine levels. There is no need to take individual amino acid supplements, which are at best useless and at worst could have harmful effects on general health.

Chromium Picolinate

Limited research shows that moderate increases in chromium, in the form of chromium picolinate, might maintain or even increase muscle mass while fat is lost. Although chromium is essential in protein and carbohydrate metabolism and thus may participate in muscle growth and function, there is no evidence that these "anabolic" effects are significant. Nine out of ten people do not consume adequate amounts of chromium, however, so increasing dietary intake to the recommended levels of 50 to 200 mcg daily is beneficial.

Putting It All Together: Dietary Recommendations

The dietary guidelines for women who strength-train, lift weights, or bodybuild are similar to recommendations for other athletes except that calories and protein might be higher depending on the frequency, intensity, and duration of the workouts. These athletes should plan their daily food intake from the Healthy Woman's Diet and should consume minimally processed carbohydrate-rich foods in small doses throughout the day, especially prior to and following a workout session.

Strength-trainers should consume more protein than the average person; however, dietary intake can easily supply adequate protein needs without using fabricated protein powders, pills, or products. Those who compete and need to lose additional body fat for good "cuts" may choose to lower dietary fat and calories slightly more during the last few weeks before a competition. Severe dieting or food restriction is not recommended, however, and can be harmful to overall health.

A moderate-dose vitamin-mineral supplement that supplies 100 percent of the U.S. RDA for all vitamins and minerals will provide more than ample nutritional insurance; there is no evidence that megadose levels (that is, ten times or more the U.S. RDA) of any nutrient improves muscle or strength gains.

Special Dietary Concerns of the Athlete and Exerciser

Several problems experienced by athletes and exercisers are related to, or can be improved with, diet.

Diarrhea: Some athletes experience diarrhea during training or competitions. These athletes should try training at different times of the day. In addition, they should examine the fiber or magnesium content of their diets since excessive intake of either could result in diarrhea. The athlete should try cutting back if intake is too high. Coffee also can increase gastrointestinal motility, and in combination with exercise, could cause diarrhea.

PMS: Athletic performance is not necessarily compromised by Premenstrual syndrome (PMS). Female athletes have won medals while performing during menstruation, and there is no evidence that menstruation limits athletic performance. The nutritional guidelines to reduce PMS symptoms are outlined on pages 364–70.

Pregnancy: Pregnant women who choose to continue training and exercising must consume a diet that meets the calorie needs of training plus the calorie and nutritional needs of pregnancy. Any nutritional deficit is harmful to the developing baby, so optimal protein, vitamin, and mineral intake must be guaranteed prior to, during, and following pregnancy. In addition, a physician should be consulted before strenuous or new forms of exercise are practiced.

Oral contraceptives: Women exercisers and athletes who take oral contraceptives might be at risk for several marginal vitamin deficiencies. For example, some oral contraceptive users have lower blood levels of folic acid and vitamins B2, B6,

B12, and C. The added demands of exercise might exacerbate these lowered levels unless dietary intake is increased.

Summary

A woman exercises for the pure enjoyment of the sport, because she is concerned about her health, because she wants to be more fit, or because she enjoys the challenge and competition. Whatever the reason, total health as well as exercise performance should be considered when choosing a nutritional plan.

Avoid any dietary practice that promises improved muscle, strength, endurance, or performance at the cost of health. The diet that will maximize athletic performance is also the diet that will ensure optimal health throughout life. The foundation of that diet is a low-fat, nutrient-dense diet such as the Healthy Woman's Diet, with its minimally processed, wholesome foods.

CHAPTER TEN

Nutrition and the Mature Woman

As a woman enters her forties and fifties, she is confronted with the first signs of aging. Granted, aging is an unavoidable and natural process that begins with conception and ends only with death, but women do have some control over how fast this natural process progresses and, in some cases, how it progresses. According to Dr. Myron Winick, "How we eat will in part determine how fast we age and what diseases we contract." Goals for a healthful life-style are to live longer, age slowly, prolong the healthy years, and improve the quality of the second half of life.

Changing life-styles in the United States reflect a shift toward these goals. The "graying of America" is largely a phenomenon of the twentieth century, with the average life expectancy at birth increasing by about twenty years during this century. For example, the rates for the leading cause of death in adults—heart disease—peaked in the mid-1960s and have declined by approximately 50 percent since then, a decline that parallels the gradual decrease in fat consumption. Death rates for cancer in women have decreased by 10 percent since the 1950s, while lung cancer incidence in women has risen. The latter is a direct result of increased marketing of cigarettes to women since World War II.

Healthful Habits Slow the Aging Process

A woman fares better than a man today when it comes to life expectancy. While women outlived men by only two to three years at the turn of the century, the span has widened in the 1990s to five to nine years. In fact, women have lower mortality rates than men for every age group and for most causes of death. The increased longevity in women is primarily a result of improved health and lower rates of heart disease and cancer in the later years.

However, although more women live longer today, many do not live healthier. Eighty percent of all nursing home residents are women—a clear reminder that the health and independence that were taken for granted in younger years must be fostered and nurtured as the body ages, or they will be lost.

Living longer is not the issue; living better is. And the longer that healthful habits are followed, the greater their beneficial effects. Following healthful nutrition and life-style habits during the middle years can have a powerful preventive effect against later disease. Although it is never too late to make changes, a lifetime of poor dietary habits cannot be totally reversed by making a few changes in the later years.

You have two choices when it comes to aging: Relinquish control of your health to the medical community and hope they can "fix" the inevitable advances of aging, or take charge of it by developing healthful habits and turn to the medical community for support of your efforts. However, except for prenatal care and antibiotics, current health and medical practices have had little impact on longevity. This is in spite of the enormous cost of medical care, which has increased from $12 billion in 1950 to the projected cost of $1 trillion in 1993. In contrast, most specialists agree that good food choices can have profound effects on the quality of life and longevity and have been a primary cause in the twentieth century for the decline in death and sickness from the "diseases of affluence."

Is Aging Inevitable?

Some evidence exists that aging is preprogrammed. "The Selfish Gene" theory states that just as puberty is an unavoidable prelude to the reproductive stages of life, so aging might be considered the "autodestructive" phase of the life cycle. In contrast, other researchers estimate that as much as 70 percent of many age-related illnesses are a result of life-style and environmental factors, not genetics, and thus are within at least partial control of the aging person. Few would disagree that there is an ultimate maximum limit to the human life span. The question is, what is that limit and how can we extend the current life span to reach it?

Theories of Aging

Aging is believed to be caused by a loss in the number of functioning cells, with muscle and nerve cells being the most affected since they are limited in their capacities to regenerate. There is also an increase in the proportion of connective tissue as a person ages. What causes these age-related changes is unknown. Many of the theories are interrelated, however, and are associated with nutritional deficiencies.

The Cross-Linkage Theory

The cross-linkage theory of aging states that body cells generate defective cell "messengers" within each cell. The defective messengers then tell the cell to produce defective or cross-linked proteins, including enzymes. The cell cannot use the cross-linked and defective proteins, so they accumulate over time and eventually reduce cell function or cause cell death. What causes the defective messengers is unknown; however, the free radical theory discussed below provides one explanation.

The Waste Products Theory

Incomplete removal of waste products within the cells also might explain how the body ages. If any of the waste removal processes malfunction, metabolic by-products could accumulate within the cells, clogging normal metabolic processes and potentially damaging or killing the cell.

The mechanisms whereby waste products accumulate are poorly understood. However, marginal deficiencies of several nutrients, such as the B vitamins and iron, have profound effects on nerve and brain tissue that result in accumulation of abnormal by-products of metabolism and reduced mental functioning.

The Immune Theory

A deterioration of the body's immune system might cause some of the changes associated with aging. For example, some immune processes malfunction as a result of aging and consequently attack body tissues rather than foreign substances, damaging or destroying them. Studies on animals support this theory of aging. Specifically, animals with a strong immunity against disease live approximately 77 percent longer than animals with poorly functioning immune systems. Other studies show that maximum life span is extended 57 percent when the immune system is strengthened.

The results of studies on animals might pertain to humans. A person's resistance to disease and infection declines with age and corresponds to poor diet and medication use that interferes with nutrient absorption. In addition, intestinal absorption and the availability of some nutrients, such as vitamin D, decrease as a person ages, thus increasing dietary requirements to maintain normal tissue concentrations. Numerous studies show improved immune function when a person consumes a low-fat, nutrient-dense diet or supplements that diet with vitamins and/or minerals.

The Free Radical Theory

A growing body of evidence supports the theory that free radicals are an underlying cause of aging. Free radicals attack the cells and impair energy production by damaging the cells' powerhouse centers (called the mitochondria). In addition, free radicals directly damage the cells' genetic code. The process results in a reduction in the number of normal-functioning cells, with a subsequent deterioration of the tissues. Eventually the cell dies and only a "clinker" remains. All of these processes have been identified as part of biological aging. In fact, the cell age of tissues is determined by the number of "clinkers" present. (See pages 240–44 for more information on free radicals and antioxidants.)

ANTIOXIDANTS AND AGING

The body's antioxidant defense against free radical damage is linked to the prevention of premature aging. Increased dietary intake and blood levels of several antioxidant nutrients, including vitamins E and C, are associated with reduced free radical damage to tissues. For example, in a study conducted at the U.S.D.A. Human Nutrition Research Center at Tufts University, vitamin E intakes of 200 IU per day reduced age-related changes in the brain. Other nutrients such as carnitine and niacin also help the cell recover from damage.

Diseases that are commonly associated with aging, such as heart disease, cancer, arthritis, and disorders that result from a suppressed immune system, also are conditions associated with free radical damage. In addition, several aspects of the body's antioxidant system decrease with advancing age, possibly because of reduced dietary intake, limited absorption, or increased nutrient needs.

A Low-Calorie, Low-Fat Diet and Longevity

Life expectancy is greater in countries where the people eat low-fat, low-calorie diets. Some people in Ecuador live to be 150 years old. Centenarians continue to work in the Hunza Valley in the Himalayas.

Research shows that calorie restriction, assuming nutrient intake remains optimal, might be one way that nutrition prolongs life. For example, the life span of rats is more than doubled by restricting calories. This extended age corresponds to 180 years in human beings. These animals live longer and are more active than their fatter, better-fed counterparts.

While leanness prolongs life and reduces the incidence of age-related disease, obesity has the opposite effect. The death rate for women who are up to 40 percent above their desirable weight is almost 50 percent higher than for slender women; for those women who are more than 40 percent above their desirable weight, it is almost 90 percent higher.

The link between low calorie intake and improved longevity might result from more than just maintaining a leaner body. Granted, calorie restriction doubles the life span despite a high fat intake; however, calorie restriction combined with a low-fat diet results in as much as fourfold increase in longevity. Apparently, maintaining a slender figure by restricting calories and eating a low-fat, nutrient-dense diet is a very effective means of ensuring a long and healthy life.

Putting It All Together: Dietary Recommendations

At this time more is unknown than is known about the aging process and how nutrition affects longevity. There is every indication, however, that optimal intake of the antioxidant nutrients, including vitamin E, vitamin C, and beta carotene, in combination with the Healthy Woman's Diet, which is low-calorie, low-fat, and nutrient-dense, will enhance the body's natural defense systems and prolong life to its genetically programmed maximum.

This means eating less fatty food, meat, and processed food, and more vegetables, fruits, whole grain breads and cereals, and cooked dried beans and peas. In addition, moderate-dose supplementation with a multivitamin-mineral preparation provides nutritional insurance when dietary practices are not optimal. See chapters 1 and 2 for more information on planning and preparing this nutritional plan and chapter 5 for information on how to design a personalized supplement program.

Exercise is another critical component of staying young and healthy during the second half of life. Exercising regularly

- increases bone density and reduces the risk of developing osteoporosis;
- prevents weight and body fat gain associated with advancing age;
- increases metabolism;
- maintains a youthful body by improving the structure and function of ligaments, tendons, and joints;
- increases muscle strength;
- maintains high HDL-cholesterol and a reduced risk of developing heart disease;
- lowers blood pressure;
- helps regulate blood sugar and prevent the development of diabetes; and
- prevents the "stiffness" and reduced physical ability associated with aging.

Women report that they feel better, look younger, and have more energy when they exercise regularly. Whereas the sedentary woman fatigues more easily, finds it increasingly more difficult to lift and carry objects, and is more prone to debilitating diseases, the physically active woman remains independent, capable, and relatively strong as she ages.

Both aerobic exercise, such as brisk walking, jogging, swimming, and cycling, as well as strength-training, such as lifting weights, help to maintain body weight, improve cardiovascular function, and maintain muscle. The following recommendations are a baseline for designing an exercise program during the middle years:

1. At least sixty minutes of physical activity during the daily routine, that is, climbing stairs, walking, or moving. This movement can be

continuous or divided into numerous "sessions" throughout the day, such as twelve minutes five times a day, or even one minute sixty times a day.

2. At least three times a week engage in a continuous exercise that lasts thirty to forty minutes and maintains an increased heart rate, such as brisk walking, aerobic dancing, skiing, or trampolining.

3. Ideally, at least once or twice a week do some form of strength-training, such as lifting light weights or working out on resistance equipment at the local gym.

Nutrition During Menopause

Menopause will soon be experienced in record proportions as the baby boomers reach middle age. In the next twenty years approximately 40 million American women will enter their mid-forties to early fifties and go through menopause; by the year 2020, 60 million women will have begun or have passed through "the change of life."

A century ago when women lived only slightly longer than their fertile ovaries, menopause was a signal of inevitable decline. Today, with women living longer, feeling better, exercising regularly, and being more active in the work force, the "change" should be viewed more as a new phase in life, a time for renewed energy, vitality, and self-assertiveness. However, it often is riddled with "old wives' tales" and social misconceptions, which can add unnecessary fear, uncertainty, and anxiety. (See table 10-1.)

Menopause: The Knowns and Unknowns

Every woman who lives beyond the age of fifty-five goes through menopause. Despite the grapevine of horror stories, however, only 15 percent suffer serious or disabling symptoms, with many of these symptoms related more to culture than to physiology. In the United States, 75 percent of women experience the hallmark symptom of hot flashes, but only 10 percent of these women suffer symptoms serious enough to require therapy. In Japan less than 20 percent of women report hot flashes. Approximately one in four women in the United States reports feeling tired or depressed, while only 5 percent of women in Japan experience these symptoms.

TABLE 10-1   When and Why Menopause Begins

The age of a woman at menopause is affected by several factors, including:

1. *Nutrition:* Malnourished women begin menopause an average of four years earlier than well-nourished women.
2. *Tobacco use:* Women who smoke begin menopause one to two years earlier than nonsmokers.
3. *Early onset of menstruation:* Women who began menstruating early are more likely to begin menopause later.
4. *Upper socioeconomic status:* Women with more money, education, and a higher standard of living also begin menopause later than other women.
5. *Oral contraceptives:* Limited evidence shows the use of birth control pills might delay the onset of menopause.

Symptoms of menopause include the following: hot flashes; night sweats; vaginal dryness; dry skin; mood swings; irritability; depression; heart palpitations; headaches; insomnia; anxiety; tiredness; poor concentration; memory loss; atrophic vaginitis; loss of sexual desire; urinary tract problems; joint pains; dry or brittle hair; brittle nails; reduced estrogen levels; and elevated FSH (follicle-stimulating hormone) levels.

Since estrogen provides a dose of protection against heart disease and osteoporosis, risk for these conditions also increases during and after menopause. Many of these menopausal symptoms and related diseases are alleviated or reduced with hormone replacement therapy (HRT).

Diet and "The Change"

Despite the confusion about what causes menopausal symptoms, there are several nutrition-related issues that can be addressed. Improved nutrition before, during, and following menopause may help prevent some disorders that plague women during these years. Improved nutrition can help avoid some drug-induced deficiencies caused by hormone replacement therapy and can help decrease some of the symptoms of menopause while maintaining a healthy, youthful body and mind.

Vitamin E or the bioflavonoids in citrus fruits might provide some relief from hot flashes. As little as 30 IU of supplemental vitamin E has decreased symptoms in some women going through natural menopause or "artificial" menopause resulting from surgical removal of the ovaries. Mood and attitude also have improved in some menopausal women when they increased vitamin E intake. This vitamin is nontoxic in doses several times recommended levels, so it is relatively safe for a woman to try vitamin E supplements as a possible solution to some menopausal symptoms.

Osteoporosis and Menopause

One in two women after menopause develops osteoporosis. More than 75 percent of the 250,000 hip fractures associated with osteoporosis cause women to lose their independence forever. For the woman who values her independence and her health, preventing this disorder is of primary importance.

Optimal calcium intake throughout life is key in the maintenance of strong, dense bones that are resistant to the development of osteoporosis. Bone mineral loss escalates during and after menopause, however, with a peak in bone loss occurring eight to ten years following menopause, thus making this a critical period in the prevention and/or treatment of osteoporosis.

Increased calcium intake (1,000 to 1,500 mg a day) during this time helps slow the loss of mineral from the bone and retard the progression of osteoporosis. Other minerals, such as manganese, fluoride, and zinc, and vitamins, such as vitamin D, also show promise in slowing the progression and helping to treat osteoporosis.

Both strength-training and weight-bearing exercise, such as brisk walking or jogging, place stress on the bones and help them remain strong. However, strenuous exercise that has resulted in amenorrhea (loss of menstruation) in the past could stimulate bone loss and speed the osteoporosis process.

Hormone replacement therapy (HRT) is the "keystone" for osteoporosis prevention and treatment. The maximum benefits are noted when HRT is initiated at the beginning of menopause; however, it is never too late to start HRT, according to researchers at the Mayo Clinic. Unfortunately, HRT also presents a health concern for many women at risk of developing certain forms of cancer and is associated with weight gain, while calcium intake poses no risk and also is effective in the prevention and treatment of this disorder. In fact, women who enter menopause with strong, dense bones do not develop osteoporosis and thus avoid the need to take additional hormones.

According to researchers at the Oregon Health Sciences University, consuming 1,500 mg of calcium daily can reduce the effective dose of HRT by half, that is, from .6 to .3 mg of Premarin, which might reduce the side effects as well. (See pages 359–64 for more information on osteoporosis.)

Calcium and Hypertension

Although optimal calcium intake is associated with a reduced risk of developing high blood pressure, there is no evidence that daily intakes of more than 1,000 mg will be any more effective in preventing hypertension prior to and following menopause.

Heart Disease and Menopause

Women are at lower risk than men of developing heart disease and suffering a heart attack—that is, until they reach menopause. In the age group that corresponds to premenopause in women, men are six times more likely to die from heart disease than are women. That ratio drops to 2.5 to 1 after menopause, and heart disease is the number one cause of death in postmenopausal women.

Since the obvious signs of atherosclerosis appear fifteen years or more after menopause, preventive measures, such as diet and exercise, ideally should begin before menopause. Two important diet-related interventions to reduce LDL-cholesterol and improve the overall cholesterol profile are weight management, in particular reducing dietary fat and increasing complex carbohydrates, and exercise.

Why is there such a large gap in risk between premenopausal and postmenopausal women? Although poorly understood, it again appears that estrogen provides a protective effect against heart disease, and with diminishing estrogen levels after menopause, heart disease risk escalates. Hormone replacement therapy (HRT) returns the lost estrogen and helps reduce some of the risk factors associated with heart disease in postmenopausal women. HRT also causes high blood pressure in some women, however, and has no effect on other risk factors such as obesity. In fact, HRT encourages weight gain in some women.

A risk-free approach to lowering the risk of heart disease after menopause is through diet, exercise, and life-style. Blood cholesterol values are improved by reducing dietary fat and increasing dietary carbohydrates, as well as by lowering the intake of cholesterol and increasing the intake of the antioxidant nutrients and some minerals such as chromium. These dietary practices combined with regular exercise, avoiding tobacco smoke, and effectively coping with stress have no side effects and are as effective, if not more so, than most medication therapies. (See pages 282–95 for more information on heart disease and diet.)

Cancer and Menopause

Two types of cancer are common in women after menopause: lung and breast cancer. Most cases of breast cancer occur in women who are fifty or older, and the risk factors for this disease include dietary fat intake, excess body weight, and alcohol consumption.

Approximately half of all women consume 40 percent of their calories from fat, a third of which comes from saturated fat. Less than half of a woman's total calorie intake comes from carbohydrate-rich foods. Switching to the low-fat, nutrient-dense Healthy Woman's Diet with less than 25 percent fat calories and more than 55 percent carbohydrate calories would have a significant effect on lowering the risk of breast cancer. A modest reduction in fat intake, from 40 percent to 30 percent of total calories, is not effective in preventing breast cancer, while cultures that consume less than 20 percent to 25 percent fat calories have a low breast cancer risk. Lung cancer is best prevented by avoiding tobacco. (See pages 272–82 for more information on cancer and diet.)

Weight Gain and Menopause

Women often gain weight after menopause and tend to deposit more fat in the abdominal area. This reshaping of a woman's figure from a pear shape to more of an apple shape could increase her risk of diabetes, heart disease, cancer, and hypertension.

Postmenopausal women have, on average, 20 percent more body fat than premenopausal women; they also have more above-the-waist fat. Abdominal fat is characterized by two locations: subcutaneous fat just under the skin (the fat that makes up "love handles") and visceral fat that is deeper, firmer, and closer to internal organs. This visceral fat results in a "metabolic syndrome" that raises blood levels of glucose, triglycerides, cholesterol, and certain hormones that, in turn, increase the risk of disease.

During and after menopause you can avoid this change in your figure and prevent an increasing risk of disease by consuming a low-fat, moderate-calorie diet and exercising on a regular basis. Although poorly understood, reducing dietary fat might affect hormone levels in women, which in turn changes fat distribution and lowers the risk of disease. In addition, one study reported that consuming too much sugar also increases the accumulation of visceral fat in the abdomen.

Hormone Replacement Therapy (HRT) and Nutrition

HRT is considered the "elixir of life" for many menopausal women. Hormone therapy reduces or eliminates many of the symptoms of menopause, from hot flashes to mood swings, and prevents the progression of osteoporosis and heart disease associated with postmenopause. Unfortunately, HRT must be continued indefinitely. When women stop taking HRT, bone loss escalates and within years the bones resemble those of women who never received HRT. (See table 10-2.)

The other stumbling block for HRT use is its side effects. HRT is associated with increased risk of developing endometrial cancer, endometriosis, uterine fibroids (fibrous growths in the uterus), and aggravating the risk of breast cancer in high-risk women or activating dormant cancer cells. There is no evidence that HRT increases the risk of cancer of the cervix, ovary, or vulva.

The combination of estrogen and progesterone might lower but not erase the increased risk of endometrial cancer; consequently, many physicians recommend cyclic therapy that combines these two female hormones. Unfortunately, progestin, a form of progesterone, might counteract the beneficial effects of estrogen in protecting against heart disease, and it also increases the risk of cyclic mood swings similar to those experienced in Premenstrual syndrome (PMS). (Women who have had a hysterectomy usually do not need to take progesterone.) Medical costs also might increase for a woman on HRT because she should have routine mammograms, liver function tests, blood cholesterol profiles, and tests for diabetes.

HRT might also affect nutritional status. Salt and fluid retention and weight gain have been reported. Some women experience abdominal cramping, loss of appetite, diarrhea, or nausea when taking estrogen. These side effects can reduce food and nutrient intake or increase the loss of nutrients from the body. (See pages 223–24 for more information on how to manage drug-induced nausea and loss of appetite.)

In fact, HRT is suspected of increasing a woman's need for several nutrients, including folic acid and vitamin B12. Other estrogen-containing drugs, such as

---

TABLE 10–2   When to Say "No" to Hormone Replacement Therapy

Hormone replacement therapy may not be advisable under the following conditions:

Previous endometrial hyperplasia (abnormal cell growth)	Family history of breast or endometrial cancers	Gallstones
	High blood pressure	Endometriosis
Previous heart attack or stroke	Active liver disease	Fibroids
Previous blood clots		

---

oral contraceptives, also might lower vitamins B1, B2, and B6, and raise blood levels of vitamin A, iron, and other minerals. Some researchers recommend a daily intake of up to 5 mg of vitamin B6 to compensate for estrogen-induced depletion of this vitamin. The Healthy Woman's Diet combined with a moderate-dose vitamin-mineral supplement would help counteract these side effects.

Putting It All Together: Dietary Recommendations

Menopause poses dramatic physical and emotional changes that are reflected in nutritional status. Some nutrient levels improve—for example, iron levels are higher in the postmenopausal woman than they are in younger women—while requirements for other nutrients, such as calcium, might increase. (See chapter 6 for dietary sources of calcium.) HRT poses additional nutritional risk, possibly increasing a woman's need for the B vitamins. The two most important nutritional considerations for the postmenopausal woman are to maintain a desirable body weight by consuming a low-fat, nutrient-dense diet, such as the Healthy Woman's Diet, and to ensure optimal dietary intake of all vitamins and minerals.

CHAPTER ELEVEN

Nutrition and Seniors

The quality of life as a woman ages depends profoundly on her capacity for physical mobility, mental alertness, independence, and health. Each of these qualities is directly related to lifelong and current nutritional habits. Many of the diseases and conditions once thought to be inevitable consequences of aging are now recognized as related to life-style, not age, and therefore preventable and often treatable.

The senior years can be a rewarding and active stage in life. Illness and poor health are not inevitable during these years if healthful life-style habits, such as nutrition and exercise, are maintained. A woman need not be an Olympic athlete or a fanatic about her diet to achieve a high level of mental and physical health in the senior years. Simple changes in diet and exercise prevent many age-related diseases and increase vitality and mental alertness. In short, you cannot prevent aging, but you do not have to feel old; seek to add life to your years, not just years to your life.

Dietary Habits

Despite the growing interest in lifelong health, many seniors continue to eat poorly, jeopardizing their health and resistance to disease and potentially shortening their life spans and diminishing the quality of their lives. It is even more difficult to design optimal diets for women living in nursing homes because of their low calorie intake.

Numerous factors in a senior's life can interfere with optimal nutrition, including reduced vision, decreased senses of smell and taste, loneliness, depression, illness, increased medications, limited income, and reduced interest in food. Altered taste can result in poor food choices if sugar is added to foods to enhance the flavor.

Digestive processes also change with age. Reduced secretion of stomach acid interferes with digestion and might reduce the absorption of certain nutrients, such as calcium, iron, and vitamin B12. Absorption of other nutrients, such as protein, carbohydrates, fats, and vitamin D, is often reduced, while kidney function may be altered, increasing or altering the excretion of other nutrients. Drugs, diarrhea, or constipation also affect the absorption of nutrients. These physiological changes suggest that some seniors might need more of certain nutrients than they did when they were younger.

The diets of seniors often fall short of optimal, while malnutrition often goes undetected. National nutrition surveys report that the diets of seniors are often low in vitamins A, C, D, E, B1, B2, B6, B12, niacin, folic acid, calcium, iron, magnesium, and zinc. Nutritional inadequacies develop slowly and insidiously or mimic changes of normal aging. Without clear-cut symptoms, diagnosis is delayed, and the harmful effects on health progress to potentially serious, yet reversible, stages. Many cases of depression, mental disorders (including memory loss and the misdiagnosis of Alzheimer's disease), poor coordination, fatigue, poor taste, and chronic infections in seniors have been successfully remedied with improved nutrition.

Other health problems associated with poor nutrition in seniors are: blood in the stools; bowel irregularities; breathlessness on exertion and/or at rest; bruising; burning, prickling, "pins and needles," or cramps in the legs; changes in skin color (gray, brown, or yellow); confusion; delayed healing of injuries, sores, or ulcers; moodiness; diarrhea; hair loss; light sensitivity; memory loss; pain or discomfort when eating or swallowing; rash unresponsive to topical medication; sore lips or tongue; swelling of the legs and ankles; thin nails; and weight loss or weight gain.

Body Weight and Longevity

More than half of all women seniors living independently are overweight, a condition that increases their risk of developing several degenerative diseases. As they age, women tend to accumulate more body fat above the waist, a type of fat associated with increased risk of diabetes, heart disease, and other degenerative disorders.

However, only obese women (those who are more than 20 percent above desirable body weight and whose fat is predominantly above the waist) should lower their body fat and weight, while moderately overweight women older than sixty-five may not be at increased risk of disease. Underweight elderly women, on the other hand, should increase their dietary intakes to achieve a desirable body weight since being too thin is associated with an increased risk of disease and death.

Protein and Calories

Protein malnutrition is common in elderly women who are ill, and it is estimated to be as high as 60 percent for patients in nursing homes. In conjunction with inadequate calorie intake, this suboptimal protein consumption can result in tissue wasting, hair loss, reduced resistance to disease and infection, loss of appetite and progressive malnutrition, depression, memory loss, and many other serious complications. The loss of appetite is often compounded by medications that decrease taste or smell acuity, or poor dentition that interferes with eating.

Calorie needs decrease with age if an active life-style that includes daily exercise is not maintained. Therefore, a sedentary woman must reduce her food intake to maintain a desirable weight; if she eats the same amount of food as she did in her younger years, she will gain weight. Even if calorie needs decrease with a more sedentary life-style, vitamin and mineral needs remain the same. So a woman must plan carefully to ensure she consumes optimal amounts of all nutrients.

Fiber and Water

Seniors who have trouble with constipation often remedy the problem by increasing their dietary intakes of fiber foods such as whole grain breads and cereals, oatmeal, fresh fruits and vegetables, and cooked dried beans and peas. A variety of fiber in foods of plant origin also helps prevent many age-related diseases such as heart disease, diabetes, high blood pressure, cancer, and diverticulitis. Increasing water intake to six or more glasses and exercising daily also helps solve bowel problems.

Fat-Soluble Vitamins

National nutrition surveys indicate that as many as 65 percent of seniors consume less than RDA levels of vitamin A. One study reports that seniors with Alzheimer's disease have low tissue levels of vitamin A and E, which could expose brain nerve cells to free radical damage and possibly speed the disease process.

Optimal vitamin D intake helps slow the development and progression of osteoporosis in older women, while a vitamin D deficiency might be a contributing factor to the high incidence of hip fractures in seniors. A prolonged deficiency causes poor bone mineralization, bone pain, and muscle weakness.

Although vitamin D is manufactured in the body when a person is exposed to sunlight, this process slows with age. Older women also may be less mobile and spend less time in the sun. As many as 75 percent of seniors consume less than two-thirds of the RDA for vitamin D, and one study reports that older women do not absorb vitamin D as well from food as they did when they were younger. Consequently, while a woman must depend even more on dietary sources of vitamin D, she often consumes less vitamin D than she did in earlier years.

Seniors who do not consume at least four glasses of fortified nonfat milk each day should take a vitamin D supplement that supplies up to, but not more than, 400 IU of the vitamin. Yogurt, cottage cheese, and other dairy products are not fortified with vitamin D and therefore are poor sources of the vitamin.

Antioxidants

Cataracts and age-related degeneration of the macula in the eye are the two most common causes of vision loss in seniors. Up to 50 percent of women over seventy-four have cataracts severe enough to interfere with vision. The antioxidant nutrients, including vitamins C and E, might protect the eyes from free radical damage associated with cataract formation and macular degeneration. Researchers at Tufts University recommend no more than 500 mg of vitamin C, 200 to 400 IU of vitamin E, and 5,000 to 10,000 IU of beta carotene each day. (See pages 315–18 for more information on diet and vision.)

Many age-related psychological disorders might be improved with increased dietary intake of vitamin E and selenium. In one study, a group of seniors received either placebos or supplements containing selenium and vitamin E. After only two months, the supplemented group showed marked improvement in depression, anxiety, mental alertness, emotional stability, motivation, initiative, hostility, interest in the environment, fatigue, appetite, and general mood. This improvement continued as long as the supplements were taken.

The antioxidant nutrients are also suspected of improving an older woman's resistance to disease and infection by strengthening the immune system. High levels of antioxidants, such as glutathione and vitamins C and E, enhance the immune response in seniors, possibly by protecting cell membranes in immune-related tissues from free radical damage. In addition, vitamin C needs for older women might be 25 percent higher than current RDAs to maintain optimal tissue levels.

B Vitamins

Low dietary intake of several B vitamins, including B1, B2, B6, B12, and folic acid, reduces mental functioning in seniors, while improved nutrition reverses these often debilitating problems and improves mental abilities. For example, as many as 47 percent of seniors consume too little vitamin B1, and at least 50 percent consume inadequate amounts of niacin. The long-term consequences of these deficiencies include skin and hair problems, depression and other emotional disorders, general weakness and suppressed immunity, and gastrointestinal problems.

Up to 80 percent of the senior population consumes less than the RDA for vitamin B6. Although a deficiency can result from poor dietary intake, it is likely that reduced absorption or utilization also contributes to this disorder. Some studies show that seniors require up to 20 percent more vitamin B6 than younger women to bring blood levels up to normal.

Inadequate vitamin B12 intake is common in seniors. In addition, approximately 20 percent of women aged sixty to sixty-nine and 40 percent of women over eighty have "atrophic gastritis," an inability to secrete sufficient stomach acid to kill bacteria. Ingested bacteria are not destroyed and, in turn, interfere with the absorption of vitamin B12 even if dietary intake is adequate. In time, the chronic low levels of vitamin B12 result in a variety of vague disorders, including tingling or abnormal gait. However, vitamin B12 deficiency also results in reduced mental capacity and other neurological disorders that can resemble Alzheimer's disease. Those who are deficient respond quickly and return to normal function when vitamin B12 intake is increased.

As many as 80 percent of seniors consume inadequate amounts of folic acid, a B vitamin essential for cell repair. Decreased absorption, altered metabolism, or increased excretion of folic acid might also contribute to the increased risk of folic acid deficiencies. Consequently, amounts greater than RDA levels might be necessary to maintain normal tissue and blood levels of this vitamin. Unfortunately, clinical signs of deficiency are seldom apparent, so malnutrition progresses undetected. Seniors who take multiple vitamin and mineral supplements that contain folic acid have higher blood values than those who do not take supplements.

Calcium

Optimal calcium intake is one of the most important nutritional considerations for all women. High calcium intake throughout life has a strong protective effect against osteoporosis later in life. Even if calcium intake has been poor in the younger years, however, it is never too late to slow the osteoporotic process. One study showed that when postmenopausal women who were consuming less than half the RDA for calcium (or 400 mg of calcium per day) increased their intake to 800 mg or more, they reduced their rates of bone loss.

A National Institutes of Health Consensus Conference recommends daily calcium intakes of 1,000 mg in postmenopausal women on hormone replacement therapy (HRT) and 1,500 mg in postmenopausal women not on HRT. Older women with reduced stomach acid should consume calcium carbonate supplements with food or select calcium citrate supplements, which are absorbed better in the low-acid digestive tract.

Zinc

Zinc is an essential factor in immune responsiveness and wound healing. In addition, inadequate consumption of zinc-rich foods results in reduced taste acuity, which leads to lowered interest in eating or increased consumption of sugary or salty foods that, in turn, aggravate malnutrition, depression, and indifference to eating.

Older women often consume zinc-poor diets and have low blood levels of this mineral. Optimal zinc intake is 12 to 15 mg. Doses far in excess of this have been linked to increased risk of heart disease and secondary deficiencies of other minerals such as copper.

Fish Oils

Both fish oil capsules and frequent inclusion of fish in the diet lower blood fat levels, help regulate blood sugar levels, and reduce the risk of numerous age-related diseases, from cancer to heart disease. Fish oils also show promise in helping to alleviate some symptoms of arthritis, asthma, and other inflammatory disorders, and enhance a woman's resistance to disease. Vitamin E–rich foods or supplements should accompany the use of fish oil capsules.

Exercise

Although the focus of this book is nutrition, the importance of exercise in the senior years cannot be underestimated. Many of the aches and pains of aging are a result of the "use it or lose it" process, also called the "disuse syndrome." Increased body fat, weak and stiff muscles, brittle or porous bones, low energy, and increased risk of numerous diseases from diabetes to heart disease are all related to a sedentary life-style.

Both aerobic activity, such as walking, bicycling, swimming, and water aerobics, and strength-training or weight lifting, increase muscle strength and flexibility and reduce the risk of disease and premature aging. Muscles and bones strengthened by exercise are less susceptible to falls and injury, and heal more quickly than nonexercised, weakened tissues. Aerobic exercise benefits the heart and blood vessels and lowers a woman's risk of developing and dying of heart disease, diabetes, and even colon cancer. Strength-training fortifies the muscles and helps slow the progression of arthritis, osteoporosis, and other age-related debilitating disorders.

The consequences of inactivity in the later years are not attractive. Women have less muscle than men throughout life, so they lose strength more rapidly after age sixty. One in two women past the age of sixty-five cannot lift 10 pounds; many cannot climb ten stairs. Many elderly women are institutionalized only because they are so profoundly weak that they are no longer capable of independent living.

Much of this suffering can be prevented by including planned exercise in the daily routine. Even elderly women who begin a moderate exercise program late in life show marked improvement in aerobic capacity within six months. They also lose body fat and improve their health status. The good news is that it is never too late to start an exercise program.

Nutrition and Specific
Age-Related Disorders

Many diseases found primarily in older persons have nutritional components. Women with rheumatoid arthritis often consume diets low in vitamins C and D, folic acid, vitamin B6, iron, and zinc. Improved dietary intake of these nutrients and/or selenium and vitamin E have shown benefits in reducing the pain and discomfort of this condition. Many of these nutrients aid in strengthening the immune system, which in turn might help lessen the severity of rheumatoid arthritis.

Medication use by seniors also can interfere with nutritional status. Excessive use of laxatives is common in older adults and can be harmful. For example, mineral oil binds to the fat-soluble vitamins—A, D, E, and K—and increases their excretion. Deficiencies of these vitamins are associated with increased risk of cancer, osteoporosis, immune problems, and blood clotting disorders.

Putting It All Together: Dietary Recommendations

Although the dietary and life-style practices that increase a woman's chances of living a healthy life past one hundred will be identified by generations to come, a wealth of information does exist showing a strong link between a low-fat, nutrient-dense diet and improved health, reduced risk of disease, and slowed progression of age-related processes.

Any age-related barriers to eating well can be remedied with a few simple guidelines for menu planning. First, older women should consume the same nutritious foods that they did when they were younger. The daily menu should be based on the Healthy Woman's Diet; however, the texture or preparation methods might change to accommodate changes in abilities to chew or digest foods.

Variety in the diet is essential. Eating a variety of foods reduces the likelihood of nutrient deficiencies and avoids excessive intake of other potentially harmful substances. Also, foods should be minimally processed since, in general, the more highly processed a food, the lower its nutrient content. (See table 11-1.)

Limiting fat to less than 30 percent of total calories and saturated fats to no more than 7 percent of total calories is very important in the senior's diet. Excessive fat intake is associated with numerous diseases, from heart disease and diabe-

TABLE 11-1   Sample Menu Ideas

MENU 1

Breakfast: Cereal and nonfat milk, toast, and fruit juice
Lunch: Peanut butter sandwich, coleslaw, fresh fruit, and milk
Dinner: Baked chicken, baked potato, steamed broccoli, salad, and gingerbread
Snacks: Crackers and cheese, applesauce, banana, or yogurt

MENU 2

Breakfast: Oatmeal and nonfat milk, toast, and fruit juice
Lunch: Tuna salad sandwich, three-bean salad, fresh fruit, and nonfat milk
Dinner: Vegetable and beef stew, cornbread, and juice
Snacks: Grated vegetables in gelatin, cottage cheese and pineapple, or fresh fruit

MENU 3

Breakfast: Peanut butter on toast, orange juice, and buttermilk
Lunch: Grilled cheese sandwich, cream of tomato soup, and fruit
Dinner: Baked fish, rice, green peas, fruit salad, and biscuits
Snacks: Yogurt, fruit, nuts, pretzels, or pudding made with nonfat milk

tes to cancer and hypertension. In addition, a high-fat diet is more likely to cause weight and body fat problems than a low-fat, nutrient-dense diet. Some fat is necessary for the proper absorption of the fat-soluble vitamins; however, diets limited to even 20 percent fat calories or less still supply ample fat for normal digestion.

Optimal intake of all vitamins and minerals is essential to reduce the risk of disease, improve immune function, and slow the aging process. The RDAs for seniors are extrapolated from requirements for younger persons and lump all women fifty-one years old and older into one category. However, the nutrient needs of a healthy fifty-one-year-old are likely to be very different from those of a ninety-one-year-old in ill health.

Because of possible reductions in the absorption and utilization of some nutrients, some researchers believe even healthy seniors "should aim for intakes about 25 percent higher than present RDAs." Most nutrients can be obtained in

TABLE 11-2 The RDAs Versus the ODAs for Seniors

The Recommended Dietary Allowances (RDAs) might not be adequate for some seniors. The Optimal Dietary Allowances (ODAs) are theoretical allowances based on the RDAs plus a 25 percent increase to account for the changes in digestion, absorption, and utilization of nutrients that often accompany the aging process. In the case of vitamin D and folic acid, the U.S. RDA levels of 400 IU and 400 mcg, respectively, are used. For nutrients where a range of intakes has been set, the upper limit of that range is used for the ODAs.

NUTRIENT	RDA	ODA
Protein	50 grams (or .8 gram per kg of body weight)	62 grams (or 1 gram per kg of body weight
Vitamin A	4,000 IU	5,000 IU
Vitamin D	200 IU	400 IU
Vitamin E	12 IU	15 IU (up to 200 IU)
Vitamin K	65 mcg	80 mcg
Vitamin C	60 mg	75 mg (up to 500 mg)
Vitamin B1	1 mg	1.25 mg
Vitamin B2	1.2 mg	1.5 mg
Niacin	13 mg	16 mg
Vitamin B6	1.6 mg	2 mg
Folic Acid	180 mcg	400 mcg
Vitamin B12	2 mcg	2.5 mcg
Calcium	800 mg	1,000–1,500 mg
Phosphorus	800 mg	1,000 mg
Magnesium	280 mg	350 mg
Iron	10 mg	12.5 mg
Iodine	150 mcg	150 mcg
Selenium	55 mcg	69 mcg
Copper	1.5–3 mg	3 mg
Manganese	2–5 mg	5 mg
Fluoride	1.5–4.0 mg	4 mg
Chromium	50–200 mcg	200 mcg
Molybdenum	75–250 mcg	250 mcg

adequate amounts from the above food intake as long as enough of these foods—at least 2,000 calories—are consumed daily. When dietary habits fall short of perfect or if calorie intake is lower than this, a moderate-dose vitamin and mineral supplement might provide nutritional insurance.

Supplementation Guidelines for Seniors

Older women are more apt to supplement their diets than are any other segment of the population, but they often choose inappropriate amounts or combinations of products, resulting in excessive intake of some nutrients and inadequate amounts of others. On the other hand, seniors who choose their supplements wisely are less likely to develop vitamin and mineral deficiencies that are otherwise common for their age.

To avoid the pitfalls of supplementation, seniors who do not consume the variety and recommended number of servings listed in the Healthy Woman's Diet should consider a supplement(s) that provides approximately 100 to 200 percent of the U.S. RDAs or 125 percent of the RDAs for vitamin D, the B vitamins, calcium, chromium, copper, iron, magnesium, manganese, selenium, and zinc. Beta carotene, vitamin C, and vitamin E can be consumed in slightly higher amounts with no known harmful effects, and, in fact, larger doses of these nutrients might be beneficial. (See table 11-2.)

Purchasing Foods

Seniors can avoid wasting food and money by practicing a few simple guidelines when purchasing foods. Seniors living alone can buy small packages of items and small amounts of fresh produce, or purchase some produce that is ripe and some that will ripen in a day or two. Produce purchased in season is usually more reasonably priced than out-of-season fruits and vegetables. Stores that carry foods in bulk bins allow a person to purchase only as much as needed.

Seniors should also read labels on packaged foods and avoid any that show fat or sugar as the first or second ingredient or that list different types of fat or sugars more than once. The meat department can often wrap individual portions of meat instead of your purchasing large packages that are likely to go to waste.

Food Preparation and Storage Ideas

Seniors who live alone can freeze leftovers or use leftover extra-lean meat, vegetables, cheese, rice, or noodles in casseroles, stews, and soups. Economy-size packages of food can be divided into smaller portions and frozen for later use. Cooking with a friend can save time and money, and the company makes eating more pleasurable. Dried nonfat milk powder can be used in soups, stews, when cooking rice, or for other dishes to increase the calcium and vitamin B2 content of the diet, especially since this type of milk is less expensive than fresh.

Casseroles, soups, and other dishes can be prepared in bulk and then divided into individual portions for easy reheating at a later time. Since cooking can be tiring for some seniors, having a chair or stool at a suitable height for the counter or stove can help.

Seniors who have trouble chewing can choose foods that are softer, such as ground meat, mashed potatoes, cottage cheese, peanut butter, oatmeal, applesauce, and soft-cooked vegetables. Meats, vegetables, and grains prepared in stews and soups are also easier to chew.

Seniors with diminished taste can season sweet potatoes, squash, and fruits with allspice, cinnamon, and ginger. Sauces, meat dishes, and other vegetables can be seasoned with nutmeg, and ham or pickled dishes with cloves. Seasonings that replace salt include basil in tomato-based soups, meat stews, and Italian sauces; dill in seafood or chicken dishes, cream sauces, and spinach; garlic for meats, seafood, chicken, mushrooms, potatoes, and tomatoes; and oregano in tomato sauces, asparagus, zucchini, and beets.

Seniors trying to avoid weight gain should be more aware of their fat intake, eat smaller portions, broil or bake foods rather than fry them, and purchase only extra-lean meats (labeled 9 percent or less fat) and trim off excess fat, use fresh or unsweetened canned fruits for dessert, and limit the use of desserts, fats, oils, and alcohol. (See chapter 7 for more information on weight management.)

Nutritious food can be simple, easy to prepare, and tasty. It also can be economical and prepared to the right texture, and still supply all the vitamins, minerals, and other nutrients essential for maintaining health throughout the senior years.

Helpful Hints for Improving the Diet

1. *Get out of a rut:* Prepare different combinations of foods to be eaten at different times. Eat breakfast foods for lunch or lunch foods for dinner. Change meal size: Eat a big breakfast and a light dinner. Eat out on occasion. Change the eating location—a different room or outside.

2. *Make it easy:* Plan one-dish meals. Freeze leftovers in single-serving sizes. Have simple canned items on hand for easy meals.

3. *Cut costs:* Plan ahead and shop only from a list. Use coupons and store specials; use unit pricing to compare costs. Buy produce in season. Shop when the store is not crowded. Always eat before shopping. Buy basic and generic foods rather than convenience or special brand products. Monitor canned goods and leftovers to reduce overpurchasing of certain items.

4. *Avoid fads:* "Health foods" in specialty stores or at the supermarket are no more healthful than regular foods but cost more. Read labels, comparison shop, and don't be fooled by fancy labels or sales slogans.

CHAPTER TWELVE

Women, Nutrition, and Drugs

Would you caution a friend against swallowing a tetracycline capsule with a glass of milk? Do you wonder about the effect two aspirin have on your red blood cells? Do you worry that your friend who takes birth control pills might not be eating enough dark green leafy vegetables and whole grain breads? Are you concerned that the diuretics your boss takes for hypertension could cause a magnesium deficiency and heart disease?

Although these concerns might seem unusual, the effects that foods and drugs have on one another can have an influence on whether the body receives the nutrients it needs and whether a medication is effective.

Medication Use and a Woman's Nutritional Status

The widespread use of prescription and over-the-counter (OTC) medications has resulted in a growing interest in how medication affects a woman's health and nutritional status. Long-term use of certain medications, such as birth control pills, aspirin, or hormone replacement therapy, might pose serious concerns for a woman's nutritional status. Even short-term use of some medications can have a temporary influence on how the body handles certain nutrients.

In turn, your nutritional status can affect the desired outcome of the medication therapy. Prescription and OTC medications can affect your nutritional status by increasing or decreasing appetite, altering the absorption of nutrients in the

Medications and Loss of Appetite

Some medications cause a temporary loss of appetite and could result in poor nutrient intake. The following suggestions help counteract drug-induced appetite changes.

- Eat when hungry, regardless of the time.
- Schedule small nutritious snacks throughout the day.
- Have nutritious snacks available, such as fresh fruit, crisp vegetables, dried fruit, cottage cheese, or sliced meat.
- Sip on nutritious beverages, such as milk shakes, juices, or milk.
- Make food appetizing. Vary the color, shape, and texture of foods.
- Eat with family and friends.
- Have nutritious snacks by the bed, such as nuts and dried fruit.
- Try new recipes.
- Exercise before eating.
- Catch up on food intake on days when eating is enjoyable.
- Take a moderate-dose, multiple vitamin-mineral supplement with the consent of a physician.
- Consult a physician if poor appetite persists.

intestines, affecting how the body uses nutrients, and increasing the excretion of certain vitamins and minerals.

Medications Alter Appetite

Some medications increase appetite and food intake, and even produce food cravings, especially for sweet foods. Long-term use of these drugs could increase the risk of obesity and other degenerative diseases related to obesity, such as cardiovascular disease, cancer, diabetes mellitus, and hypertension.

In contrast, other medications reduce appetite and result in weight loss. Although this may sound attractive to you if you are trying to lose weight, loss of appetite (anorexia) means a reduced food and nutrient intake and the potential for nutrient deficiencies, malnutrition, and loss of lean body mass. Many drugs alter taste, which can reduce your interest in eating. In addition, some medications can alter your mood, which in turn reduces your desire to eat. Weight loss often occurs in women who are already underweight, thus compounding borderline malnutrition. Poor nutrition also suppresses the immune system, which interferes with the body's ability to defend itself against disease. In many cases it is not the medication but the underlying disease or disorder that causes the anorexia. However, creating one disorder while treating another is a common problem with medication use.

Medications Affect Nutrient Absorption

Medications can interfere with nutrient absorption in numerous ways. They can bind to a nutrient in the intestinal tract and limit its absorption. For example, nondigestible mineral oil binds to the fat-soluble vitamins—vitamins A, D, E, and K—and limits their absorption; consequently, secondary deficiencies of these vitamins are a side effect of long-term mineral oil use.

Drugs can reduce the time that food is in the intestine, thus limiting the absorption time of nutrients. Some drugs that increase intestinal movement decrease the absorption of vitamin B2 because of reduced exposure time of the vitamin to the absorption sites along the digestive tract.

Medications can also change the structure or function of a nutrient so it is not absorbed in the intestines. Drugs such as antacids change the acidity of the intestinal tract and might interfere with the absorption of nutrients that depend on a specific acidity for absorption, such as iron. Drugs also can physically or chemically block absorption sites in the digestive tract or reduce the absorption capabilities of the intestinal lining. For example, neomycin alters the intestinal lining and blocks the absorption of vitamins A and B12.

Drugs can interfere with the digestive juices so that dietary fat and the fat-soluble vitamins, which require these emulsifiers for absorption, are poorly absorbed. Finally, drugs can interfere with the functioning of the pancreas and its digestive enzymes that are required for the absorption of other nutrients, such as protein and carbohydrate.

Medications Affect How the Body Uses Nutrients

How medications affect nutrients within the body is complicated and poorly understood. In the body, some drugs mimic the shape of, and are mistaken for, vitamins, and block any real vitamins from participating in metabolic reactions. The drug has no nutritional activity, however, and thus halts or hinders metabolic processes.

Medications Increase Nutrient Excretion

Medications such as diuretics and laxatives increase the excretion of nutrients, especially minerals. Since minerals coexist in a delicate balance with one another, loss of one mineral could result in secondary deficiencies of others.

Nutritional status is affected by long-term or multiple use of medications. The consequences of using medications will vary depending on a variety of factors, including nutrient stores; age, size, and medical condition; the diet's nutritional adequacy; and the quantity or duration of medication use.

It is always best to take a medication for the prescribed amount of time and no longer. In addition, optimal nutrition prior to, during, and following long-term use of a medication minimizes the potential drug-induced effects on nutritional status. A woman who is marginally nourished prior to taking a medication, who continues to consume a nutrient-poor diet while on the medication, and who takes several medications or takes one medication for long periods of time is placing herself at risk for developing medication-induced malnutrition.

Who Is at Risk for Drug-Induced Nutrient Deficiencies?

Although every woman should be aware of how medications affect her nutritional status, there are some who are at greater risk for drug-induced deficiencies. First, seniors account for the greatest amount of medication use; they also frequently take several medications and often long-term, for chronic ailments. Since seniors are a high-risk group for suboptimal nutritional status because of poor diet, reduced nutrient absorption, and other reasons, the combination of medication use and poor nutritional status can result in malnutrition.

Second, women who abuse alcohol are also a high-risk population. Alcohol reduces nutrient absorption, increases nutrient needs, reduces appetite and food intake, and is often accompanied by a poor diet.

Third, women who have long-term health problems, such as cancer, diabetes, epilepsy, disorders of the digestive tract, emotional disorders, or heart disease, are also at high risk for drug-induced nutrient deficiencies because of chronic use and multiple use of medications. Dosages also contribute to the potential for nutrient deficiencies, with high-dose therapies affecting nutritional status more than low-dose therapies.

Fourth, women who should be extra careful to ensure optimal nutrient intake are those on weight-reduction or food-restricted diets, such as strict vegetarians, those who eat sporadically, and pregnant or breast-feeding women with high nutritional needs who also must take medication.

Alcohol

Malnutrition is a common result of alcohol abuse. Alcohol either replaces other nutritious foods and thus limits nutrient intake or, less often, is consumed in conjunction with adequate food intake and thus contributes to obesity. Alcohol also increases a woman's requirements for several nutrients, including vitamins B1 and B6, biotin, and niacin, which aid in detoxification of alcohol in the liver. Alcohol is suspected of increasing free radical damage to tissues, which increases the body's need for the antioxidant nutrients to repair and rebuild damaged tissues.

Alcohol irritates and damages the digestive tract and inhibits the absorption of several nutrients, including vitamins C, B1, B12, folic acid, the fat-soluble vitamins, protein, calcium, and other nutrients. In turn, deficiencies of these nutrients affect the absorptive capability of the digestive tract and can contribute to malnutrition.

Alcohol interferes with the body's use of many nutrients, so even if the diet is adequate, the nutrients are unavailable for normal metabolic processes. Consequently, symptoms of malnutrition develop. For example, excessive alcohol interferes with the conversion of vitamins D, B1, B6, and folic acid to their biologically active forms, so malnutrition develops even when dietary intake of these nutrients is adequate.

Alcohol also depletes the body's tissue stores of several nutrients, including vitamins A and E, and selenium. Many of these nutrients function as antioxidants, and alcohol-induced depletion of these nutrients can leave the body defenseless against disease and infection.

One study by the Westchester County Medical Center in Valhalla, New

York, reported that selenium concentrations are depleted before clinical signs of liver damage are noted in alcoholics, which suggests limited antioxidant status might contribute to alcohol-induced liver damage.

Women might suffer the effects of alcohol more than men. Compared to men, women maintain higher blood levels of alcohol after drinking the equivalent amount of alcohol. One study showed that the lining of a man's stomach has higher concentrations of enzymes to inactivate alcohol, while more alcohol remains intact in a woman's stomach and enters the bloodstream. These higher blood levels over time could place women at higher risk for liver disease, pancreas problems, nerve damage, and nutritional deficiencies.

The best things you can do for your health are stop abusing alcohol, and consume a low-fat, nutrient-dense diet as outlined in the Healthy Woman's Diet. Even the best diet combined with vitamin-mineral supplements cannot protect the body's organs from the damage caused by alcohol abuse. However, diet and supplementation might help replenish lost nutrients and thus slow the progression of some nutritional problems related to alcoholism. For example, pantothenic acid and vitamin B1 might help prevent the alcohol-induced reduction in certain brain chemicals associated with memory and thought processes. In addition, the toxic effects of chronic alcohol consumption on the liver might be attenuated by vitamin C. The diet should also supply ample amounts of all nutrients, including the B vitamins, vitamin A, vitamin D, calcium, copper, iron, magnesium, potassium, selenium, and zinc.

Antacids

Many women consume antacids as a supplemental source of calcium. In addition, antacids are a quick remedy for stomach upsets caused by stress or excessive intake of coffee, spicy or fatty foods, or alcohol. While antacids might provide quick relief for stomach discomfort, they could also contribute to nutrient deficiencies if consumed in excess.

Antacids that contain magnesium or aluminum hydroxides inhibit calcium absorption and increase the risk of developing bone disorders and osteoporosis. Aluminum is toxic to the nerves and bones, and absorption of this metal from an antacid could pose a problem if it is consumed with citrus fruits or juices. Sodium bicarbonate (baking soda) used as a "stomach settler" also interferes with calcium absorption; however, a woman is at risk only if she drinks a sodium bicarbonate mixture daily while also consuming a low-calcium diet.

Antacids reduce stomach acidity, which is useful to someone with excessive stomach acid or a "nervous stomach," but their use can result in anemia or nutrient deficiencies if they are consumed frequently and for long periods of time. Neutralizing stomach acid also reduces the absorption of the vitamins and minerals—such as iron, calcium, folic acid, vitamin A, and vitamin B12—that require an acid digestive system for maximum absorption. This effect can be minimized if the antacid is taken on an empty stomach rather than with meals or with vitamin-mineral supplements where it can interact with dietary nutrients.

Researchers at Oklahoma State University report that the use of calcium carbonate antacids might compromise chromium absorption and aggravate a pre-existing marginal chromium deficiency. Chromium absorption and tissue levels of chromium decrease when the diets of animals are supplemented with calcium carbonate. The antacids might form undigestible complexes with chromium or alter the acidity of the digestive tract.

Antibiotics

Antibiotics are effective because they destroy disease-causing bacteria in the digestive tract; however, they indiscriminately destroy beneficial bacteria that help maintain health. Several nutrients are manufactured by bacteria in the large intestine, including biotin, vitamin K, and other vitamins. Antibiotics upset the delicate balance in the digestive tract and reduce or halt the manufacture of these nutrients.

Long-term use of antibiotics produces a vitamin K deficiency and might deplete the small amount of vitamin C stored in the body. In addition, consuming some antibiotics, such as tetracycline, with a meal or with milk reduces the absorption of both the medication and several minerals, including calcium, iron, and magnesium. Reduced absorption of vitamin B12 and potassium also have been reported with long-term antibiotic use. These deficiencies are prevented if a nutrient-dense diet is consumed that contains ample amounts of vitamins and minerals and if antibiotic therapy is temporary.

In contrast, vitamin C might reduce bacterial resistance to antibiotic therapy and improve recovery from infection, according to researchers at the Harvard

School of Public Health in Boston. In this study the combined effect of vitamin C and antibiotics was more effective in destroying bacteria than medication alone. In fact, the effective antibiotic dose could be reduced when vitamin C intake was increased.

Antidepressants

Some women on long-term antidepressant medications lose their desire to eat, stop eating or eat sporadically, choose nutrient-poor foods, and experience reduced absorption or increased urinary excretion of several nutrients, including calcium, magnesium, the B vitamins, and vitamin C. Some antidepressant medications produce nausea, dry mouth, diarrhea, reduced salivation, or stomach upsets that also interfere with optimal nutrition. In fact, some patients on long-term antidepressant medication therapy show low blood levels of B vitamins and respond favorably with improvements in mood and anxiety levels when vitamin supplements are added to the diet.

The monoamine oxidase inhibitors (MAOI) used in the treatment of depression can cause several unpleasant and potentially harmful effects, including hypertension, when consumed with foods that contain a substance called tyramine. Aged and fermented cheeses, sour cream, fermented sausages, beer, red wine, and soy sauce are a few examples of tyramine-containing foods. These foods should be limited or avoided when taking MAOI medications.

Nutrient deficiencies are rare, however, even when therapy continues for some time, if you consume a low-fat, nutrient-dense diet as outlined in the Healthy Woman's Diet, which contains ample amounts of all vitamins, minerals, protein, fiber, essential fats, and carbohydrates, or if you take a moderate-dose vitamin-mineral supplement when dietary intake is poor.

Arthritis Medications

A common medication used in the treatment of rheumatoid arthritis is d-penicillamine, or Cuprimine. This medication sometimes reduces food intake by producing nausea, mouth sores, stomach pain, and tongue inflammation, and it also reduces the absorption of several nutrients, including zinc, iron, and other minerals. The drug-nutrient interactions are minimized if this medication is taken on an empty stomach one to two hours following a meal. Vitamin B6 requirements also might increase if you take this medication. Any vitamin or mineral supplements should be taken at least two or more hours before or after the medication and should always be monitored by a physician.

Aspirin

Aspirin is used for everything from headaches and athletic injuries to the treatment of heart disease. However, this panacealike over-the-counter medication can also increase the risk of developing nutrient deficiencies if taken repetitively and for long periods of time.

Since aspirin can cause bleeding in the digestive tract, long-term use could result in iron deficiency, reduced formation of red blood cells, and anemia, especially if you have preexisting stomach problems. Long-term use of aspirin might also cause deficiencies of folic acid and vitamins B12 and C, which can be prevented by consuming more foods rich in these nutrients or by taking a moderate-dose multiple vitamin and mineral supplement at opposite times of the day from aspirin intake.

Birth Control Pills

The use of birth control pills has been linked to several diseases including heart disease, although this link is controversial. The female hormone progestin is associated with an elevated risk of heart disease, and birth control pills with either low doses or an alternate form of this hormone might help improve heart disease risk. Suspicion that birth control pills increased the risk of developing breast cancer has not been substantiated, but a potential link to cervical cancer is still being investigated.

Long-term use of birth control pills can affect the absorption and use of several nutrients. The pills are associated with weight gain, increased appetite, reduced absorption of folic acid and other vitamins, and altered distribution of several nutrients within the body's tissues.

High blood levels of some nutrients, such as vitamin A, copper, and iron, are noted in some women, while low blood levels of vitamins E, C, B1, B2, B6, folic acid, and zinc are noted in others on birth control pills. These fluctuations in nutrient levels are only partially attributed to the medication, with other factors such as dietary habits also influencing the nutritional status. Although increased dietary intake of foods rich in these nutrients or a moderate-dose vitamin and mineral supplement are practical approaches to the prevention of drug-induced deficiencies, there is no evidence that large supplemental doses of these nutrients improve the nutritional status of women taking birth control pills.

Numerous studies report that these pills lower blood and tissue levels and increase the dietary requirements for vitamin B6. This nutrient is particularly interesting since even moderate deficiencies of vitamin B6 produce many of the mood disorders associated with the use of birth control pills, such as depression, irritability, and insomnia.

Vitamin B6 is an essential component in the production of the brain chemical serotonin that regulates pain, mood, some eating behaviors, and sleep. Low vitamin B6 levels reduce serotonin levels, which could produce mild depression and the other symptoms mentioned above. Birth control pills affect the status of vitamin B6 only in those who are already consuming a marginal amount of this vitamin. Improvements in mood and sleep are reported when vitamin B6 intake is increased. Often all that is needed to ensure optimal nutrient intake and reduced mood or sleep problems is improved dietary habits and increased dietary intake of vitamin B6–rich foods.

Cigarettes

Tobacco smoke influences the nutritional status of both smokers and people who inhale other people's tobacco smoke (also called passive smokers). Inhaling tobacco smoke removes vitamin C from the tissues and blood and increases requirements to more than 200 mg per day for this vitamin (the RDA is 60 mg). Blood levels of vitamin C decrease as cigarette consumption increases and are as much as 30 percent lower in smokers compared to nonsmokers. Smokers tend to consume less, absorb less, and use more vitamin C than do nonsmokers, while requirements are higher not only to counteract these adverse effects of tobacco but also to reduce free radical damage to tissues generated by tobacco smoke.

Dietary intakes and tissue levels of vitamin A and beta carotene are also low in smokers and passive smokers. In contrast, when tissue levels of vitamin A, beta carotene, and vitamin E are high, the risk of developing lung and oral cancers and other respiratory disorders is reduced. Since tobacco smoke increases free radical damage to tissues, the reduced cancer risk associated with these vitamins is probably a result of their antioxidant abilities to destroy and deactivate free radicals. (See pages 240–44 for more information on free radicals and antioxidants.)

B vitamins are also affected by smoking. Cigarette use alters vitamin B6 metabolism, and the residual effects might last as long as two years after cessation of smoking. One study found that blood levels of vitamin B6 were significantly lower in smokers than in nonsmokers. Although the long-term effects of this sustained decrease in vitamin B6 metabolism are unknown, increasing dietary intake of this vitamin is harmless and potentially useful.

Increased intake of folic acid and vitamin B12 also might help prevent some of the damage caused by tobacco use. Researchers at the University of Alabama in Birmingham reported that smokers who supplement their diets with these two B vitamins have significantly fewer precancerous cells than do other smokers.

The best advice is to stop smoking and avoid all forms of tobacco smoke, including cigarettes, pipes, and cigars. Since women who smoke during pregnancy have low blood zinc levels and are more likely than nonsmokers to give birth to zinc-deficient babies who are at high risk for birth defects and disease, it is even more important that women who are considering pregnancy should avoid cigarette smoke from all sources. In addition, optimal dietary intake of the antioxidant nutrients (that is, vitamin C, beta carotene, and vitamin E), the B vitamins, and some minerals might help counteract some of the harmful effects of tobacco smoke.

Coffee, Tea, and Caffeine

Coffee and caffeine have been accused of contributing to many degenerative disorders, including heart disease and cancer; however, the effects of coffee or caffeine on these disorders remain inconclusive. A study from the University of California, San Diego, reported that it is not coffee but the habits associated with coffee drinking that predispose a woman to heart disease. Coffee drinkers are more likely than nondrinkers to consume more alcohol, dietary saturated fat, and cholesterol; they are more likely to smoke and not exercise regularly. In addition, smoking and exercise are "dose-related" to coffee consumption. That is, the more a woman

Java Junkies: Looking for Alternatives?

To reduce but not eliminate one of life's little pleasures, gradually cut down the number of cups of coffee by one or two a day. Switch to instant coffee or an instant blended with chicory or grain. (These coffees contain half the caffeine of regular brews.) Blend regular with decaffeinated coffee before brewing or have your local coffee shop prepare a blend of regular and decaffeinated coffees. The grain-based beverages, such as Pero, Postum, and Cafix, are hearty substitutes that contain no caffeine and only 7 to 12 calories per serving.

smokes and the less she exercises, the greater her coffee consumption and her risk of developing heart disease. These associations between coffee consumption and heart disease behaviors hold true for both drinkers of caffeinated and decaffeinated coffee.

Unfortunately, the evidence is not clear-cut. Other studies have reported a significant association between coffee consumption and the risk of heart attack. Again, the more coffee a person consumed, the greater the risk. In addition, the chance of having a fatal heart attack rises steadily in men who drink three or more cups of coffee a day; however, the effects on women have not been adequately studied. Switching from regular to decaffeinated coffee might not be the answer, either, since both caffeinated and decaffeinated coffees have been implicated in heart disease risk.

How does coffee increase a person's risk of heart disease? Caffeine in doses greater than five cups of coffee a day might increase total blood cholesterol and LDL-cholesterol levels, blood pressure, and heart arrhythmias—all factors that increase a person's risk of developing heart disease. It is not well substantiated, however, whether this is caused by caffeine, one or more of the three hundred other compounds in coffee, or related behaviors associated with coffee consumption. Drip-filtered coffee, the type consumed by 75 percent of Americans, has no effect on cholesterol levels, so coffee may influence heart disease risk by other unknown mechanisms besides raising blood fat levels.

In short, coffee and/or caffeine consumption is associated with an increased risk of heart disease only when a person consumes more than three to five cups a day. Moderate intake appears safe, while tea consumption at any dose has not been linked to heart disease risk.

TABLE 12-1   The Caffeine Content of Selected Beverages and Over-the-Counter Medications

ITEM	MG	ITEM	MG
Coffee (5-ounce cup)*		Dark chocolate, semisweet (1 ounce)	5–35
Brewed, drip method	60–180	Soft drinks—colas (12-ounce serving)	36–59
Instant	30–120	Nonprescription Drugs	
Decaffeinated	1–5	Dexatrim	200
Tea (5-ounce cup)*		Prolamine	140
Brewed	20–110	No Doz	100
Instant	25–50	Anacin, Midol, Vanquish	33
Iced (12-ounce glass)	67–76	Excedrin	65
Cocoa beverage (5-ounce cup)	2–20	Dristan	30
Chocolate milk (8 ounces)	2–7		

*Caffeine content will vary depending on the strength of the brew.

The scientific evidence linking coffee with cancer is also confusing. Caffeine might encourage the growth of tumors depending on a person's exposure to cancer-causing substances in the environment, the type of cell affected, and the stage of cell replication. One study on rats showed that caffeine increased the risk of cancer fivefold when the animals were also deficient in the B vitamin folic acid. The amount of caffeine used in this study approached typical doses consumed by some adults. If coffee does have cancer-promoting effects, it might be a result of other compounds in the brew rather than the caffeine since cola (another caffeine-containing beverage) is not associated with an increased cancer risk. Tea consumption also shows little or no increased risk of cancer.

Tannins and other compounds in coffee and tea reduce mineral absorption, especially iron, by as much as 90 percent and can rob the body of other minerals, such as calcium. Two cups or less each day apparently pose no health risk, but one study reported that intakes greater than this could cause calcium imbalances and increase the risk of developing osteoporosis. Consequently, women should drink coffee and tea between meals rather than with food to minimize the effects of these beverages on mineral status and the risk of anemia and osteoporosis. Consuming extra vitamin C at a meal helps counteract the effects of coffee on iron absorption. (See table 12-1.)

High Blood Pressure Medications

Diuretic medications used in the treatment of hypertension increase urinary excretion of magnesium and might increase a person's resistance to medication therapy and the risk of cardiovascular disease (CVD). Thus, this medication therapy lowers blood pressure but increases other risk factors for cardiovascular disease. In addition, potassium supplementation, which often accompanies hypertensive medications, increases magnesium loss. Magnesium supplementation in combination with diuretic treatment is associated with reduced medication dosages and improved cardiovascular risk.

Two other hypertensive medications, called captopril and enalapril, might reduce zinc levels. A study from Tel Aviv University reported that these medications, especially captopril, increased urinary loss of zinc and reduced zinc levels in red blood cells. Depletion of zinc from the tissues could compromise the immune function, reduce a woman's resistance to colds and infection, and delay wound healing. Other studies report diuretic medications such as clopamide, used in the treatment of hypertension, alter tissue levels of copper and zinc.

Hormone Replacement Therapy (HRT)

HRT might affect nutritional status. Some women taking HRT retain salt and water and complain of weight gain. HRT also can affect nutrition if you experience abdominal cramping, loss of appetite, diarrhea, or nausea. These side effects can reduce food and nutrient intake. HRT might also increase the risk of several nutrient deficiencies, including folic acid and vitamin B12. Other estrogen-containing drugs, such as birth control pills, lower blood levels of vitamins B1, B2, and B6, and raise blood levels of vitamin A, iron, and other minerals. However, it is poorly understood whether HRT also affects these nutrients. (See pages 207–8 for more information on HRT.)

Weight Control ("Diet") Pills

Until recently the consensus in the scientific community was that prescription weight control medications, also called "anorexiants," had little or no effect on long-term weight management. In addition, some of these medications, such as phentermine and fenfluramine, have negative side effects, including insomnia, nervousness, and irritability in the case of phentermine, and sedation and depression with fenfluramine. Dizziness, increased blood pressure, diarrhea, and irregular heartbeat also have been reported.

Research at the University of Rochester School of Medicine and Dentistry refuted these findings and stated that the combination of phentermine and fenfluramine—plus behavior modification, calorie restriction, and exercise—resulted in significant weight loss. According to this study, this combined therapy also produced fewer side effects. However, people had difficulty maintaining the weight loss unless they continued to take the weight-loss medications.

Phenylpropanolamine is an over-the-counter appetite suppressant with inconsistent effects on weight loss. Many studies have reported that this drug produced minimal weight loss, and its side effects can be serious. One study reported a slight improvement in weight loss when people combined phenylpropanolamine with a low-calorie diet; however, the drug did not reduce appetite, so it is unclear what effect it had on weight loss.

The combined effects of the drug ephedrine and caffeine might help weight-loss efforts, according to a study conducted at the Harvard Medical School in Boston. The results of this study showed that, unlike food restriction, the ephedrine-caffeine mixture prevented or stopped the development of obesity in genetically predisposed animals by normalizing energy metabolism to resemble that of lean animals.

Dehydroepiandrosterone (DHEA) has shown some anti-obesity effects in animals but also could be dangerous, which resulted in its ban from food supplements by the Food and Drug Administration in 1985. This hormonelike substance might alter the deposition or mobilization of fat from fat tissues and interfere with calorie-induced increases in fat-cell numbers; however, the long-term effects of DHEA use are unknown.

PART THREE

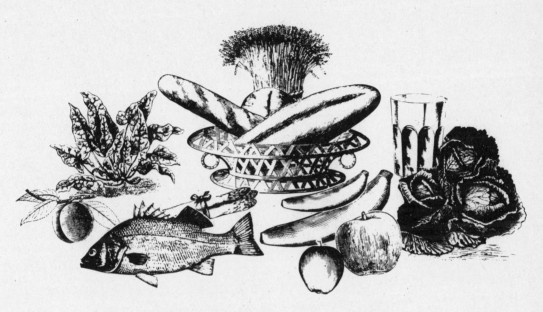

Nutrition and
Women's Health Issues

Introduction

In this century, nutrition research is estimated to double every eighteen months. The emphasis has shifted from mere survival to avoiding clinical nutrient deficiencies. By the middle of this century, clinical nutrient deficiencies such as beriberi and scurvy were rare in the United States; they had been replaced by the revolutionary concept of a "balanced diet." By the 1970s the health consciousness of the nation shifted from treatment to prevention, and research investigated optimal levels of specific nutrients needed to prevent chronic disease and premature aging.

Since the 1970s, the science of nutrition has pushed beyond the prevention and treatment of disease. Nutrition is now recognized as playing a fundamental role in health, aging, intelligence, mental health, and behavior. For example, the emotional roller coaster that sometimes precedes menstruation might result partially from nutrient imbalances, and some forms of depression and insomnia are known to be diet-related.

Nutritional pharmacology has emerged as a new branch of nutrition, and the well-balanced diet has been redefined as one that meets the unique nutrient needs of each woman for the optimal health of both body and mind. Researchers now understand that nutrition strengthens the body's defense systems, including the antioxidant and immune systems, and plays a primary role in fundamental life processes. Nutrition is recognized as the most powerful factor in maximizing your body's health potential throughout life.

Free Radicals, Antioxidants, and Other Liberators

"Free radicals" sounds like the name of a terrorist group, and for your body, they are terrorists. These cellular rebels wage war on health and could be the fundamental cause of numerous diseases, from cancer to heart disease, reduced resistance to colds and infection, and compromised athletic ability.

Free radicals are highly reactive molecules. To stabilize themselves, they seek out and grab onto chemically stable compounds such as fats, proteins, and the genetic material in the body's cells. Unfortunately, this initial attack, while stabilizing the first free radical, damages the cell and generates a new free radical, producing a destructive chain reaction.

Free radicals are unavoidable. These reactive compounds are formed by radiation and herbicides; they are found in air pollution, ozone, and tobacco smoke; and they are consumed in rancid fats. Some environmental pollutants react within the body to form free radicals. Many biological processes generate free radicals in and of themselves, including hormonelike substances called prostaglandins, normal oxygen metabolism, and reactions involving certain metals.

THE OXYGEN PARADOX

Oxygen is the most critical "nutrient" for life. A person can survive for months without adequate vitamins or minerals, weeks without protein or carbohydrate, and days without water, but the human body cannot survive for more than a few moments without oxygen. Oxygen is also the primary source of free radicals. Oxygen fragments—called oxygen free radicals, oxidants, and "singlet" oxygen—are involved in numerous degenerative processes. This type of free radical activity is called oxidative damage.

FREE RADICAL ATTACK

Free radicals react indiscriminately with vulnerable sites on cells. Although the targets are numerous, the most important ones include fats, enzymes, and DNA.

The fatty membranes that surround every cell in the body are the prime targets for free radical attack. The shape and function of the polyunsaturated fats in membranes are changed when a free radical attacks them. The damaged membrane is unable to transport nutrients, oxygen, and water into the cell or regulate the removal of waste products from the cell. Extensive free radical damage causes the membrane to rupture and release cellular components into surrounding tissues, which further damages tissues and generates additional free radicals. In effect, free radical attacks on cell membranes result in damage to the cell, destroy important cell enzymes, and often cause cell mutation and death.

Free radicals also attack the fats floating in the blood. They react with low-density lipoproteins (LDL), the carriers of blood cholesterol associated with an increased risk for atherosclerosis and heart disease. Free radical–damaged LDL-cholesterol lingers longer in the blood and raises LDL-cholesterol levels. In addition, "oxidized" LDL-cholesterol is more damaging than normal LDL-cholesterol, which further increases the risk of developing atherosclerosis and heart disease.

The "powerhouses" of the cell are surrounded by a cell membrane comprised of polyunsaturated fats that are also vulnerable to free radical attack. These powerhouses, called mitochondria, are the site of the cell's energy production. Free radical damage to these centers shuts down energy production and protein synthesis. The cell dies and only a cell remnant, or "clinker," remains in the body. The age of tissues is determined by the number of clinkers present, thus linking free radical damage to premature aging.

Free radicals attack and alter cellular enzymes, the protein-derived catalysts that speed all metabolic processes. The damaged enzyme is inactivated, which slows or halts all processes dependent on that enzyme. Other protein compounds in the body, in addition to enzymes, are also altered by free radical attack. In addition, free radicals activate dormant enzymes that, in turn, cause tissue damage and disease, such as emphysema. Free radicals also release neurotoxins that affect nerve and brain function.

The cell's genetic code is susceptible to free radical damage, causing "breaks" or "tears" in the DNA. DNA regulates cell reproduction and the growth and repair of all body processes. These breaks have important implications in the development of disease because they must be repaired or the cell cannot function properly. At best, the cell dies when the genetic code is so altered that its messages can no longer be read by the cell. Excessive cell death is associated with premature aging. At worst, the cell mutates and begins a line of renegade cells that could be cancerous or at least disease-promoting. The enzymes that repair damaged DNA are not accurate, and there is a high probability that the wrong DNA unit will be incorporated into the repaired DNA strand. This alters the cell's blueprint and increases the risk of abnormal cell growth and cancer.

In summary, free radical damage to the body is implicated in the initiation and progression of numerous diseases, including the following:

1. destruction of the cells that line the blood vessels, which increases the risk of developing atherosclerosis, hypertension, and cardiovascular disease;
2. the inflammatory response observed in rheumatoid arthritis;
3. lung injury, irreversible respiratory damage, and asthma;
4. cancer;
5. eye damage, cataract formation, and vision loss;
6. premature aging;
7. duodenal ulcers and other digestive tract disorders;
8. liver damage;
9. multiple sclerosis; and
10. reduced resistance to infection and disease.

ANTIOXIDANTS: ARMED FORCES AGAINST FREE RADICALS

Fortunately, the body has a complex defense system against free radicals. If it were not for this system, the chain reactions generated from free radical attack might quickly cripple and destroy the body. This defense system is called the body's antioxidant system and includes enzymes, such as superoxide dismutase and xanthine oxidase; vitamins, such as beta carotene, vitamin C, and vitamin E; and minerals, such as selenium, manganese, and zinc. In addition, certain dietary bioflavonoids, some amino acids such as cystine, and a variety of other diet-related compounds might have antioxidant capabilities. (See table on page 243.)

Vitamin E is the first line of defense; it destroys free radicals when they first attack the cells. Optimal vitamin E intake protects against ozone-generated free radicals in smog and protects the tissues from most forms of free radical damage. In contrast, inadequate vitamin E intake increases the risk of disease and might reduce athletic performance because of unchecked free radical damage.

Vitamin C is the primary antioxidant in the body's watery compartments. Vitamin C reduces the risk of developing numerous free radical–associated diseases, from cataracts to cancer. Beta carotene is also a potent antioxidant. In fact, one molecule of beta carotene can wipe out up to one thousand free radicals. Beta carotene is especially effective in preventing free radicals from forming and

A Partial List of Antioxidant-Rich Foods

VITAMIN C	BETA CAROTENE	VITAMIN E	SELENIUM
Asparagus	Apple	Almonds	Chicken without the
Beet greens	Apricots	Avocado	skin
Broccoli	Asparagus	Broccoli	Lean meat
Brussels sprouts	Beet greens	Cottonseed oil	Nonfat milk
Cabbage	Brussels sprouts	Safflower oil (preferably	Organ meats
Cantaloupe	Cantaloupe	cold-pressed)	Seafood
Collard greens	Carrot and carrot juice	Wheat germ and	Vegetables
Grapefruit and grape-	Celery	wheat germ oil	100% whole grain
fruit juice	Collard greens	100% whole grain	cereal
Green peas	Peach	cereal	100% whole wheat
Green pepper	Romaine lettuce	100% whole wheat	bread
Orange and orange	Spinach	bread	
juice	Sweet potato		
Red bell peppers	Winter squash		
Strawberries			
Tomato juice			

BIOFLAVONOIDS

Bioflavonoids also act as antioxidants. These compounds are pigments in fruits and vegetables and are concentrated in the peel, skin, and outer layers of plants or the white core of green peppers. Oranges and other citrus fruits contain approximately 50 to 100 mg of bioflavonoids per 100 grams (3½ ounces) of fruit.

---

strengthens the immune system, which might explain the effectiveness of this nutrient in helping to prevent cancer.

Other antioxidants, such as selenium and the bioflavonoids in citrus fruits, also defend against free radical damage. For example, optimal selenium intake reduces cancer risk and strengthens the immune system, while low dietary intake of selenium results in increased free radical levels in the tissues.

Several antioxidants function as teams to deactivate free radicals. Vitamin E and the enzyme superoxide dismutase intercede at the first stage when free radicals attack polyunsaturated fats and convert them to more free radicals. Any free radicals that escape this attack are recognized by the combined efforts of selenium and the enzyme glutathione peroxidase and are converted back into polyunsaturated fats before they can attack other fat molecules. Some antioxidants, such as vitamin C, protect other antioxidants, such as vitamin E, from premature destruction and therefore strengthen and self-preserve the antioxidant system.

Numerous studies show that elevated intakes or blood levels of antioxidants reduce the risk of free radical damage to tissues and reduce the incidence of disease. For example, optimal dietary intake or supplementation with selenium, vitamin C, and vitamin E improves the antioxidant capabilities of patients with multiple sclerosis. In contrast, low levels of antioxidants are found in diseased organs and tissues and increase a person's risk of developing disease, including cancer, cardiovascular disease, duodenal ulcer, lung disease, and hyperthyroidism. The role of antioxidants in the prevention and treatment of specific diseases will be discussed in detail in the chapters that follow.

Fight Back! Your Immune System

If you seldom get a cold, have never had a serious illness, and bounce back quickly even when you are sick, chances are your body has built up a strong defense system against invading bacteria, viruses, and other hostile microorganisms. You also probably eat a diet composed of nutrient-dense, immune-protective foods. In contrast, the impact of even marginal nutrient deficiencies on the body's fundamental ability to defend itself against infection and disease could have profound and far-reaching effects on health and the quality of life.

The body is under constant attack. Air, water, food, other people, and any aspect of the environment exposes a person to bacteria, viruses, and other microorganisms that either aid in the maintenance of health or are potentially harmful. However, science now recognizes that the body is not as much a victim as an accomplice to disease and infection.

The immune system, a complex system that includes numerous specialized chemicals, cells, tissues, and organs, is the body's fundamental defense against both invasion by foreign substances that cause infection and internal generation of abnormal cell growth, such as cancer. A well-functioning immune system can successfully combat the repeated onslaught of disease-causing microorganisms; a poorly functioning immune system cannot fight off infection and can unleash a variety of diseases from allergies and arthritis to cancer and the common cold.

The Immune System: A Brief Overview

The immune system is composed of millions of cells that pass information back and forth. This complex defense system provides constant feedback on the "state of the body." The result is a sensitive and intricate system of checks and balances that, in the presence of optimal nutrient intake and moderate to low stress, guarantees an immune response that is efficient, quick, and specific.

ORGANS, CELLS, AND CHEMICALS OF THE IMMUNE SYSTEM

Your skin and the mucous linings in the nose and lungs are the body's first lines of defense against routine invasions from bacteria, viruses, and other microorganisms. Within the body, the immune system includes several specific organs strategically located and generally referred to as "lymphoid organs," which include the bone marrow, thymus, lymph nodes, spleen, tonsils, appendix, and clusters of lymphoid tissue in the small intestine (also called Peyer's patches).

The immune system stockpiles an enormous arsenal of weapons and signals for fighting foreign invasion. Specialized white blood cells, called B-cells, are the hub of the immune system outside the body's cells. They circulate in the blood and other body fluids where they neutralize the toxins produced by bacteria. B-cells secrete chemicals called antibodies. In contrast, T-cells are the hub of immune function within the cells. Among other things, T-cells produce chemicals called lymphokines, such as interferon (a protein that defends cells from viruses). Other specialized cells in the immune system include natural killer cells, macrophages, monocytes, and other white blood cells.

NUTRITION AND IMMUNITY

The relationship between nutrition and immunity is cyclical. Inadequate availability of protein or almost any vitamin or mineral jeopardizes optimal immune function, while every infection impinges sooner or later on nutritional status in some manner. Severely malnourished people are at high risk for disease and death primarily because of nutritional deficiencies that impair immune function.

In the past, most studies on humans focused on how protein malnutrition affected immune function. These studies showed unequivocally that all aspects of immune function—including the size, structure, and composition of the immune system's organs, cells, and chemicals—were dramatically and negatively affected by poor nutrition. More recently, the effects of even marginal vitamin and mineral deficiencies on immune function have surfaced. In comparison, optimal intake of protein, vitamins, and minerals, and consumption of a low-fat diet enhance the immune system and reduce the risk of infection and disease.

For example, a person's resistance to disease declines with age. At the same time, nutrient deficiencies often develop that coincide with depressed immune function. When seniors eat better, they score better on immune tests. Many times, however, apparently healthy people actually have impaired immunity. Marginal nutrient deficiencies can depress immune function long before clinical signs of deficiency have developed.

ANTIOXIDANT NUTRIENTS AND IMMUNITY

Almost every vitamin and mineral plays a role in the immune system. However, some nutrients appear to have a more important role than others. The antioxidant nutrients, such as vitamin E, beta carotene, and vitamin C, are especially important in maintaining optimal immune function. For example, the initiation of the immune response probably occurs at the cell membrane. Vitamin E, the primary fat-soluble antioxidant, is an essential component of all cell membranes, including the outer membrane and those that surround the cell's nucleus (which houses the genetic material) and the cell's powerhouse centers called mitochondria. Vitamin E and other antioxidants prevent free radical damage to, and help maintain, the normal structure and function of immune cells and tissues.

Beta carotene is a powerful immune-enhancing nutrient that both affects the activity of immune cells and acts directly to inhibit abnormal cell growth (tumors). For example, optimal dietary intake of beta carotene increases the production and activity of both B-cells and T-cells, macrophages, and natural killer cells, and slows or halts the growth of tumors.

Even marginal dietary intake of vitamin C can have far-reaching effects on a person's resistance to infection and disease. Vitamin C strengthens the immune system by increasing the production and activity of lymphocytes and other white blood cells. This antioxidant vitamin also increases the ability of white blood cells to destroy disease-causing microorganisms, stimulates the speed and aggressiveness of white blood cells, deactivates harmful substances produced when immune cells attack bacteria, and increases the production of interferon. In contrast, white blood cell formation and wound healing are suppressed when vitamin C intake is suboptimal.

Selenium is another antioxidant that strengthens the immune system. Optimal selenium intake increases antibody production, accelerates the production and effectiveness of white blood cells to attack and destroy harmful microorganisms, and strengths the body's surveillance of abnormal cell growth and cancer.

IMMUNITY AND OTHER VITAMINS AND MINERALS

In addition to the antioxidants, other vitamins and minerals also strengthen the body's resistance to infection and disease. These nutrients include the B vitamins—B1, B2, B6, B12, niacin, folic acid, biotin, pantothenic acid; vitamin D; vitamin A; and the minerals copper, iron, and magnesium.

Marginal dietary intake of vitamin B6 reduces resistance to infection and disease, while increased vitamin B6 intake strengthens the immune response. Zinc deficiency is also associated with a poorly functioning immune system. If you are diagnosed with impaired immunity, you probably also have low blood levels of zinc. By increasing your zinc intake, you often can improve your immune response. Vitamin A deficiency, among other things, weakens the mucous linings of the lungs and allows bacteria and viruses to attack more freely.

OTHER DIETARY FACTORS AND IMMUNITY

An increasingly large number of dietary factors, other than vitamins, minerals, and protein, alters immunity. Many of these dietary factors do not correct or prevent a nutrient deficiency but rather produce what is called a "pharmacological" effect; that is, they function more like a natural druglike substance than a nutrient.

For example, the nonessential amino acid arginine might enhance immune function in patients recovering from burns, injury, or surgery. Garlic also contains compounds, including allicin, the substance responsible for garlic's smell, that inhibit the growth of or kill two dozen kinds of bacteria and at least sixty types of fungi and yeast. Garlic extracts also enhance immune function and strengthen the body's defense against cancer.

A low-fat diet stimulates the immune system, while a high-fat diet increases the susceptibility to infection and disease. Interestingly, the type of fat also influences immune function. For example, polyunsaturated fats in vegetable oils (linoleic acid), evening primrose oil or borage oil (gamma linolenic acid or GLA), and fish oils (eicosapentaenoic acid or EPA) might suppress immunity when consumed in large amounts. Other aspects of a healthful life-style, such as maintaining desirable weight, moderate exercise, and effective stress management, also improve resistance to infection and disease.

DISPELLING THE MYTH: MORE IS BETTER

While moderate doses of some nutrients stimulate the body's defense system, larger doses might impair the immune response. Several studies on vitamin C, zinc, and copper reported that these nutrients consumed in excessive amounts might suppress certain aspects of immunity. For example, in one study, 2 grams of vitamin C taken daily impaired the immune system's ability to kill bacteria. Immune function returned to normal within four weeks of discontinuing the megadose therapy.

The mechanisms for this possible immune-suppressive effect are unknown; however, one researcher speculated that high blood levels of vitamin C might stimulate the stress hormones (the corticosteroids), which in turn suppress immunity. Supplemental doses of zinc that exceed Recommended Dietary Allowance levels (15 mg) by ten- to twentyfold also might reduce immunity and increase a person's risk of disease.

Apparently the body might have a feedback system whereby up to optimal intakes of vitamin C and zinc progressively strengthen the immune system, while too much of these nutrients consumed over long periods of time might suppress it.

HOW MUCH IS ENOUGH?

The optimal range of nutrient intakes to maximize the body's defense system is unknown. The Food and Nutrition Board did not consider the effects of specific vitamins and minerals when it established the Recommended Dietary Allowances (RDAs). In most cases consuming RDA levels of a nutrient is sufficient to strengthen immunity. In some cases, however, immune function progressively improves with increasing amounts of a nutrient, even to amounts far in excess of RDA values. Until more is known about vitamin and mineral tolerances and the effects of these nutrients on immunity, it is best to stay within the safe zone and limit dietary intake of most nutrients to within 300 percent of the RDAs.

At this time there are no inexpensive, accurate, or accessible tests that determine a person's unique nutritional status. Traditionally, poor nutrition was assessed by overt clinical symptoms, such as a low value on a hematocrit test (indicator of advanced iron deficiency). These measures are crude and incomplete. More important, immunity can be strikingly affected by even marginal nutrient status long before clinical deficiency symptoms are detected. Since even marginal nutrient deficiencies uniformly depress specific aspects of the immune system, it is

---

Dietary Guidelines for Maintaining a Strong Immune System

1. Limit fat to no more than 30 percent of total calories.

2. Consume 3 to 5 servings daily of protein-rich foods such as cooked dried beans and peas, fish, nonfat or low-fat dairy products, chicken without the skin, or extra-lean meat. (A serving is ½ cup beans; 1 cup nonfat milk; or 2 ounces meat, fish, or poultry.)

3. Consume 5 or more servings daily of fresh fruits and vegetables. At least 2 servings should be a dark green vegetable, such as broccoli, spinach, or Romaine lettuce, and/or dark orange vegetables, such as carrots and winter squash. At least 2 servings should be a food high in vitamin C, such as citrus fruits and green peppers. Several times a week consume cruciferous vegetables, such as cabbage, asparagus, cauliflower, broccoli, or Brussels sprouts. Select only the freshest produce, and eat one-third to one-half of your selections raw (that is, in salads or as crunchy snacks).

4. Consume 6 or more servings of whole grain breads and cereals and starchy vegetables. Add wheat germ to hot cereals, peanut butter, or other foods whenever possible. (One serving is a slice of bread, ½ cup cooked pasta or rice, or 1 medium baked potato.)

5. Use garlic in cooking whenever possible. (See chapter 2 for more information on menu planning and meal preparation.)

---

likely that immune function tests will someday serve as indicators of nutritional status and disease susceptibility. (See table above.)

The Good News

Granted, more is unknown than is known about how vitamins, minerals, and other nutrients affect health and disease processes or how they interact in the body. The good news is that what is known about nutrition repeatedly shows that what you eat can have a strong and far-reaching effect on your health today and your susceptibility to disease and premature aging in the future.

An optimal diet such as the Healthy Woman's Diet, not just an adequate one, can counteract many of the processes once thought to be the inevitable consequence of aging. Even a minor nuisance such as the common cold or flu may be prevented, or at least the severity reduced, with proper diet. As nutrition grows beyond the "balanced diet" and into the realm of nutritional pharmacology, you can make informed decisions about what to eat and how to supplement to maximize your body's health potential.

WHERE DO I TURN FOR ACCURATE NUTRITION INFORMATION?

A registered dietitian (R.D.) is one who has been trained in nutrition science. An R.D. who has kept abreast of the current research or who has a Ph.D. from an accredited university is the best source of accurate and up-to-date nutrition information. A medical doctor (M.D.) may have selected nutrition as a specialty, but for the most part an M.D. has minimal training in nutrition.

Other individuals who have professional training in nutrition may call themselves "nutritionists," but there are no legal definitions or standards of education and experience for these people. The accuracy of their information can therefore range from excellent to very poor.

Among the groups you can contact in your community are the Dietetic Association, the American Society for Clinical Nutrition (Bethesda, Maryland), the American College of Nutrition (Wilmington, North Carolina), the American Heart Association (your local chapter), and the American Diabetic Association (local chapters or the national office in Chicago, Illinois). They can provide information or refer you to other qualified sources. Your city, county, or state health departments or state extension services often have R.D.s on staff; however, you should always interview them about how well they keep up with current research. Government agencies that provide accurate nutrition information include the U.S. Department of Agriculture and the U.S. Department of Health and Human Services.

There are no absolute rules for accurate information because the science of nutrition is growing so rapidly. Always consult several sources before making a personal decision regarding nutrition, and make sure one of those sources is professionally trained and is well versed in the current research.

Acquired Immunodeficiency Syndrome (AIDS)

AIDS is a progressive disease associated with suppressed immune function and a high incidence of a cancer called Karposi's sarcoma. People do not die from

AIDS but from secondary infections or diseases related to compromised immunity.

Nutrition and AIDS

The mechanisms of malnutrition in the development and progression of AIDS are poorly understood. It has been theorized that people with compromised immunity, such as occurs with marginal intake of many vitamins and minerals, are more susceptible to contracting the AIDS virus and progressing to advanced stages in the infection. Nutritional status progressively deteriorates in patients with human immunodeficiency virus (HIV) infection, which results in weight loss, tissue wasting (associated with protein-calorie malnutrition), and reduced immune function.

Clinical nutrient deficiencies also develop as the disease progresses. These conditions develop as a result of limited food intake, increased nutrient requirements, and reduced absorption of nutrients. Malnutrition, in turn, interferes with the recovery from secondary illness or encourages the progression of AIDS disease primarily by suppressing the immune response and altering other essential body defenses.

ANTIOXIDANTS

HIV infection is the early stage in a process that can progress to a symptomatic later stage known as AIDS. Although the factors that encourage replication of the virus, therefore determining the length of the latency period, are poorly understood, Dr. David H. Baker at the University of Illinois reported that HIV activity was affected by the concentration of antioxidants. In particular, vitamin C and glutathione (an antioxidant produced in the body or consumed in foods such as spinach and parsley and supplements) inhibited the growth of HIV. Laboratory studies supported global reports of glutathione deficiency in nonsymptomatic HIV-positive people, which might reflect an association between the antioxidant levels in cells and the latency period of HIV infection.

Limited evidence supports Dr. Baker's associations between antioxidants and AIDS. For example, measurements of selenium status in AIDS patients show that blood selenium levels are low and are correlated with other symptoms of malnutrition, impaired immunity, and overall poor health. Another study showed that beta carotene supplements improved immunity in AIDS patients. Since HIV is associated with a progressive decline in immune function, the immune-stimulating effects of beta carotene could have a profound influence on progression of the disease.

B VITAMINS

B vitamin deficiencies are common in AIDS patients but as yet show no implications in the development of AIDS; however, deficiencies might explain some symptoms of AIDS-related nerve dysfunction. As many as one in every five AIDS patients tested are vitamin B12 deficient and often show numbness, tingling in the toes and hands, and other disorders of the spinal cord. Patients treated with vitamin B12 often showed improvements in these symptoms within days of beginning supplements. Unfortunately, the evidence is not clear, and other studies have reported no differences between vitamin B12 intake of AIDS patients and healthy controls.

Folic acid status is also poor in many AIDS patients, which might be the result of poor dietary intake or the use of medications that interfere with folic acid use in the body. Finally, one study from the Hospital Saint-Luc in Montreal reported that vitamin B1 deficiency was relatively common in AIDS patients and might be responsible for some of the neurological changes associated with advanced stages of this condition.

ZINC

Zinc deficiency might aggravate the symptoms of AIDS and speed the progress of the disease. Zinc plays an important role in the immune system and the maintenance of the body's natural defense against viral infection, and optimal zinc status might help prevent or correct immune disorders associated with HIV infection.

FISH OILS

Researchers at the Efamol Research Institute in Kentville, Nova Scotia, speculated that relative deficiencies of certain fats, in particular fish oils and gamma linolenic acid (GLA), might contribute to the development of AIDS. The researchers proposed that fish oils and GLA acted as antiviral agents that prevented the spread of infection and destroyed the virus, which would be an effective defense in both the prevention and treatment of AIDS. However, these associations are purely speculative, and more research is needed before dietary or supplemental recommendations can be made.

Putting It All Together: Dietary Recommendations

Until more is known about how nutrition affects the development and progression of AIDS, it is wise to consume optimal amounts of the nutrients known to strengthen immune function, including the antioxidant nutrients, B vitamins, trace elements such as selenium and zinc, vitamin A, and glutathione.

In addition, consume a low-fat, nutrient-dense diet as outlined in chapter 1 to ensure optimal dietary intake of all nutrients and food components (such as indoles in some vegetables that help prevent cancer). Make sure to consume frequent servings of dark green leafy vegetables, such as spinach and parsley. In addition, calorie intake should be adequate to maintain a desirable body weight.

Researchers at the New York University Medical Center state that nutrition supplementation is necessary for people at risk for developing AIDS. Because of the high mortality rate of patients with AIDS and the lack of a clearly defined treatment, any therapy that shows a potential effectiveness should be considered.

The immune-suppressive state associated with AIDS is believed to be preceded by malnutrition, which increases susceptibility to the AIDS virus. Nutritional supplementation with calories, protein, vitamins, and minerals might improve immune resistance to infection in people with or at risk for AIDS, especially those people who are asymptomatic.

Finally, and most important, practicing safe sex helps reduce the risk for contracting the HIV virus and developing AIDS. This disease is irreversible and its primary transmission is through sexual conduct (also, blood transfusion and drug injections). Anyone is a candidate, regardless of age, gender, life-style, income, or race. Therefore, potential sexual partners should have an AIDS test prior to sexual contact and verify that they have had no other sexual contact since that test. Some evidence shows that the test should follow a six-month period of abstinence to ensure an accurate reading. A condom plus spermicidal jelly or cream also should be used.

A healthful life-style for the prevention of AIDS includes regular exercise, effective stress management, frequent periods of relaxation, avoidance of alcohol and tobacco, and a strong social support system.

Anemia

Anemia is the most common disorder of the blood. It is characterized by a deficiency in the size or number of red blood cells or the amount of hemoglobin (the oxygen-carrying protein) they contain. Since the body's oxygen supply is dependent on red blood cells, anything that limits their number or size also limits the body's capacity to transport oxygen and carbon dioxide. The tissues are consequently "starved" for oxygen. Without oxygen they cannot "breathe" or use energy.

A woman who is anemic might experience one or more of the following symptoms: lethargy; apathy; weakness; poor concentration and reduced alertness; out of breath after minor exertion, such as walking up a flight of stairs; increased susceptibility to colds, flu, and infection; loss of appetite or craving for nonfood items such as ice; headaches; clumsiness; irritability; pale or sallow complexion; reduced work or athletic performance; poor body temperature regulation (complains of being cold); thin or flat fingernails; and stomach disorders.

All symptoms of anemia are related to the reduced oxygen-carrying capacity of the blood. Many of these symptoms are subtle but become more pronounced during times of stress (for example, during a 10K race or while vacationing at high altitudes).

Anemia can result from numerous conditions, including blood loss, infection and inflammation, and kidney disease. However, by far the most common causes are related to diet. Nutritional anemia results from an inadequate supply of iron, protein, B vitamins (B12, B6, and folic acid), vitamin C, vitamin E, and/or copper. The deficiency develops because of inadequate dietary intake, poor absorption, faulty use of the nutrient within the body, or increased nutrient requirements, such as in pregnancy or during periods of rapid growth.

Nutrition and Anemia

IRON

Iron deficiency is the most common cause of anemia, and iron deficiency anemia is the most common form of malnutrition in women. Why is one of the earth's most abundant minerals also the most likely cause of nutritional deficiency? The answer is high requirements, poor intake, and limited absorption.

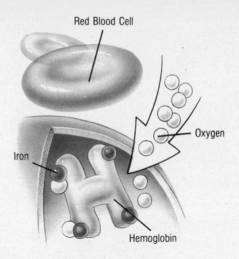

Red Blood Cell

Oxygen

Iron

Hemoglobin

The Red Blood Cell

Within each red blood cell are protein molecules called hemoglobin. Embedded in each hemoglobin are four iron particles that give the red blood cells their ability to transport oxygen. Iron binds to oxygen in the lungs; it carries and then releases that oxygen to the tissues. In addition, iron is the functional component of a hemoglobinlike molecule within the muscle cells called myoglobin. Iron is responsible for storing and transporting oxygen within the cells of the heart and working muscles. Inadequate availability of iron results in reduced production of red blood cells and myoglobin. The red blood cells that do form are small, with less hemoglobin and a reduced oxygen-carrying capacity. (See figure above.)

Anemia is the final stage of iron deficiency. Long before the reduction in red blood cells, the tissue stores of iron have been drained, enzymes dependent on iron have been affected, and immune functions requiring iron have been suppressed. Although a patient might feel weak or apathetic, common tests, such as the hemoglobin and hematocrit blood tests, will show no evidence of anemia.

The serum ferritin and total iron binding capacity (TIBC) tests are the best and most sensitive indicators of iron deficiency. In addition, iron levels vary from day to day, so the average values from multiple tests provide the most reliable information on iron status. (See the following sections for more information on marginal iron deficiency: Common Cold, Fatigue, Headaches, Mood and Emotions, Skin, and Stress.) (See table on page 256.)

Tests for Iron Deficiency and Iron-Deficiency Anemia

PLASMA FERRITIN:

Normal values, 40 to 160 mcg per liter
Iron depletion, 20 mcg per liter
Iron-deficiency anemia, less than 12 mcg per liter

IRON BINDING CAPACITY (TIBC):

Normal values, 300 to 360 mcg per deciliter
Iron depletion, 360 mcg per deciliter
Iron-deficiency anemia, 410 mcg per deciliter

TRANSFERRIN SATURATION:

Normal value, 20% to 50%
Iron depletion, 30%
Iron-deficiency anemia, less than 10%

HEMOGLOBIN:

Normal value, 12 to 16 grams per deciliter
Iron-deficiency anemia, less than 12 grams per deciliter

HEMATOCRIT:

Normal value, 37% to 47%
Iron-deficiency anemia, less than 37%

The body recycles iron. When red blood cells die, the iron is reused to make new cells. Consequently, iron requirements are minimal (10 mg per day) for healthy men and postmenopausal women. However, menstrual blood loss places a monthly drain on iron in premenopausal women. In fact, menstrual blood loss is a better indicator of a woman's iron need than dietary iron intake. Women with heavy menstrual bleeding lose more iron and have higher iron requirements than women with light menstrual flow. Unfortunately, women with heavy menstrual bleeding (called menorrhagia) usually are unaware that their blood loss is unusual. Consequently, iron depletion can progress undetected for months or years until a routine blood test uncovers anemia.

Women's Recommended Dietary Allowance for iron is based on a 1966 study by Dr. L. Hallberg of menstrual iron losses in women. However, this study was conducted prior to the popular use of the intrauterine device (IUD). In 1991, Dr. Hallberg reported that because the IUD substantially increases blood loss during menstruation, a woman's iron need is increased by as much as fourfold. In contrast, women on the birth control pill might have lower iron requirements since this form of birth control often reduces menstrual flow. (See chapter 8 for more information on iron needs during pregnancy.)

The RDA for iron varies between 15 mg and 18 mg for nonpregnant women. However, to maintain optimal iron stores Dr. Hallberg recommends a daily intake of at least 19 mg for adult women and 22 mg for menstruating teenagers. Women using the IUD or with heavy menstrual flow require even greater daily intakes. Considering that a well-balanced diet provides approximately 6 mg of iron for every 1,000 calories, a woman must consume at least 2,500 to 3,000 calories to meet even minimal RDA levels. It is not surprising, therefore, that many major national nutrition surveys report that 90 percent of women do not consume enough iron.

In addition, dietary iron is poorly absorbed. The iron in meats (called "heme" iron) is best absorbed, with from 20 percent to 34 percent of dietary intake actually entering the bloodstream. Iron in plants, such as grains, vegetables, and cooked dried beans and peas, is called nonheme or inorganic iron. Only 2 percent to 5 percent of this type of iron is absorbed. The average iron absorption from a mixed diet containing heme and nonheme iron is estimated at only 10 percent of total intake.

Consuming a vitamin C–rich food (such as orange juice) with an iron-rich food (such as whole grain cereal) increases the percentage of iron absorbed. In addition, combining a small amount of heme-iron (lean red meat) with a large amount of nonheme iron (cooked dried beans and peas), such as chili with meat and beans, also improves iron absorption.

Iron absorption is susceptible to many other dietary factors. It is reduced by calcium supplements, oxalates in spinach, and phytates in unleavened whole grain breads, such as whole wheat tortillas or muffins. Compounds called "tannins" in tea and coffee can reduce iron absorption by as much as 90 percent. Some researchers recommend that tea and coffee be consumed between rather than with meals to maximize iron retention. Fortunately, vitamin C consumed with many of these dietary substances, including coffee, tea, and phytates, helps counteract their negative effects on iron absorption. (See table on page 258)

SELENIUM

Although not directly related to anemia, poor dietary intake of selenium might aggravate a preexisting risk of developing anemia. Blood levels of selenium are low in anemic animals, while increasing selenium intake sometimes corrects the condition. Selenium, a component of the antioxidant enzyme glutathione peroxidase, protects red blood cells from free radical damage and destruction.

The Iron Content of Selected Foods

FOOD	QUANTITY	TOTAL IRON (MG)	HEME IRON (MG)	NONHEME IRON (MG)
Meatless spaghetti sauce (cooked in cast-iron skillet)	6 ounces	11.5	—	11.5
Applesauce (homemade in cast-iron skillet)	½ cup	9.8	—	9.8
Apricots, dried	½ cup	3.6	—	3.6
Molasses, blackstrap	1 tablespoon	3.2	—	3.2
Beef, lean	3 ounces	2.7	1.1	1.6
Beans, cooked	½ cup	2.6	—	2.6
Raisins	½ cup	2.6	—	2.6
Prune juice	¼ cup	2.6	—	2.6
Lima beans	½ cup	2.4	—	2.4
Chicken, meat only	3½ ounces	1.5	.8	.7
Green peas	½ cup	1.5	—	1.5
Meatless spaghetti sauce (cooked in noniron skillet)	6 ounces	1.4	—	1.4
Cookies, molasses	2 medium	1.4	—	1.4
Greens, mustard	½ cup	1.3	—	1.3
Tuna, water-packed	2 ounces	1.2	.4	.8
Strawberries	¾ cup	1.1	—	1.1
Tomato juice	½ cup	1.1	—	1.1
Brussels sprouts	½ cup	0.9	—	.9
Broccoli	⅔ cup	.9	—	.8
Bread, whole wheat	1 slice	.8	—	.8
Peanut butter	2 tablespoons	.6	—	.6
Applesauce	½ cup	.4	—	.4

VITAMIN B12

Inadequate intake or poor absorption of vitamin B12 results in a form of anemia called macrocytic (large cell) or megaloblastic anemia. As compared to the small, pale red blood cells noted in iron-deficiency anemia, the cells are large, fragile, and reduced in numbers. Despite these microscopic differences, the symptoms in both forms of anemia are the same and include lethargy, weakness, and poor concentration. In addition, iron deficiency may accompany vitamin B12 deficiency and mask the underlying secondary anemia.

A vitamin B12 deficiency is the result of either inadequate dietary intake or poor absorption. Vitamin B12 is found only in foods of animal origin, such as meat, chicken, fish, and milk products, or fermented foods such as miso. The amount required to maintain health is very small, only 2 mcg a day; therefore, even small amounts of lean meat or fish (such as 3 ounces of tuna or 2 cups of milk or yogurt) provide more than enough vitamin B12. People who avoid all these foods, such as strict vegetarians, could develop vitamin B12 deficiency and its associated anemia unless fortified soy milk or vitamin supplements are included in their daily diet. Low blood levels of vitamin B12, however, are found in nonvegetarians and people of all ages.

Poor absorption, not dietary intake, is usually the cause of vitamin B12–related anemia, in which case the condition is called pernicious anemia. Vitamin B12 requires a substance in digestive juices called "intrinsic factor." Reduced production of intrinsic factor results in poor vitamin B12 absorption and deficiency, resulting in pernicious anemia.

Vitamin B12 is also affected by other nutrients in the diet. For example, a vitamin E deficiency limits the usefulness of vitamin B12 in the body. Absorption of vitamin B12 is affected by the levels of vitamin B6, calcium, and iron in the body. The effects of megadose vitamin C on vitamin B12 absorption are contradictory; some studies show large doses of supplemental vitamin C reduce the vitamin B12 content of foods, while other studies show no effect. The Food and Drug Administration limits the amount of folic acid allowed in supplements because a high dietary intake of folic acid masks vitamin B12 anemia.

FOLIC ACID

Folic acid is essential for the normal development and maintenance of all body cells. Consequently, folic acid deficiency produces a macrocytic anemia similar to a vitamin B12 deficiency. The most common causes of folic acid–induced anemia are poor dietary habits; reduced absorption; prolonged use of folic acid–competing medications such as anticonvulsants, aspirin, and birth control pills; and/or increased requirements during growth periods such as pregnancy. (See chapter 12 for more information on how medications affect folic acid status and chapter 8 for information on folic acid before and during pregnancy.)

The body maintains limited tissue stores of folic acid, so a deficiency, characterized first by low blood levels and then by anemia, can develop within months. It is important to diagnose this form of anemia properly. Supplementing with folic acid would correct the anemia but would not correct a possible concurrent vitamin B12 deficiency, which would continue and cause progressive nerve damage.

Poor dietary intake of folic acid is common. Surveys show that many women eat only limited amounts of folic acid–rich foods, consuming only half the recommended daily amounts of this B vitamin. Processing removes as much as 68 percent of the folic acid in foods, while overcooking further reduces its availability. The most recent Recommended Dietary Allowances for folic acid have been significantly reduced from 400 mcg per day to only 180 mcg per day for nonpregnant women. This reduction is based on typical rather than optimal dietary intakes and has met with considerable controversy in the scientific community. The previous RDAs of 400 mcg have been used as a baseline for making dietary recommendations in this book.

VITAMIN E

Several hereditary diseases including sickle cell anemia are characterized by destruction of red blood cells, called hemolytic anemia. An important function of vitamin E is to protect cell membranes from destruction by free radicals. Low blood levels of vitamin E, suggesting increased susceptibility to free radical damage, often accompany these diseases. In many cases, treating patients with supplemental vitamin E produces promising results. In addition, vitamin E supplementation might be an effective treatment for hemolytic anemia in kidney patients undergoing hemodialysis.

Interestingly, high iron intake for the treatment of iron-deficiency anemia and/or substituting vegetable oils for saturated fats might increase free radical damage and place increased demands on the body's vitamin E needs. Iron in large quantities can produce free radicals, while the polyunsaturated fats are the primary targets and generators of free radicals. Therefore, a diet or supplemental program that is high in either polyunsaturated fats (such as vegetable oils) or iron increases the daily requirement for vitamin E.

Other Nutrients and Anemia

Other nutrients, including vitamin B6, vitamin C, copper, and protein, are important in the formation of hemoglobin and red blood cells. A deficiency of one or more of these nutrients and other nutrients, such as biotin, molybdenum, and zinc, could result in anemia.

A vitamin B6 deficiency results in an anemia that resembles iron deficiency. Iron levels in the blood are normal, but hemoglobin and red blood cells are not formed properly in the absence of optimal vitamin B6 intake. After treatment under a physician's supervision that usually includes therapeutic doses of 50 mg to 200 mg of vitamin B6 daily, symptoms subside within a few weeks.

Vitamin C is necessary for the proper absorption and metabolic function of iron. One of the symptoms of vitamin C deficiency is anemia related to the vitamin's role in iron metabolism.

Anemia was the first identified symptom of a copper deficiency. Results of animal studies in the 1930s showed that anemia associated with excess milk consumption responded to iron supplementation only after the animals had first received copper supplements. Copper stimulates hemoglobin synthesis, while poor copper intake results in impaired red blood cell formation even in the presence of adequate iron stores. In addition, copper releases iron from storage and increases intestinal absorption of iron when the two minerals are consumed in moderate amounts.

Recommended intakes for copper are 1.5 mg to 3 mg per day. The average daily amount of copper reported in one study was only .8 mg. Thus, some women may be consuming below recommended levels of this mineral. Despite potentially low dietary intake, symptoms of copper deficiency in healthy adults are rare.

Protein is essential for the normal formation of hemoglobin and red blood cells. However, protein deficiency seldom occurs alone. In most cases a diet inadequate in protein is also suboptimal in many nutrients, including iron, vitamin B12, and vitamin B6.

Protein deficiency is rare in the United States because consumption is often two to three times the recommended daily amounts. Protein deficiency does occur, however, in elderly women who do not eat properly (the "tea and toast" syndrome) or who suffer from long-standing illnesses that interfere with optimal dietary intake.

Putting It All Together: Dietary Guidelines

A nutritious diet containing at least 2,500 calories of nutrient-dense foods will help ensure optimal intake of most nutrients related to anemia. Multiple nutrient deficiencies often contribute to the development of anemia, and it should never be assumed that only iron is needed until a thorough investigation of dietary intake is conducted. (See chapters 1 and 2 for a detailed description of the Healthy Woman's Diet.)

The primary treatment for diagnosed iron-deficiency anemia is iron supplementation, usually combined with increased vitamin C. The best absorbed forms of iron are ferrous succinate and ferrous sulfate. Other iron compounds that are absorbed well include ferrous lactate, fumarate, glycine sulfate, glutamate, and gluconate. Iron is best absorbed on an empty stomach; however, large supplemental doses of iron can cause digestive tract upset, diarrhea, or constipation. These symptoms might be relieved by beginning supplementation with a small dose and increasing it over several days or weeks.

Although time-release supplements reduce stomach upset, they might not be absorbed as well as traditional forms of iron. The optimal dose depends on the severity of the anemia and other compounding factors and should always be determined after proper diagnostic tests and consultation with a physician. Iron supplementation usually produces improvements within one to three weeks but should be continued for six to twelve months to ensure that tissue iron levels are restored.

In addition to iron supplements, the nutrient content of the diet should be carefully reviewed. Several servings daily of iron-rich foods should be included in the diet, preferably combining lean meats and vitamin C–rich foods with iron-rich plants. Women who consume less than 2,500 calories daily, especially those using the IUD or who experience heavy menstrual flow, are likely candidates for iron depletion and deficiency and might consider low-dose supplementation (18 mg of iron daily) as nutritional insurance.

One of the best sources of dietary iron is cooking in cast-iron skillets. Replacing coated or glass cookware with cast iron can increase the iron content of a meal by as much as twenty-six-fold. Acidic foods, such as spaghetti sauce, chili with meat and beans, and beef-vegetable stew, are especially good at leaching the iron out of the pot and into the food. In addition, the longer the food simmers, the higher its iron content. In contrast, the iron in fortified foods, such as ready-to-eat cereals and "enriched" bread, is poorly absorbed.

Pernicious anemia is treated by vitamin B12 injections (administered by a physician), which bypass the intestinal failure to absorb it. Macrocytic or megaloblastic anemia associated with poor dietary intake of either vitamin B12 or folic acid is treated with improved diet and oral supplements. Symptoms may improve before changes are noted in the blood.

Several servings of vitamin B12 and folic acid–rich foods should be included daily in the diet. Two to three servings daily of protein-rich foods from animal sources will supply ample amounts of vitamin B12. Folic acid is found primarily in dark green leafy vegetables (foliage), orange juice, and wheat germ. This B vitamin is destroyed by heat, prolonged storage, and reheating of leftovers. A folic acid–rich food that is stored in the refrigerator for three or four days, is overcooked or reheated, or is allowed to sit on a serving table for long periods of time contains little or no folic acid by the time it is eaten.

Fruits and vegetables should be chosen fresh, stored for limited amounts of time, eaten raw or only slightly cooked, and prepared in a minimum amount of water. Minimally processed foods should be selected to ensure optimal dietary intake of vitamin E, the trace minerals such as copper, and vitamin B6.

PRECAUTIONS

Concerns about iron overload (also called "hemochromatosis") in women appear to be unfounded. This rare condition is most likely to occur in men after age fifty. There is no strong evidence of an increase in this condition corresponding to iron fortification of food or moderate iron supplementation.

Large supplemental doses of iron for prolonged periods of time could result in secondary deficiencies of other trace minerals such as zinc or copper. To help avoid this potential interaction, iron supplements should be taken alone and/or zinc and copper intake should be increased slightly, either by increased consumption of foods high in these nutrients or by low- to moderate-dose supplementation taken at opposite times from the iron supplement.

Arthritis

The most common forms of arthritis are rheumatoid arthritis, osteoarthritis, and gout. Rheumatoid arthritis is the most serious because it is the most crippling of the three. Inflammation and thickening of the lining and tissues surrounding the joints damage the bones, causing deformity and disability. Although the cause is poorly understood, some scientists believe that rheumatoid arthritis is linked to disruption of the body's immune system and/or free radical damage to the tissues surrounding joints. (See pages 240–44 for more information on free radicals and antioxidants.)

Osteoarthritis is the "wear and tear" disease associated with degeneration of the cartilage. Long-term irritation of the joints caused by overweight, poor posture, injury, or strain is the primary contributor to this form of arthritis. Women are more affected than men, and older women are more prone to osteoarthritis than younger women.

Gout, the easiest form of arthritis to diagnose and treat, is most common in men. In gout, one of the body's waste products, called uric acid, accumulates and forms crystals that lodge in areas of the body, such as the joints, where the blood supply is slow or insufficient to remove the uric acid crystals.

Nutrition and Arthritis

No diet or nutrient is known to prevent or cure rheumatoid arthritis. However, several dietary habits contribute to a person's optimal health and possibly reduction of some symptoms.

People with rheumatoid arthritis often eat suboptimal diets, have low blood levels of several vitamins and minerals, and are overweight. Because they often consume suboptimal amounts of complex carbohydrate–rich foods and nonfat dairy foods, their poor nutrition aggravates disease symptoms.

For example, pain and stiffness increase when a person is malnourished. Rheumatoid arthritis is an inflammatory disease that increases nutrient needs but at the same time alters the intestinal lining, which interferes with the absorption of nutrients. The disease and some medications used in its treatment cause peptic ulcers and gastritis, which further reduce digestion and a person's desire to eat.

Deficiencies of folic acid, vitamin D, vitamin B6, copper, iron, and zinc are frequently found in people with rheumatoid arthritis. Symptoms often improve when patients increase their intake of one or more of these nutrients. Preliminary reports also show improvement when patients consume vitamin A, selenium-rich yeast, vitamin E, and calcium. Although altered levels of vitamins and minerals could be a result rather than a cause of the disease, maintaining optimal nutrition provides the immune system with tools to fend off infection and disease.

In addition, nutrition counteracts the adverse effects of medication. Steroids used in the treatment of rheumatoid arthritis can cause bone loss. Daily supplementation with calcium and vitamin D help prevent this loss. Anti-inflammatory medications and aspirin increase vitamin C excretion and can result in bruising, while adequate intake of this vitamin prevents these symptoms.

IRON

Researchers at the London Hospital Medical College theorize that high iron intake might worsen the joint inflammation associated with rheumatoid arthritis. Excessive iron intake might encourage free radical damage to joint tissues, encouraging persistent and locally destructive inflammatory processes. Moderate to low iron intake might suppress joint inflammation and improve symptoms.

ANTIOXIDANTS

Antioxidant nutrients are often low in the diets of rheumatoid arthritis patients. Since free radical damage to the immune system and to the joint tissues is thought to contribute to rheumatoid arthritis, optimal intake of antioxidant nutrients might help counteract this tissue damage.

Several studies report improvement in symptoms when antioxidant nutrient intake is increased. For example, blood levels of selenium are low in rheumatoid arthritis patients, while the severity of the disease increases as selenium levels decrease. Pain and morning stiffness improve with increased intake of selenium and vitamin E. Researchers speculate that antioxidant nutrients deactivate the free radicals called peroxides that might encourage inflammatory processes, while strengthening the body's immune system.

Vitamin C helps reduce the inflammation of rheumatoid arthritis and might lessen the pain associated with osteoarthritis. Low dietary intake of vitamin C promotes the development of osteoarthritis in experimental animals and inhibits inflammation in rheumatoid arthritis. Treatment of osteoarthritis with vitamin C might help slow the deterioration of cartilage, resulting in less pain and likelihood of surgical intervention.

DIETARY FATS

Two families of hormone-like substances called prostaglandins and leukotrienes are related to both suppression and escalation of inflammatory processes in rheumatoid arthritis. Dietary fats are building blocks for these compounds. For example, vegetable oils encourage inflammation by serving as building blocks for harmful prostaglandins and leukotrienes. In contrast, fish oils (also called the omega-3 fatty acids) are building blocks for other prostaglandins and leukotrienes that inhibit inflammation.

Repeatedly, fish oils from either dietary sources or capsules have reduced the pain, stiffness, and swelling of rheumatoid arthritis by reducing levels of harmful hormone-like substances, altering inflammatory processes, and strengthening the immune response. In addition, anti-inflammatory medication dosage is sometimes reduced when patients increase their consumption of fish oils. The effectiveness of fish oils is greatest when vegetable oil consumption is low. One study reported, however, that long-term supplementation with fish oils might increase the risk of developing osteoarthritis.

A VEGETARIAN DIET

Rheumatoid arthritis symptoms improve when people fast, which strongly suggests a diet-induced component to the disease. In addition, some people are hypersensitive to milk products and have fewer arthritis symptoms when these foods are removed from the diet.

Researchers at the University of Oslo in Norway placed patients on a fast followed by a vegetarian diet, while another group (the control group) fasted and then returned to normal dietary intakes. Within four weeks, the vegetarians showed significant improvements in the number of tender and swollen joints, pain, duration of morning stiffness, grip strength, and immune function, while the control group showed no improvements other than slightly less pain.

Putting It All Together: Dietary Recommendations

The various forms of arthritis have different causes and symptoms, and require different types of treatment. In addition, any form of arthritis can vary from person to person, and thus treatment must be tailored to the individual.

Some rheumatoid arthritis symptoms might be the result of food intolerances, allergies, or problems with digestion or absorption of foods. An elimination diet may be effective but must be carefully monitored by a physician and/or a dietitian. With this diet, suspected aggravating foods (such as wheat or milk products, black walnuts, alfalfa, and nitrite-containing foods) are eliminated from the diet and gradually added back one at a time to monitor adverse reactions. (See pages 329–33 for more information on food intolerances.)

Osteoarthritis and gout frequently occur in overweight people. Maintaining a desirable weight throughout life helps prevent these two forms of arthritis, while losing weight lowers the blood uric acid level in gout patients and helps in the treatment of osteoarthritis.

Make sure consumption of all antioxidant nutrients is at least at Recommended Dietary Allowance levels and possibly higher for vitamin C, beta carotene, and vitamin E. Include two or more servings of fish in the weekly diet. If symptoms do not improve, try a nutrient-dense vegetarian diet (see guidelines on pages 85–92) for one month or more to see if this dietary change is effective.

Overconsumption of iron or vitamin D might aggravate arthritis symptoms or result in other disorders, including secondary deficiencies of zinc or irreversible calcium deposition in heart and other soft tissues. Finally, frequent, moderate exercise increases the blood flow and therefore oxygen and nutrient supply to all body tissues and can retard the aging processes of all tissues, including bones and joints.

Arthritis sufferers are susceptible to quick, easy, secret, or special cures. Many fads, from copper bracelets to a vryllium tube hung from the lapel, appear to work when in reality the disease disappeared on its own. Many "popular" diets for arthritis are not effective and might contribute to malnutrition and aggravation of arthritis symptoms. These diets include those that eliminate acidic fruits and vegetables, eating only one type of food at each meal (altering the acid-base balance of the diet), low-protein diets, low-calorie diets (except for weight management), and low-carbohydrate diets.

The belief that overconsumption of calcium causes osteoarthritis is also unfounded. Optimal calcium intake improves bone density and strength but has no effect on abnormal calcification of joints associated with osteoarthritis.

The fact that more than half of all cases of rheumatoid arthritis spontaneously cure themselves suggests the immune system can often overcome the disorder if supplied with the necessary nutritional ammunition to stage a full-scale "war."

Bowel Problems

Disorders of the bowel, including the small and large intestine, are numerous. This section discusses nutritional concerns for the most common, including flatulence (gas), constipation, diarrhea, irritable bowel syndrome (spastic colon), diverticular disease, and inflammatory bowel disease.

Flatulence (Gas)

The average person generates 1 to 3 pints of gas each day, which consists of nitrogen, oxygen, hydrogen, and small amounts of methane. The causes of gas include swallowing air while eating or drinking, increased intestinal activity, and excessive bacterial fermentation of food components in the bowel. People with too much gas often produce the same amount as other people, but because of increased movement of food through the bowel, the gas is not reabsorbed through the colon wall as it is in other people. Increasing the fiber content of the diet also can cause temporary gas.

The following vegetables and fruits produce gas:

Vegetables:

Beans—kidney, lima, navy
Broccoli
Brussels sprouts
Cabbage
Cauliflower
Corn
Cucumber
Kohlrabi
Leeks
Lentils
Onions

Peas, split or black-eyed
Peppers, green
Pimentos
Radishes
Rutabagas
Sauerkraut
Scallions
Shallots
Soybeans
Turnips

Fruits:

Apples, raw
Apple juice
Avocados
Cantaloupe
Honeydew melon
Prune juice
Raisins
Watermelon

Carbohydrate-rich foods are often the worst offenders. Most gas results from sugars, starches, and fibers that reach the large intestine without being digested and absorbed. Colonies of harmless bacteria in the colon eat the carbohydrates, giving off the by-products—hydrogen, carbon dioxide, and methane in some people. Gas production can be reduced or avoided by gradually replacing low-fiber foods with high-fiber foods during a two- to four-week period.

A special type of sugar called raffinose is found in beans and, in smaller amounts, some vegetables and grains. The human body lacks the enzyme (alpha-galactosidase) to digest this sugar, so bacteria in the colon have a feast. Flatulence from beans can be prevented or reduced by following these preparation guidelines:

1. Soak the beans overnight and discard the water.
2. Add fresh water, cook for half an hour, and again throw away the water. Add 9 cups of water for every cup of beans.
3. Cook beans thoroughly to avoid raw starch granules that also produce gas.
4. Discard the liquid from canned beans; it is loaded with raffinose.

A product on the market called Beano contains the digestive enzyme alpha-galactosidase. A few drops added to a bowl of beans essentially stops the gas-producing bacteria in the colon and reduces the bloating and distension that trouble many people. (If Beano is not available in your area, call AkPharma at 1-800-257-8650 for a free sample.)

Dietary recommendations for gas sufferers include eating more slowly, chewing with the mouth closed, and avoiding gulping food. Avoid the gas-forming foods and then add back those that are tolerated well. People vary in their reactions to foods, so don't assume that what is "gassy" for someone else will be "gassy" for you.

Excessive gas could be a sign of lactose intolerance (inability to digest milk sugar) or a deficiency of another intestinal enzyme. As a trial, omit milk and milk products from the diet, including ice cream, yogurt, milk, cheese, puddings, and custard, and observe any improvements in symptoms.

Constipation

Constipation is a very subjective complaint. Ideally, a person should have a bowel movement each day; however, constipation is objectively defined as less than three stools per week or when three or more days go by without a bowel movement. The causes of constipation are numerous and include lack of exercise, side effects of medication, disease, crash dieting, obesity, dehydration, and a low-fiber diet.

The primary dietary recommendation is to increase the fiber content of the diet by eating more fresh fruits and vegetables, whole grain breads and cereals, and cooked dried beans and peas. The diet should contain at least five servings of fruits and vegetables, six servings of whole grains, and one serving of cooked beans.

Avoid highly refined foods, such as white rice and bread, cream of wheat, pastries, pies, cakes, enriched noodles, and commercial snack foods. Prunes and prune juice are high in fiber and also stimulate intestinal movement. (See pages 42–47 for a listing of high-, moderate-, and low-fiber foods.) In addition,

- Drink at least eight to ten glasses of water daily.
- Avoid excessive intake of iron or calcium carbonate supplements.
- Consume optimal amounts of vitamin B1.
- Avoid using large amounts of bran cereals as a source of fiber. Excessive amounts of this processed fiber can be irritating to the intestinal tract and cause flatulence or intestinal blockage.
- The regular use of laxatives is discouraged since this practice causes dependence and possibly spastic constipation.
- Regular aerobic exercise improves bowel function and often cures constipation.

Diarrhea

Diarrhea is a symptom, not a disease. Food passes rapidly through the intestine, resulting in potential nutrient deficiencies if the condition persists. Diarrhea should be differentiated from more serious conditions such as dysentery and is caused by a variety of conditions, including lactose intolerance or other intestinal disorders, bacterial and viral infections, laxatives such as castor oil, ulcerative colitis, and Crohn's disease. Coffee or caffeine consumption, even in moderate amounts of one to two cups each day, can cause diarrhea in sensitive people. Iron and/or calcium supplements can also cause diarrhea in some individuals.

The primary nutritional goal in the treatment of diarrhea is to remove the cause. A low-fiber diet is often used temporarily to reduce the undigestible bulk in the intestine. This diet consists of potatoes without the skin, enriched white bread and rice, strained fruit juices, plain crackers without seeds, milk (unless the person is lactose intolerant), creamed or broth-based soups, fish or chicken, and enriched pastas.

In contrast to the treatment for constipation, vegetables, fruits, whole grains, cooked dried beans and peas, seeds, and other fiber-rich foods are avoided in treating diarrhea. Drink at least ten glasses of water daily to replace fluids. Pectin in applesauce provides some therapeutic benefits, but never use concentrated canning pectin as a source of this fiber. Fiber foods are gradually reintroduced when the diarrhea subsides and food tolerance is restored. Chronic diarrhea requires physician monitoring and may require vitamin and mineral supplementation to avoid deficiencies from poor food absorption.

Irritable Bowel Syndrome

Irritable bowel syndrome (IBS), also called spastic colitis or spastic colon, probably results from disturbances in intestinal activity, stress, and dietary deficiencies or intolerances. Overstimulation of the nerves that trigger bowel activity results in excessive bowel contractions, abdominal pain, diarrhea or constipation, and nausea. Contributing causes vary but often include the use of laxatives, tobacco, caffeine, alcohol, antibiotic therapy, digestive tract infections, and irregularities in sleep, fluid intake, and bowel movements. People with IBS are frequently tense, underweight, and upset. From past experiences they are afraid to eat because of anticipated pain.

The goal of nutritional therapy is to relieve the condition, regain optimal nutritional status, and increase body weight. A low-fat, nutrient-dense, high-fiber diet helps relieve constricting pressure in the bowel and promotes normal bowel activity. Avoid large supplemental doses of vitamins and minerals that might irritate the intestinal tract. Relaxation and stress management are also essential in the long-term management of this bowel problem.

Diverticular Disease

Diverticula are pouches in the weakened intestinal wall. The disease might go unnoticed, or you may experience discomfort, cramping, painful bowel movements, diarrhea or constipation, or nausea.

Diverticulitis is inflammation and infection of the pouches resulting from accumulation of fecal matter in these pockets. The incidence of diverticular disease increases with age, possibly because of reduced strength of the intestinal wall or lifelong poor eating and exercise habits.

The first line of nutritional defense is to increase the fiber content of the diet, which reduces the pressure within the intestines that is thought to cause the pockets, decreases the pain, and speeds the movement of food through the bowel. Even 2 teaspoons of bran three times a day relieves the symptoms of diverticular disease in most people. The high-fiber diet may produce temporary gas, which subsides within a few weeks.

Inflammatory Bowel Disease

Inflammatory bowel disease (IBD) is classified according to the section of the bowel that is affected. Inflammation of the small intestine is usually called Crohn's disease, while inflammation of the rectum and right portions of the colon is called ulcerative colitis. Symptoms include diarrhea, bleeding, abdominal pain, fever, and weight loss. Viral infections, suppressed immunity, and nutrient deficiencies have been implicated in the development and progression of inflammatory bowel diseases; however, the exact cause(s) is unknown.

Nutrient deficiencies are common in people with IBD. Fever and infection increase nutrient requirements, while the pain and inflammatory processes reduce food intake and absorption. Common symptoms of IBD such as impaired taste, reduced appetite, and suppressed immunity might result from zinc deficiency and sometimes respond favorably to zinc supplementation.

Vitamin A is essential for the development and maintenance of the intestinal lining, but as yet no evidence links this vitamin with the prevention or treatment of bowel disease. Dietary management of Crohn's disease and ulcerative colitis requires singular counseling and monitoring by a physician and a dietitian.

Cancer in Women

Cancer is an umbrella term for a variety of diseases characterized by the uncontrolled growth and spread of abnormal cells. The American Cancer Society estimates that one in every three people will eventually have cancer, while approximately fourteen hundred people die every day from the disease. Despite these distressing statistics, many cancers in women can be cured if detected and treated promptly. Even more important, up to 70 percent of all cancers are preventable through diet, exercise, and other life-style habits.

The causes of cancer are only partially understood. Both environmental factors, such as chemicals, radiation, and viruses, and internal factors, such as hormones, immune conditions, and inherited mutations, are implicated in the development and progression of cancer. After exposure to these factors, either acting alone or working together, it may take ten or more years before clinical signs of cancer develop.

Under normal conditions, body cell growth is monitored so that cell death balances with cell reproduction and growth. The random cell that mutates is identified and destroyed by the immune and antioxidant systems. With cancer, the process is left unchecked and consists of two stages: the initiation stage and the promotion stage.

Initially, a normal cell is exposed to a cancer-promoting substance called a mutagen or a carcinogen that converts it into an abnormal cell. During the promotion stage, the abnormal cell is encouraged to multiply and spread into surrounding tissues. Both stages must be present for a normal cell to develop into cancer. Other processes are also necessary for cancer development, such as a compromised immune system, since many normal cells convert to abnormal cells and die or multiply into masses called benign tumors that are relatively harmless. (See figure on page 274.) (See pages 376–77 for information on skin cancer.)

Breast Cancer

Approximately one in every nine women will develop breast cancer, with the incidence increasing at a rate of 3 percent per year. Many factors beyond a woman's control contribute to risk, including having a mother or sister with breast cancer, having a first child after age thirty, beginning menstruation at an early age, or having a special type of fibrocystic breast disease (FBD) called atypical hyperplasia. (See pages 324–27 for more information on FBD.) Early detection and prompt treatment have greatly reduced mortality rates for breast cancer in this country; however, diet and life-style can be altered to help prevent this disease.

DIETARY FAT

According to Dr. Leonard Cohen, head of the section of nutritional endocrinology at Naylor Dana Institute of the American Health Foundation, the initiation stage in breast cancer occurs during puberty when the mammary glands are developing. This stage is not diet-related but probably results from hereditary factors. These precancerous "lesions" develop into cancer only if they are stimulated by a promoting agent such as dietary fat.

Dietary fat favors fat accumulation in breast tissue and alters the female hormones, such as estrogen and prolactin, so they promote cancer formation. In addition, dietary fat might suppress the immune system so that the body fails to reject the abnormal cells. Another set of hormone-like compounds, called prostaglandins, might stimulate the growth of cancer and are also regulated by dietary fat intake.

The risk of developing breast cancer increases as fat and animal protein intake increases and fiber, vegetable, and fruit intake decreases. Both total dietary

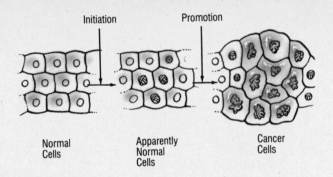

Initiation   Promotion

Normal
Cells

Apparently
Normal
Cells

Cancer
Cells

**The Two Stages of Cancer Growth Are
Initiation and Promotion**

fat (which includes fat from both animal and plant sources) and saturated fat from meats and dairy products increase breast cancer risk.

Women living in Japan consume a very low fat diet (11 to 15 percent fat calories) and have one-tenth the breast cancer risk of American women. However, when Japanese women migrate to Hawaii and California and consume a diet containing 40 percent fat calories, the second generation's breast cancer rates approach those of Americans. In the United States, young women who consume a low-fat, meatless diet have hormonal levels associated with a low risk for later breast cancer as compared to young women who eat a typical American diet. (The link between dietary fat and breast cancer remains controversial, however, and may be associated with pesticides and other toxins that are carried in fat, rather than fat per se.)

In short, it is not genetics but diet and life-style that determine the amount of risk. Apparently the risk increases as a woman ages, with postmenopausal women who consume high-fat diets more likely to develop breast cancer than younger women. This correlates with breast cancer rates since more than two-thirds of all cancers occur in women over age fifty.

According to a landmark study that investigated the link between breast cancer and dietary fat in eighty-nine thousand nurses, a reduction in fat intake from 40 percent to 30 percent of total calories is not sufficient to lower risk. It is likely that fat intake must be below 25 percent of total calories before breast cancer risk is reduced. This requires considerable changes in the typical American diet.

Two dietary fats that appear protective against breast cancer are fish oils and olive oils. Fish oils slow tumor growth and prolong survival in animals with mammary (breast) cancer. Although poorly understood, fish and olive oils might alter prostaglandins that otherwise encourage the development of cancer.

BODY FAT

Although excess body fat increases a woman's risk of developing breast cancer and of having the cancer progress to more serious stages, recent evidence suggests that where the fat is deposited has the greatest impact on health. A woman who carries most of her extra fat above the waist in her abdomen and chest (an apple-shaped body) is at greater risk of breast cancer than a woman with hefty thighs and hips (a pear-shaped body).

Researchers at Syracuse University monitored body measurements in overweight women who lost weight. They found that apple-shaped women lost more of their weight in the chest and abdomen; consequently, their body shape changed noticeably as they lost weight. Other studies have confirmed these results. Losing weight lowers what is called the waist-to-hip ratio (WHR), the proportion of fat above the waist compared to the fat at hip and thigh level. (An apple has a high WHR, while a pear has a low WHR.) When it comes to health, "apples" derive the greatest benefits from weight loss because they lose more weight from the upper body; even a 10 percent reduction in weight significantly decreases the apple's risk of developing breast cancer.

CALORIES

Calorie level and total dietary fat are implicated in breast cancer. Animals fed high-calorie diets, regardless of the fat content, developed breast cancer at a much higher rate than animals fed moderate- to low-calorie diets. It is difficult to isolate the separate effects of total calories, dietary fat, and body weight in the development of breast cancer; however, total calories and body fat usually decrease when dietary fat is reduced.

FIBER

There is general agreement that the female hormone estrogen is involved in the development and progression of breast cancer. Once cancerous breast tumors have developed, approximately one-third have been found to regress when estrogen levels are reduced.

Fiber may be one way of lowering estrogen levels, therefore helping to prevent breast cancer. Within even two months of consuming a high-fiber diet, especially wheat fiber, blood estrogen levels fall. The combined effect of raising fiber and lowering fat intake is most effective in reducing the risk of breast cancer.

VITAMIN E

Most of the evidence linking vitamin E with breast cancer comes from studies on animals. A deficiency of vitamin E increased the incidence of mammary tumors in animals. Tumor formation, growth, and quantity decreased when animals were given supplements of this fat-soluble vitamin; they also lived longer. In studies on humans, women with breast cancer showed improvement when their diets were supplemented with vitamin E. Women with low blood levels of vitamin E had a fivefold increase in risk of breast cancer compared to women with normal or high blood levels of the vitamin.

The most accepted role of vitamin E in the prevention of breast cancer is as an antioxidant. Vitamin E also might help protect the cells' genetic code from mutation. A few studies indicated that vitamin E converted cancer cells back to normal cells. Dr. R. S. London at North Charles General Hospital in Baltimore suspects that a woman must consume considerably more than the Recommended Dietary Allowance to maintain optimal vitamin E levels and prevent cancer.

MINERALS: SELENIUM AND CALCIUM

Several minerals have been implicated in decreasing breast cancer risk. Increased supplemental or dietary intake of selenium might reduce the risk of developing breast cancer. Women with low blood selenium levels have two times the cancer risk of women with high selenium levels. In addition, current low blood selenium levels might be an indicator of the risk of cancer in the future. The link between selenium intake and breast cancer is not conclusive, and more research is needed. It could be that selenium works in conjunction with vitamins E and C for maximum effectiveness.

Since selenium is potentially toxic, total diet and supplemental intakes should not exceed 200 mcg per day. However, a potentially nontoxic method of increasing selenium intake is to consume selenium-enriched garlic, which contains both the mineral and other cancer-preventing compounds that might help protect against breast cancer.

Low dietary intake of calcium and vitamin D coupled with a high intake of phosphorus might increase a woman's susceptibility to some forms of breast cancer, according to researchers at Sloan-Kettering Cancer Center in New York. In two studies on animals, dietary intakes of phosphorus and vitamin D altered calcium availability while reducing phosphorus intake. In contrast, increased calcium and vitamin D intakes reduced breast cancer risk.

FIBER AND VITAMINS

Women who consume several servings daily of fresh fruits and vegetables have as much as a tenfold reduction in breast cancer risk compared to women who avoid these foods. It is unclear why fruits and vegetables are protective; however, the high fiber and vitamin content is likely to at least contribute to the reduced risk.

As fat intake decreases and fiber intake increases, the risk of breast cancer drops. Vitamin C has a consistent and significant inverse relationship with cancer; as vitamin C intake increases, the risk of breast cancer decreases. In fact, some researchers speculate that as many as 25 percent of breast cancer cases are preventable by increasing vitamin C–rich foods in the diet.

Both vitamin A and beta carotene (the building block of vitamin A found in fruits and vegetables) help protect against breast cancer; however, the two nutrients provide different means of protection, and both should be consumed in the diet. Beta carotene also stimulates the immune system and might have a secondary effect in cancer prevention. Breast cancer risk increases as consumption of beta carotene decreases. One study found that breast cancer risk was highest in women consuming the least amount of beta carotene–rich foods, while vitamin A was not associated with cancer risk. Daily intake of beta carotene–rich foods is necessary since recent evidence shows that blood levels of beta carotene drop quickly when dietary intake is inadequate.

Colorectal Cancer

Although not exclusively a women's disease, colorectal cancer is the third most common form of cancer in women and is responsible for 14 percent of all deaths from cancer in women. A family history of colorectal cancer is a risk factor; however, diet plays a fundamental role in the development and progression of this form of cancer.

DIETARY FAT

Substantial evidence indicates that differences in colorectal cancer incidence between countries is related to dietary fat intake. Dietary fat enhances cholesterol and bile acid production by the liver and results in greater amounts of these substances in the colon. Bacteria in the colon, in turn, convert these fatty substances into cancer-causing compounds. In studies on animals and on humans, bile acids and other fats in the intestine damaged the lining of the colon and increased abnormal cell growth.

A westernized diet high in animal fat from meat and dairy products and low in fiber and calcium increases colorectal cancer rates in animals. In fact, a high-fat diet combined with a sedentary life-style might be responsible for as much as 40 percent of the colorectal cancer rate in women.

FIBER

Studies have repeatedly shown that a fiber-rich diet composed primarily of whole grain breads and cereals, fresh fruits and vegetables, and other fiber foods reduces a woman's risk of developing precancerous polyps in the colon and colorectal cancer. A high-fiber diet speeds the removal of cancer-causing substances such as bile acid and cholesterol by-products and reduces the risk of developing colorectal cancer. Because these foods are also excellent sources of vitamins and minerals, it is difficult to separate the effects of one nutrient. Insoluble fiber, such as the fiber in wheat bran, is the most protective against colorectal cancers.

CALCIUM AND VITAMIN D

Increased dietary intake of calcium and possibly vitamin D reduces a woman's risk of developing colon cancer. Tumor incidence is 50 percent to 70 percent lower in those who consume high-calcium diets, possibly because calcium binds to the cancer-causing fats in the colon and converts them into harmless substances that the body excretes.

The optimal calcium intake is unknown; however, researchers at Rutgers University College of Pharmacy recommend intakes of 1,500 mg to 1,800 mg per day for maximum benefit. Vitamin D can be toxic, so intake should not exceed two times the Recommended Dietary Allowance, or no more than 800 IU.

PROTEIN

Dietary protein from animal sources is linked to colorectal cancer risk. In one study, protein was associated with a risk of colon and rectal cancers in women that was two to three times greater. The risk of colon cancer is highest in women who eat approximately 5 ounces or more of red meat daily, while women who limit red meat to no more than 2 ounces per day have the lowest risk. However, the less the better. Women who eat red meat infrequently, that is, once a week or once a month, still have a 40 percent higher risk of developing colon cancer than women who eat meat less often.

CALORIES AND SUGAR

People with colorectal cancer consume more calories and more sugar than healthy people, and it is likely that excessive calorie and sugar intake might increase a woman's risk of developing bowel cancer. Highly refined carbohydrates might be fermented by bacteria in the colon, and these by-products might contribute to the development or progression of cancer. In addition, excessive calories could result in overweight, and as body fat increases above desirable levels, colorectal cancer risk also increases.

VITAMINS

The antioxidants—vitamin C, vitamin E, and beta carotene—might protect against developing colon cancer. People who supplement their diets with these vitamins show fewer precancerous conditions in the colon. However, the anti-oxidant vitamins are most effective when consumed with a low-fat, high-fiber diet.

OTHER SUBSTANCES IN PLANT FOODS

A diet high in foods of plant origin also helps reduce the risk of colon cancer. Besides being high in vitamins, fiber, and minerals, these foods also contain a family of compounds called the phytosterols, which are similar to cholesterol but have a protective rather than a harmful effect on the digestive tract. They possibly increase the excretion of cholesterol, inhibit the conversion of cholesterol to cancer-causing substances, and reduce cancer initiation and growth in the colon. Foods high in phytosterols include wheat germ, vegetable oils, corn, soybeans, peas, kidney beans, and rice bran.

Ovarian Cancer

Ovarian cancer is the fifth leading cause of cancer-related death in women. One in every seventy women will develop this form of cancer, and more than thirteen thousand died as a result of it in 1992. Risk increases with age, and also at greater risk are women who have never had children, who are at an early age at their first pregnancy, have a family history of ovarian cancer, experience an early menopause, are obese, or are users of oral contraceptives. A woman with breast cancer has a twofold increased risk of developing ovarian cancer. Unfortunately, the disease typically remains silent until it is far advanced, making treatment difficult and the prognosis poor. When ovarian cancer is diagnosed and treated early, 85 percent of women live five years or longer.

DIETARY FAT

The major dietary difference between ovarian cancer rates in different countries is that in countries where women eat a high-fat, high-meat, high-milk diet, ovarian cancer rates are also high. It is unlikely that milk, per se, is a contributor, but saturated fat in milk may be the culprit since no association has been found between nonfat milk intake and ovarian cancer risk.

Another study found a strong association between ovarian cancer risk and the high intake of eggs and fried foods. Women who ate eggs three or more times a week had a three times greater risk of fatal ovarian cancer than women who ate eggs less than once a week. Women who ate fried foods five or more days a week had a 2.9 times greater risk of developing cancer than women who ate fried foods less than three times a week.

VITAMIN A AND BETA CAROTENE

In nearly 90 percent of cases, cancer originates in the lining or epithelial tissue of the ovaries. Vitamin A is well known for its fundamental role in the maintenance of epithelial tissue, including the lining of the ovaries, and the cancer-preventive effects of vitamin A and beta carotene are well documented. Blood levels of these two nutrients, which reflect dietary intake, are inversely related to the risk of ovarian cancer; as blood levels decrease, the risk of ovarian cancer increases.

Cervical, Uterine, and Endometrial Cancers

Although precancerous conditions of the cervix are more common today, invasive cervical cancer has steadily decreased in the past few years. Women at highest risk of cervical cancer were at an early age for first intercourse, have multiple sex partners, smoke cigarettes, or have contracted genital herpes or certain other sexually transmitted diseases. Uterine cancers are most common in women over the age of fifty. The death rate for uterine and cervical cancer has decreased more than 70 percent in the past forty years, primarily because women have routine Pap smears, which detect cervical cancer at an early stage.

Endometrial cancer is cancer in the lining (endometrium) of the uterus. Endometrial cancer risk increases if a woman has a history of infertility, fails to ovulate, is obese, or has been on prolonged estrogen therapy. Researchers at the University of South Florida College of Medicine also report that accumulation of excess body fat in the upper body significantly increases the risk of endometrial cancer.

VITAMINS

Blood levels of the antioxidant nutrients, including beta carotene, vitamin E, and vitamin C, are inversely related to cervical cancer risk. Women with cervical cancer have low blood levels and cervical tissue levels of these nutrients and the B vitamin folic acid compared to healthy women. Smokers also have lower blood levels of vitamin C and beta carotene, thus further increasing their risk of developing cervical cancer.

The low blood levels reflect poor dietary intake since women at risk for cervical cancer also consume fewer fruits and vegetables high in these nutrients, such as carrots, spinach, broccoli, cantaloupe, and leaf lettuce. Studies have reported that calcium intake is low in women with endometrial cancer, and frequent consumption of yogurt is associated with a reduced risk.

BODY FAT AND CALORIES

Body weight is associated with postmenopausal endometrial cancer and also might be associated with cancer in younger women. Women with high body fat percentages have increased levels of a type of estrogen (a female hormone) that is more "biologically active" and is associated with cancer risk. Researchers at the University of Hawaii reported that women who gain weight later in life are at the highest risk of developing endometrial cancer after age sixty. In addition, restricting calories reduces the risk of breast and uterine cancers.

Putting It All Together: Dietary Recommendations

The National Academy of Sciences report, "Diet, Nutrition, and Cancer," states that diet alone is responsible for 60 percent or more of all cancers in women. The most important dietary change you can make to protect against these diseases is to reduce dietary fat to less than 30 percent of total calories, preferably to less than 25 percent.

This requires dramatic dietary changes if you are currently consuming a typical American diet that contains 37 percent to 40 percent fat calories. Review the guidelines for the low-fat, nutrient-dense Healthy Woman's Diet. Make sure that two or three vegetables are orange or green to ensure optimal beta carotene intake (at least 5,000 IU per day), and consume two or more vitamin C-rich foods, such as citrus fruits, to guarantee at least 200 mg of this vitamin daily.

Limit red meat to once a month (or avoid altogether) and replace with more servings of fish. Increase vitamin E intake to at least 100 IU, and vitamin A to 2,500 to 5,000 IU. Supplementing with the antioxidant vitamins is useful only if combined with a low-fat, high-fiber diet.

The cruciferous vegetables, including Brussels sprouts, broccoli, cabbage, asparagus, and kohlrabi, contain additional anticancer substances called indoles. Include five or more servings of these vegetables in the weekly menu.

Avoid obesity, especially if you store excess fat in the upper body (apple-shaped body type). Women who are 40 percent or more overweight have a 55 percent greater risk of developing cancer. However, since losing and regaining weight is more harmful to health than maintaining a slightly overweight body size, take dieting seriously and commit to weight loss only if you are sure you can devote the time and effort to maintain the loss for life. (See chapter 7 for guidelines on weight management.)

Beyond diet, other life-style factors that help reduce cancer risk include relaxation and stress management, monthly breast self exams, daily exercise, avoidance of tobacco smoke, moderate alcohol intake, and routine screening such as a mammogram and a Pap smear. Even people exposed to cigarette smoke (passive smokers) are at increased risk of developing several types of cancers. Early detection and treatment are paramount to cancer survival.

Hormone replacement therapy (HRT) for women after menopause also increases the risk of developing reproductive cancers, especially endometrial cancer. This risk is reduced when progesterone is added to estrogen therapy. The association between HRT and breast cancer is poorly understood. Studies showing a small but significant increased risk indicate that this occurs after five years or more of HRT, and progesterone does not have the protective effect for breast cancer that it does for endometrial cancer.

Cardiovascular Disease

Cardiovascular disease (CVD) is epidemic in the United States. It is the leading cause of death and disease, accounting for one in every two deaths. Of the more than 512,000 people who die of heart attacks each year, approximately 244,000 are women. In fact, half of all women eventually develop some form of heart disease.

A recurring theme in most reviews about diet and CVD is the lack of information on women. For example, a handful of studies on CVD have been conducted on women, and only three of the major cholesterol-lowering drug studies included women. Preliminary research has provided evidence indicating that the risk factors for women are similar to men, with small differences. Compared to men, women at risk for CVD smoke less, have higher blood cholesterol levels, and are more apt to be obese.

Heart attacks usually strike women after age sixty-five, or ten to fifteen years later than men. Blood cholesterol levels are on average thirteen "points" higher in postmenopausal women compared to younger women (20 mg per deciliter higher in women with natural menopause and 11 mg per deciliter higher in women with hysterectomies). The lower risk prior to menopause suggests that the female hormone estrogen provides protection against heart disease.

However, younger women with certain risk factors, such as smoking, diabetes, hypertension, high cholesterol, or a family history of heart disease, are also targets for premature heart disease. Hypertension is a major health problem among women. The prevalence of hypertension in women is 26.8 percent compared to 33 percent in men. Age influences these numbers, however, since hypertension is more prevalent in men prior to sixty-four and more prevalent in women from sixty-five onward. Women are also more prone to other types of cardiovascular diseases, such as heart valve disorders and blood clots (venous thrombosis), and are more likely to die following the onset of cardiovascular illness.

The dietary and life-style research and recommendations given below are primarily based on studies done on men with reference to women whenever the information was available.

What Causes Heart Disease?

The initiation and progression of CVD is a complex, multifaceted process that begins in early childhood. It progresses at varying rates throughout a person's life span. Blood cholesterol and triglyceride levels are the primary indicator of risk. In addition, free radical damage to both the artery walls and blood cholesterol; abnormal "clumping" of blood cell fragments called platelets; release of a hormonelike substance called thromboxane and white blood cells called monocytes; and enlargement and engorgement with cholesterol of the muscle cells lining the

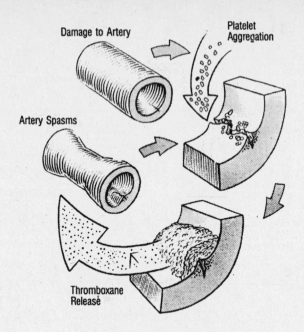

**A Possible Theory for the Beginning
of Atherosclerosis**

The damaged artery attracts blood cell fragments called platelets. These platelets release a substance called thromboxane that causes the artery to spasm, which causes more damage to the artery. A cycle develops that causes more and more damage to the artery, the accumulation of cholesterol, and the development of atherosclerosis.

arteries are a few of the factors in the development of atherosclerosis and CVD. (See figure above.)

In the blood, cholesterol is packaged in water-soluble "bubbles" called lipoproteins. "Total cholesterol" refers to all cholesterol in the blood, including cholesterol in LDLs and HDLs. The greater the proportion of total cholesterol packaged in low-density lipoproteins (LDL-cholesterol), the greater a woman's risk of developing atherosclerosis, heart disease, and stroke. The more total cholesterol packaged in high-density lipoproteins (HDL-cholesterol), the lower a woman's risk of CVD. Cholesterol is found only in the blood, not in food. However, both LDL- and HDL-cholesterol are influenced by diet.

The female hormone estrogen alters the metabolism of blood cholesterol and

---

THE GENDER GAP

Until recently, heart disease was thought to be a "man's disease." Some physicians apply different sets of standards when diagnosing and treating the sexes, and there is some suspicion that physicians do not always take a woman's symptoms seriously.

Women are less likely than men to be diagnosed or treated aggressively for heart disease. Women experience more complications from treatment and are three times more likely than men to die on the operating table and to die within the first year following bypass surgery. Although this is partially because the heart and coronary arteries in women are smaller than men's, it also is because women wait longer before choosing surgery. As a result, women are often older, sicker, heavier, and more out of shape than men at the time of surgery.

---

helps to maintain lower LDL-cholesterol in women than is common in men. How this process works is not entirely understood, and why oral contraceptives raise blood LDL-cholesterol levels, increase blood clotting, and double the rate of heart attack is unclear. In contrast, hormone replacement therapy (HRT) during menopause lowers LDL-cholesterol, raises HDL-cholesterol (known as the "good" cholesterol), and maintains a reduced CVD risk.

The National Cholesterol Education Program states that total cholesterol levels greater than 200 mg per deciliter or LDL levels greater than 130 mg per deciliter reflect moderate risk, while levels of 220 mg per deciliter and 160 mg per deciliter or greater, respectively, reflect high risk of heart disease. A ratio of total cholesterol to HDL-cholesterol below 3.5 to 1 represents a low risk for heart disease, a ratio of 4.5 to 1 is moderate risk, and a ratio of 6.5 to 1 or greater is indicative of high risk. Recently, a new lipoprotein called Lipoprotein (a), or Lp(a), has been implicated in heart disease. High levels of Lp(a), even in the presence of low total cholesterol, could increase your disease risk.

The factors that increase the risk of developing heart disease are as follows (risk increases substantially when two or more factors are present):

- Elevated blood cholesterol levels (greater than 200 mg per deciliter)
- Elevated low-density lipoprotein cholesterol (an LDL-cholesterol greater than 130 mg per deciliter)
- Low high-density lipoprotein cholesterol (a ratio of total cholesterol to HDL-cholesterol greater than 4.5 to 1)

- Elevated triglyceride levels (a "red flag" indicator that fat metabolism is abnormal)
- Cigarette smoking
- High blood pressure
- Diabetes
- A sedentary life-style
- Obesity, especially if body fat is primarily accumulated above the waist
- Stress
- A family history of heart disease
- Female gender after menopause

It is best to keep an eye on all blood cholesterol levels. HDL values are not routinely checked, so ask specifically for this test. More important, ask for a copy of the blood lipid panel sheet; do not settle for a vague statement such as "Your cholesterol is normal." Remember, "normal" in the United States means you have a fifty-fifty chance of dying from heart disease. Women at low risk should repeat the blood test every five years, while women with "red-flag" values should make dietary and life-style changes immediately and be rechecked annually or even more frequently. (See table on page 287.)

Nutrition and CVD

The most important piece in the diet–heart disease puzzle is cholesterol. Anything that raises total cholesterol or LDL-cholesterol or lowers HDL-cholesterol increases the risk of developing heart disease.

DIETARY FAT AND CHOLESTEROL

Reducing dietary fat has the greatest impact on lowering blood cholesterol and the risk of developing CVD. As dietary fat, especially saturated fat, intake increases, so do blood cholesterol and LDL-cholesterol levels and the risk of developing atherosclerosis and heart disease. Dietary cholesterol also increases blood cholesterol levels, but not as dramatically as saturated fats. In contrast, as saturated fat intake is reduced, blood cholesterol levels and risk of heart disease drop.

The dietary protectors against heart disease include the polyunsaturated fats found in liquid vegetable oils, the monounsaturated fats found in olive and canola

Blood Cholesterol Levels and the Risk of Heart Disease

The risk of developing heart disease depends on blood cholesterol levels, the ratio of total cholesterol to HDL-cholesterol, and age. The following blood cholesterol levels are guidelines for heart disease risk.

AGE	MODERATE RISK (MG PER DECILITER OF BLOOD)	HIGH RISK (MG PER DECILITER OF BLOOD)
Less than 20 years	170	185
20–39	200	220
30–39	220	240
40+	240	260

The amount of total cholesterol packaged in HDL-cholesterol is also important in establishing risk. HDL cholesterol is not routinely measured and must be specifically requested. The information obtained from a blood cholesterol test can be used to determine the ratio of total cholesterol to HDL-cholesterol. A ratio of 3.5 to 1 reflects a very low risk of developing heart disease. A ratio that ranges from 4.5 to 1 to 6.5 to 1 is a moderate risk category, and a ratio greater than 6.6 to 1 reflects a high risk.

$$\frac{\text{TOTAL CHOLESTEROL (MG PER DECILITER)}}{\text{HDL-CHOLESTEROL (MG PER DECILITER)}}$$

Example 1: $\dfrac{260}{40}$ = 6.5 to 1, or high risk

Example 2: $\dfrac{180}{55}$ = 3.3 to 1, or low risk

oils, and fish oils. Unfortunately, most polyunsaturated vegetable oils also lower the "good" HDL cholesterol. In addition, they are susceptible to free radicals, the highly reactive compounds suspected to initiate and promote the development of heart disease. In contrast, the monounsaturated oils lower total blood cholesterol, do not lower HDL-cholesterol, and slow the progression of atherosclerosis by generating a special kind of cholesterol that is resistant to free radical damage.

Fish oils also play a protective role in CVD. Fish oils contain a type of polyunsaturated fat called eicosapentaenoic acid, or EPA, which is one of several fats called omega-3 fatty acids. EPA and other omega-3 fatty acids are more effective than other polyunsaturated fats in lowering blood triglyceride and cholesterol levels, reducing platelet clumping, and decreasing the production of thromboxane, which damages artery walls. Although not a panacea, fish combined with a low-fat, high-fiber diet is very effective in reducing the risk of developing CVD in people who have moderate to seriously high blood fat levels.

PROTEIN

How frequently you eat red meat is strongly linked to your risk of having heart disease. The association is strongest after menopause, which suggests that the female hormones somehow counteract the harmful effects in meat, and that risk increases when these hormone levels drop after menopause.

Blood cholesterol levels are also reduced when meat protein is replaced with soy milk or soybeans. The fiber and other substances in soy products help reduce cholesterol and CVD risk.

FIBER

The soluble fibers in oat bran, fruits, some vegetables, and cooked dried beans and peas lower blood cholesterol levels, and thus reduce the risk of developing CVD. The insoluble fibers found in wheat bran have little effect on CVD risk. (See table III-6.)

SUGAR

Limited evidence suggests that a high-sugar diet alters insulin levels and predisposes a person to heart disease. Dr. J. Yudkin at St. John's Wood in London theorizes that it is sugar, not dietary fat, that triggers the metabolic syndrome associated with heart disease.

BODY WEIGHT

Women with excess body fat, especially if it is stored primarily in the chest and abdomen (the apple-shaped body, or a gynoid body fat distribution), are at high risk of developing CVD. In fact, researchers at Brigham and Women's Hospital in Boston have reported that being overweight is associated with 40 percent of all heart disease in women, and gaining an additional 20 pounds during adult life doubles the risk. Losing weight lowers blood cholesterol levels and reduces CVD risk; however, repeated weight loss and gain is more harmful to cardiovascular health than never dieting and remaining slightly overweight.

A Fiber Quiz

Test your fiber IQ by answering the following questions True or False.

_____ **1.** Only foods of plant origin, such as vegetables, grains, and nuts, have fiber.

_____ **2.** Fiber decreases the risk of heart disease by binding to blood cholesterol and removing it from the body.

_____ **3.** All of the fiber in a fruit is in the skin or the peel.

_____ **4.** Crunchiness is a good indicator of a food's fiber content.

_____ **5.** The terms "crude fiber," "dietary fiber," and "edible fiber" all refer to the total fiber content of the diet.

_____ **6.** Wheat bran is approximately 40% to 50% fiber and also contains protein and some starch, sugar, and fat.

_____ **7.** Vegetables and fruits should be eaten raw because cooking destroys fiber.

_____ **8.** Always check the label on commercial fiber foods since some products contain the equivalent of a pat of butter in highly saturated coconut oil per serving.

_____ **9.** When it comes to fiber, the old saying, "Just because something is good doesn't mean more is better," applies.

ANSWERS:

1. True.

2. False. Fiber never enters the bloodstream, so it has no direct effect on blood cholesterol. Instead, fiber lowers blood cholesterol by binding to cholesterol-rich bile acids in the digestive tract, thus reducing their reabsorption and helping to drain cholesterol from the body.

3. False. Although the skin and peel are rich sources of fiber, fiber is also in the rest of the fruit.

4. False. Crunch does not always equate with fiber. The crunchy crust on French bread has no more fiber than plain white bread, while soft cooked carrots have the same fiber content as crunchy raw carrots.

5. False. Crude fiber is what remains after foods are chemically treated with strong acids or alkalis, but it is only a small portion of the fiber in foods. Dietary fiber includes all substances that are resistant to the body's digestive enzymes but does not include fiber compounds that are broken down by bacteria in the colon; it is therefore a low estimate of the total fiber intake. However, dietary fiber is a more precise measurement

(continues)

A Fiber Quiz *(continued)*

than crude fiber values and can be as much as three times higher. Edible fiber is difficult to measure but includes all fiber consumed in the diet.

6. True.

7. False. Cooking softens the cell walls of vegetables, but the fiber content remains the same.

8. True.

9. True. Excessive fiber intake (greater than 50 grams per day) is associated with diarrhea, bloating, and possibly a reduced absorption of minerals such as zinc, iron, and manganese.

The higher risk of heart disease noted in men might be more a result of men's greater likelihood to store fat in their chest abdominal areas. Women are more likely to store fat in their hips and thighs, a type of fat less likely to cause heart disease. According to research from the University of Sweden, body fat distribution, or a high amount of fat above the waist compared to fat below the waist, might explain the differences in heart disease rates between the sexes.

ANTIOXIDANTS

Paramount to understanding and potentially preventing CVD is determining what initially damages the arteries and instigates atherosclerosis. A current and compelling theory links CVD with free radicals and the body's antioxidant system. (See pages 240–44 for a description of free radicals and the antioxidants.)

Free radical damage to cells might be initiating and promoting factors in the development of atherosclerosis and CVD. Repeated free radical attack and damage to both the arteries' endothelium (lining) and other cells associated with the atherosclerotic process, such as platelets, could instigate the events that lead to cholesterol accumulation in the arteries (called plaque). Therefore, antioxidant protection of the artery lining from free radical damage could be essential to reducing the risk of developing atherosclerosis and CVD.

Several antioxidant nutrients have been implicated in the control of atherosclerosis. For example, antioxidant levels are low in tissues that later show signs of free radical damage.

Women who consume selenium-poor diets develop heart damage called cardiomyopathy, which is associated with the high incidence of heart attack. One study reported that women with low blood selenium levels had a six- to sevenfold increased risk of a heart attack. Selenium's antioxidant functions probably explain, at least partially, how this trace mineral protects the heart and blood vessels.

Free radical damage is an underlying link to tobacco use and CVD since smoking is a major risk factor for CVD and is also a source of free radicals. The free radicals in tobacco smoke damage cell membranes and the genetic material within the cells lining the blood vessels. Normal dietary levels of antioxidants are not adequate to counteract the harmful effects of these free radicals or maintain optimal blood levels of some antioxidant nutrients.

Free radicals also play a role in cholesterol and lipoprotein metabolism. Apparently, free radical–damaged LDL-cholesterol, also called oxidized LDL or Ox-LDL, in the blood is more likely to cause atherosclerosis and heart disease than normal LDL-cholesterol. In addition, Ox-LDL increases artery spasms and constriction, thus increasing artery damage and the risk of developing atherosclerosis. Normal LDL has no effect on artery constriction. Vitamins C and E might provide protection against the formation of Ox-LDL by preventing free radicals from damaging LDL-cholesterol.

Free radicals also damage cholesterol in foods to produce an altered type of dietary cholesterol called cholesterol oxides, which are more likely to damage arteries and the heart. Cholesterol oxides have been found in deep-fat-fried foods, powdered eggs, and processed meats, and in human blood. In laboratory studies, cholesterol oxides injected into artery cells produced defects in the artery lining, platelet clumping, and cholesterol accumulation associated with the initiation of atherosclerosis. If dietary cholesterol oxides are key factors in the initiation of atherosclerosis, then dietary intake of the antioxidant nutrients, including vitamin C, beta carotene, vitamin E, selenium, and manganese, becomes even more important in the prevention and treatment of heart disease.

NIACIN

As nicotinic acid, niacin lowers total cholesterol, raises HDL, thwarts the atherosclerotic process, and might aid in the regression of atherosclerosis. Niacin lowers blood fat levels, relaxes artery walls, reduces platelet clumping, and helps remove cholesterol from artery walls, thus aiding in the regression of atherosclerosis.

Therapeutic doses of niacin cause flushing, which can be reduced if the supplements are taken in divided doses throughout the day, half an aspirin is taken a half hour before the niacin, and the niacin dose begins small and is gradually increased over several weeks. Niacin in doses greater than 500 mg should be taken only with the supervision of a physician since large doses can produce liver damage.

CHROMIUM

Chromium is an essential element in the regulation of fat metabolism, and insufficient dietary chromium is linked to an increased risk of developing CVD. Low chromium intake and blood chromium levels are associated with elevated blood cholesterol levels and increased risk of atherosclerosis. In contrast, an increased intake of chromium results in reductions in total cholesterol, LDL-cholesterol, and plaque formation in the arteries, and an increase in HDL-cholesterol.

Dietary intake of chromium is suboptimal. Dr. Richard Anderson of the U.S.D.A. Human Nutrition Research Center in Beltsville, Maryland, reported that 90 percent of self-selected diets contain less than the recommended lower limit of 50 mcg (the upper limit is 200 mcg). Chromium intake averages 15 mcg per 1,000 calories, while calorie intake averages less than 1,600 calories for women. Consequently, most women are likely to be marginally deficient in chromium, consuming less than 25 mcg per day.

COPPER

Copper deficiency increases blood cholesterol and LDL-cholesterol and decreases HDL-cholesterol, thus increasing the risk of developing CVD. Poor dietary intake of copper also damages the structure and function of the heart, increasing the risk of a heart attack. On the other hand, excessive dietary intake of copper and elevated blood copper levels are also linked to an increased risk of developing CVD. Consequently, dietary intake should remain within the safe and adequate zone of 2 mg to 4 mg per day.

IRON

The University of Kuopio in Finland reported that men with high blood iron levels are at increased risk of suffering a heart attack. The researchers speculated that excessive iron generated free radicals that predisposed a person to increased risk of heart disease. These findings are preliminary, however, and may reflect abnormalities in iron metabolism, rather than dietary intake. In addition, at this time there is no evidence that high iron levels in women increase the risk of heart disease.

MAGNESIUM

A marginal magnesium deficiency might be one of the most common contributors to heart disease complications. Magnesium deficiency is associated with irregular heartbeat, angina or chest pain associated with heart disease, heart muscle damage, coronary artery spasms, and increased risk of atherosclerosis and heart attack. Blood magnesium levels are low in patients suffering heart attacks, and tissue levels of magnesium are suboptimal prior to, during, and following a heart attack. Finally, evidence has suggested that a magnesium deficiency contributes to, rather than results from, the development of heart disease. In contrast, increased magnesium intake normalizes the heartbeat, relaxes the coronary arteries, and reduces a person's likelihood of suffering a heart attack.

The ratio of calcium to magnesium is also important. Supplementing with calcium but failing to increase magnesium intake might increase the risk of heart damage. Consequently, the two minerals should be supplied together in a ratio of approximately 1.5 to 2 parts calcium to every 1 part magnesium (such as 1,000 mg of calcium and 500 mg magnesium). The dose is best utilized when divided into several small doses daily since the body can effectively digest and absorb only approximately 100 mg of magnesium at a time.

ZINC

Marginal zinc deficiency is associated with elevated total blood cholesterol and LDL-cholesterol, and decreased HDL-cholesterol, thus increasing a woman's CVD risk. In contrast, optimal zinc intake reduces total and LDL-cholesterol, raises HDL-cholesterol, and is associated with a lowered CVD risk. Limited evidence also shows that zinc might strengthen the lining of the arteries so they are less susceptible to damage and the initiation of atherosclerosis.

As with copper, excessive zinc intake (160 mg per day) has the reverse effect—lowering HDL-cholesterol and increasing the risk of developing CVD. Consequently, zinc intake should not exceed two to three times the recommended guidelines or between 15 mg and 45 mg per day unless monitored by a physician.

GARLIC

Garlic and garlic oil might protect the heart against disease. Garlic dissolves blood clots, inhibits clot formation, and lowers blood cholesterol levels. Garlic has been shown to reverse atherosclerosis in rabbits. A sulfur-containing compound in garlic called ajoene is at least partially responsible for garlic's ability to reduce platelet clumping, thereby reducing the risk of developing atherosclerosis and heart disease. Unfortunately, the optimal dietary intake is approximately eight cloves of garlic per day, but a daily consumption of two to three cloves or a high-quality garlic supplement might produce beneficial effects.

COFFEE

Some studies have reported that coffee increases a person's risk of developing heart disease, while others have shown no association. Researchers at Stanford University's School of Medicine found that even decaffeinated coffee raised LDL-cholesterol levels, suggesting that another compound in coffee besides caffeine might affect heart disease risk.

Putting It All Together: Dietary Recommendations

In most cases, atherosclerosis and cardiovascular disease can be prevented, their progress halted, and the damage reversed if dietary and life-style patterns are modified and medication therapy is followed in diet-resistant cases. The low-fat, high-fiber Healthy Woman's Diet coupled with regular aerobic exercise remains the primary defense.

In addition to these low-fat, high-fiber guidelines, you should limit eggs to three a week, including eggs in baked goods, custard, processed foods, and pastries. Use two egg whites for every whole egg in recipes. Use olive and canola oils rather than other vegetable oils or processed oils such as margarine and shortening. Also, cook with fresh garlic whenever possible.

Divide food intake into four to six small meals and snacks throughout the day. Research has shown that several "mini-meals," as opposed to the "three square meals a day" food pattern, lowers blood cholesterol levels, helps maintain a desirable weight, and reduces the risk of developing CVD. Other controversial dietary factors that might help reduce a person's risk of developing CVD include Brewer's yeast, charcoal supplements, wheat germ, saponins found in cooked dried beans and peas, taking a moderate-dose multivitamin-mineral supplement (containing vitamin E, vitamin C, beta carotene, chromium, copper, magnesium, selenium, and zinc), and following a vegetarian diet.

In addition to diet, a woman's risk of CVD is reduced when she maintains a desirable weight, avoids tobacco smoke, maintains a normal blood pressure, effectively handles stress, maintains a strong social support network, and prevents or controls diabetes. Even living or working with a smoker can increase a non-smoker's risk of heart disease.

The association between personality and heart disease risk (that is, a more aggressive or hostile personality, Type A personality, having a higher risk of heart disease) might be the result of health behaviors associated with an angry personality. "Uptight" personalities in both men and women are also most likely to smoke cigarettes, drink too much alcohol, eat too much, and accumulate body fat above the waist.

Estrogen replacement therapy after menopause helps protect against cardiovascular disease and stroke, providing as much as a 60 percent reduction in CVD incidence. However, the cardiovascular effects of adding progesterone to the estrogen therapy, which reduces the risk of developing endometrial cancer, are unknown. Some widely used progesterones have adverse effects on blood cholesterol levels and might increase CVD risk and blood pressure. Carefully consider all the risks and benefits of hormone replacement therapy before making a decision.

Family history is an important factor. Those with a father, mother, uncle, aunt, grandparent, or other immediate family members who have had heart disease are at high risk and should pay close attention to the risk factors that are within their control. Also, women begin to lose their inborn protection against heart attacks after menopause, and since risk increases in later years, life-style choices are even more important.

Carpal Tunnel Syndrome

A major nerve that carries signals from the brain to the hands passes through a confined tunnel in the wrist formed by the wrist bones, known as the carpals. The tunnel is rigid, so anything that causes swelling or inflammation of the encased tissues will result in pressure and pinching on that nerve. The condition is called carpal tunnel syndrome (CTS).

Symptoms of CTS, which can affect one or both hands at the same time, include intermittent numbness, pain that shoots up the arm from the wrist, and a sensation of tingling or burning in the hands and fingers. These may increase throughout the day, may be severe enough to cause sleeplessness, and can become worse over time.

CTS is fairly common in women engaged in sports, such as volleyball or racquetball, or in jobs that place stress on the wrist, and minor injuries, such as falling backward on your hand, might also cause the tendons to swell. A change in the balance of hormones during pregnancy and menopause may result in an accumulation of fluid and subsequent swelling of the wrists, which might explain the increased prevalence of CTS in these women.

In some cases CTS clears up without treatment. In others, a splint worn on the wrist at night helps relieve the pain. The usual treatment is anti-inflammatory or diuretic medications or cortisone injections to reduce the swelling. Conditions unresponsive to medication require surgery to cut through the tough membrane and create a larger space for the encased nerve.

Nutrition and Carpal Tunnel Syndrome

Vitamin B6 has been linked to the development and treatment of CTS. People with long-term inadequate intake of this B vitamin have an increased likelihood of developing CTS, and the symptoms of CTS are often reduced or relieved when vitamin B6 intake is increased. Several case studies have reported that vitamin B6 supplementation eliminated the need for surgery.

How a vitamin B6 deficiency affects the development of CTS is poorly understood. The vitamin is involved in the development and maintenance of healthy nerve tissue, while a deficiency can cause inflammation of the nerve tissue resembling that seen in CTS.

Vitamin B6 is typically low in women's diets. According to estimates by the U.S. Department of Agriculture, half of all women consume less than two-thirds of the RDA for this vitamin. However, vitamin B6 therapy is effective in some but not all cases of CTS. Researchers speculate that this discrepancy might be explained by differences in vitamin B6 requirements among women, as some require unusually high levels of the vitamin to maintain normal metabolic process.

Sometimes vitamin B6 therapy is effective despite normal blood vitamin levels prior to treatment. In these cases it is conceivable that reduced blood flow in the cartilage and bone tissue involved in CTS results in a localized deficiency of vitamin B6, whereas other tissues with increased circulation have an adequate supply of the vitamin.

Putting It All Together: Dietary Recommendations

If the muscles of the hands have begun to atrophy and weaken, then surgery is probably necessary. In most cases, however, a CTS patient might benefit from a three- to four-month trial of vitamin B6 supplementation. Most studies that reported success used daily supplements containing 50 mg to 200 mg of vitamin B6. The daily dose can drop to 25 mg after several months if the symptoms respond to this therapy.

If the symptoms are not relieved, do not increase the dosage thinking that more will be better. In some people, large doses of vitamin B6 cause poor coordination and numbness and tingling in the hands, a condition called peripheral neuropathy. Megadose vitamin B6 therapy has also caused permanent nerve damage. The threshold above which toxic symptoms occur appears to be between 300 mg and 500 mg of vitamin B6 a day. Never self-medicate; a physician should always monitor the use of large supplemental doses of vitamin B6 for the treatment of CTS.

Cervical Dysplasia

Cervical dysplasia is an abnormal growth of tissue in the cervix. Most cases are apparently harmless; in some cases, however, abnormal cells progress to cancer. Cervical cancer is largely preventable if this precancerous tissue is detected and treated at an early stage.

Although the causes of cervical dysplasia are poorly understood, evidence shows that this condition is associated with a sexually transmitted viral infection. This virus is also found in healthy women, however, which implies that a "host" factor makes some women more susceptible to infection than others. Several factors have been identified as possibly increasing the chances of developing dysplasia, including sexual and reproductive history, socioeconomic status, cigarette smoking, lowered immunity, and nutrition.

Nutrition and Cervical Dysplasia

Studies have shown that vitamin deficiencies, especially of folic acid and possibly vitamin C, beta carotene, and vitamin E, are linked to increased risk of developing cervical dysplasia. These links are particularly interesting since deficiencies of these nutrients are also associated with other risk factors of cervical dysplasia, including oral contraceptive use, pregnancy, and cigarette smoking.

Folic Acid

For more than ten years researchers have reported a link between cervical dysplasia and low folic acid intake. A study at the University of Alabama investigated folic acid status in 294 women with cervical dysplasia and found that risk increased as blood levels of folic acid dropped. The researchers speculated that a marginal folic acid deficiency might make the cervical cells' genetic material more vulnerable to attack by the virus, while normal to optimal folic acid intake might keep genetic material within the cells resistant to viral attack.

Other studies have found the same connection between poor folic acid intake and/or low blood levels of the B vitamin and increased risk for dysplasia. In addition, women with dysplasia who subsequently supplement their diets with folic acid increase their blood folic acid levels and sometimes convert the abnormal tissue back to healthy normal tissue.

Unfortunately, not all studies have shown a therapeutic effect. Dr. C. E. Butterworth at the University of Alabama has reported that folic acid deficiency encourages the development of cervical dysplasia but that supplements do not always alter the course of the condition once it has developed.

Interestingly, some women with cervical dysplasia have normal blood folic acid levels, yet their cervical tissues are low in folic acid. Nutrient requirements have traditionally been considered in terms of the whole person and have been measured by blood levels. It now appears likely that localized nutrient deficiencies can also occur, sometimes triggered by medication (for example, oral contraceptives). In these cases the blood levels of a vitamin such as folic acid were normal, while specific tissues remained deficient. These tissues appeared to respond when greater than normal amounts of a nutrient were consumed.

Even a marginal folic acid deficiency causes breaks and damage to the genetic code that resemble the initial stages of dysplasia and eventually cancer. This folic acid–induced damage to the cells' DNA is affected by other dietary components. Researchers at the University of California at Berkeley and at Harvard School of Public Health reported that consuming coffee or other caffeine-containing beverages in the presence of a folic acid deficiency might escalate by as much as fivefold the risk of developing dysplasia or cancer. In contrast, caffeine had no effect on cell growth when folic acid intake was optimal.

ANTIOXIDANTS: VITAMIN C, VITAMIN E, AND BETA CAROTENE

Vitamin C intake is lower among women with cervical dysplasia than healthy women and is related to as much as a tenfold higher risk of developing dysplasia. The risk of developing cervical dysplasia increases as blood levels of both vitamin E and beta carotene decrease.

It is hard to decipher the effects of either vitamin C or beta carotene alone since these vitamins are often found in the same foods as folic acid. Consequently, a deficiency of one is likely to result in deficiencies of the other vitamins. Dietary intake and blood levels of both vitamin C and beta carotene are low in people who smoke, which is another risk factor for cervical dysplasia. Other antioxidants, such as selenium, have been linked to an increased risk of cervical cancer, but as yet there is no evidence that they affect the risk of developing cervical dysplasia.

Putting It All Together: Dietary Recommendations

The Healthy Woman's Diet is the foundation for the prevention of cervical dysplasia. Make sure to include two to three folic acid–rich foods in the daily menu. Choose very fresh produce such as crispy dark green leafy vegetables, avoid long-term storage, and eat vegetables raw or only slightly cooked.

Make sure vitamin C and beta carotene intakes are optimal by consuming an additional citrus fruit and dark orange vegetable along with the folic acid–rich foods. A supplement that supplies moderate levels of these nutrients and vitamin E can also provide nutritional insurance.

You should avoid consuming more than 400 mcg of supplemental folic acid (pregnant women can consume 800 mcg) unless supervised by a physician. Large doses of folic acid can mask a vitamin B12 deficiency, which although very rare can cause permanent nerve damage if allowed to progress. Finally and most important, schedule routine Pap smears and have your physician closely monitor any abnormal cell growth.

Chronic Fatigue Syndrome

Chronic fatigue syndrome (CFS) is a collection of symptoms that includes muscle fatigue, sore throat, depression, insomnia, poor concentration, exhaustion, and joint aches. Upper respiratory infections, swollen lymph nodes, and night sweats may develop. The symptoms are not dramatic, but what makes this disorder unique is that the symptoms linger for months and sometimes never resolve but merely come and go. It has also been called the "yuppie disease" since most of the people who develop symptoms are white, educated professionals in their twenties and thirties. Women with CFS outnumber men two to one.

The symptoms are thought to be a result of a viral infection, in particular the Epstein-Barr virus. Consequently, chronic fatigue syndrome has also been called chronic Epstein-Barr virus or CEBV. Like chicken pox, however, the Epstein-Barr virus is very common. As many as 95 percent of all people have been exposed to this virus, but only a few developed CFS. Chronic fatigue sufferers often have high levels of antibodies to the Epstein-Barr virus, but that does not signify infection; antibodies are also high in energetic people with no symptoms. Consequently, the link between CFS and this virus remains controversial.

Accumulating evidence shows that CFS patients can be classified into at least three categories: those with a previous history of psychological problems, those with underlying disorders that exhibit similar symptoms to CFS, and patients with no history of emotional problems but who exhibit all the symptoms of CFS. This latter group might be suffering from a compromised immune system.

Since antibodies to the Epstein-Barr virus are found in both healthy and fatigued subjects, it is most likely that an abnormal immune system, not just exposure to the virus, has led to infection. Several studies have shown that CFS patients have lower numbers of white blood cells, such as T lymphocytes, and these immune cells are less active than those found in healthy individuals. It is not known at this time whether the possible suppressed immunity is a cause or a result of CFS.

Interestingly, the integral links between mood, stress, and immunity are exemplified in CFS. Researchers have reported that depression is common in people with CFS, and antidepressant medications and sleep therapy appear to produce favorable results for CFS patients.

Putting It All Together: Dietary Recommendations

Until more is known about the causes of CFS, the best dietary advice is to consume ample amounts of all the nutrients associated with a strong immune system. This would include a low-fat, nutrient-dense diet as outlined in the Healthy Woman's

Diet, composed primarily of fresh fruits and vegetables, whole grain breads and cereals, cooked dried beans and peas, with small amounts of nonfat milk or yogurt and fish or chicken. (See chapter 1 and more information on nutrition and the immune system on pages 244–49.) Amounts greater than RDA levels for the antioxidant nutrients might be required.

One study from the University of Southampton in England reported that CFS sufferers have low blood levels of magnesium and respond favorably to magnesium supplementation. How magnesium might exert its effects is poorly understood. The improvements in energy levels and mood reported in this study corresponded with findings of other investigators who used magnesium at RDA levels to treat anxiety, insomnia, and organic mental disorders.

Habits such as smoking, crash dieting, a sedentary life-style, and alcohol abuse aggravate the symptoms of CFS. In addition, it is likely that a psychological component contributes to the condition. The fact that professional women are at the highest risk of CFS implies that the added stresses of career, maintaining a healthy marriage, and raising children give women "more to be sick and tired about."

Married women spend 4 to 8 hours a day on housework in addition to time spent on the job. In contrast, a typical husband spends 1.6 hours on domestic tasks. In another study, the average working mother spent 40 hours at work and 37 hours doing housework each week. In order to accomplish this schedule, women typically give up personal time, sleep, and playtime. It is likely that this race to "do it all" contributes to the increased risk of developing CFS. If this is the case, then delegating responsibilities or letting go of the "superwoman" complex might be the best treatment of all.

The Common Cold

The common cold is actually a group of minor infections caused by any one of almost two hundred different viruses. Symptoms are usually limited to congestion in the nose and a sore throat, but some viruses also affect the larynx (causing laryngitis) and the lungs (causing bronchitis). Sometimes a viral infection is followed by a more serious bacterial infection of the throat, lungs, or ears. Although colds are most common in infancy and early childhood when the immune system is still maturing, anyone at any time can "catch a cold."

Nutrition and the Common Cold

The link between nutrition and the common cold was made famous when Nobel Laureate Linus Pauling theorized that megadoses of vitamin C would prevent or cure the common cold. Since that time, research on nutrition and the immune system has uncovered a wealth of evidence linking most vitamins and minerals to prevention of the common cold, the flu, other infections, and disease. In fact, all nutrients associated with strengthening the immune system, including beta carotene, vitamin E, the B vitamins, vitamin C, selenium, zinc, iron, and other minerals, are important for both the prevention and treatment of the common cold or any infection. (See pages 244–49 for more information on nutrition and immunity.) Specific research on the common cold is limited to vitamin C and zinc.

VITAMIN C

Vitamin C has an antiviral effect in preventing or limiting the severity of the common cold. Results of studies on vitamin C supplementation and the common cold have produced varying results. Some studies have reported that 1 gram daily of vitamin C does not limit the number of colds a person contracts but does reduce the duration and severity of the illness.

Other studies have shown that vitamin C supplementation does not affect the duration but does help prevent the common cold and limit the severity of those colds that do develop. In addition, maintaining high blood levels of vitamin C by consuming moderate doses every one to two hours might reduce the severity of the common cold and other viral infections.

Although more research is needed to clarify vitamin C's role in the prevention and treatment of the common cold, it is likely that the vitamin is at least somewhat effective since it also promotes and potentiates the production of interferon, the body's natural antiviral agent. The effective dose appears to be higher than typical dietary intakes; thus, moderate supplementation might be useful prior to, at the first sign of, and during a cold.

ZINC

Zinc plays a fundamental role in maintaining a healthy immune system. Zinc deficiency impairs many aspects of immunity, while optimal intake of this trace mineral enhances immune function even in healthy people. Zinc also has a direct effect on limiting the growth of microorganisms, such as bacteria and possibly viruses. For example, certain viruses cannot survive in a zinc-rich environment. This antiviral effect was the basis for the development of zinc lozenges that dissolve in the mouth and coat the lining of the throat.

One study showed that zinc gluconate lozenges shortened the duration of colds, with some people becoming asymptomatic within hours after taking the lozenges. Further research is needed before recommendations for the optimal dose of zinc in the treatment of the common cold can be made, especially since zinc is an example of more not necessarily being better.

Although optimal dietary intake of zinc stimulates the immune system and might help in the prevention of the common cold, excessive intake of zinc—that is 150 mg to 200 mg (the RDA for zinc is 12 mg per day)—might suppress certain immune processes and increase a person's susceptibility to colds and infection.

Putting It All Together: Dietary Recommendations

The Healthy Woman's Diet is the foundation for nutritional prevention and management of the common cold. In addition, you should make sure that your diet contains optimal amounts of the vitamins and minerals essential for maintaining a strong immune system. (See pages 244–49 for more information on nutrition and the immune system, and chapter 5 for guidelines on choosing a vitamin-mineral supplement.)

Extra nutritional insurance in the form of a moderate-dose vitamin C supplement also might help prevent or curb the severity and/or duration of the common cold. For maximum effectiveness take a low-dose vitamin C supplement (or better yet, drink a glass of orange juice) every two hours after the first sign of a cold and throughout the duration of the infection. Orange juice, oranges, and other citrus fruits high in vitamin C have an added advantage in that they also contain compounds called bioflavonoids that might help stimulate the immune system.

Other health habits that help prevent the common cold and aid in a speedy recovery include effective stress management, relaxation, seven to eight hours of sleep each night, six to seven glasses of water daily, staying warm, increasing the moisture in the air with a vaporizer or humidifier, and possibly taking an aspirin at night to relieve aches and pains.

Consult a physician if the cold lasts more than ten days, if symptoms show that the infection has spread beyond the nose and throat, or if you are susceptible to bronchitis or ear infections. Earaches, pain in the face or forehead, a temperature exceeding 102 degrees Fahrenheit, persistent hoarseness or sore throat, shortness of breath and wheeziness, and/or a dry, painful cough are symptoms that require immediate medical attention.

Cuts, Scratches, Bruises, and Burns

In most cases the healing of a wound requires a complex interplay of numerous body systems, including the immune system, the circulatory system, and cellular mechanisms responsible for the repair of damaged tissue and the growth of new tissue. Nutrition plays a fundamental role in each of these processes.

Nutrition and Wounds

Nutritional needs for healing minor cuts and bruises are probably not different from those needed for maintaining health. However, even marginal deficiencies of some nutrients, such as vitamin C and zinc, which are relatively common in some segments of the population, can interfere with optimal recovery from everyday tissue damage, including athletic injuries, minor burns and cuts, or even sunburn. Nutrient needs before and following surgery increase to meet the demands of stress and wound healing. Supplementing the diet with pantothenic acid (a B vitamin) prior to and after surgery improves tissue strength and speeds the healing of wounds. In contrast, poor healing of skin ulcers is associated with low blood levels of several trace minerals, such as zinc.

In general, all nutrients related to the immune function (see pages 244–49), the antioxidant system (see pages 240–44), and circulation, including protein, iron, the B vitamins, vitamin C, vitamin E, calcium, copper, and zinc, are needed in moderate amounts for optimal healing of cuts, burns, and bruises. In addition, several of these nutrients also function directly in the healing process.

PROTEIN

When tissues are damaged, the body rallies several systems to repair and build new ones. This process is called anabolism. Since skin and underlying tissues are composed primarily of protein, optimal dietary intake is essential for quick and complete healing of cuts, scrapes, burns, and other injuries. Trauma and disease also increase protein requirements above normal needs. Consumption of high-quality protein, such as milk, meat, fish, chicken, or a combination of grains and legumes, is necessary to ensure production of specific tissue proteins or other nitrogen-containing compounds during healing and recovery from surgery or minor wounds.

VITAMIN A

The most well defined role of vitamin A (and its building block, beta carotene) is to maintain healthy epithelial tissues of the skin, eyes, lungs, stomach, and other internal and external body surfaces. For years vitamin A was called the "anti-infection" vitamin because it promotes the healing of infected tissues. More important, vitamin A maintains healthy skin so that it is less susceptible to infection and damage. (See pages 376–77 for more information on nutrition and skin cancer.)

VITAMIN E

Limited evidence shows that vitamin E might be important in wound healing. One study reported that vitamin E supplements reduced free radical damage to tissues, including skin grafts. Other studies have reported that vitamin E is helpful in recovering from burns and other wounds.

VITAMIN C

Skin, blood vessel walls, and all body tissues are held together by connective tissue, of which collagen is a major component. Repairing tissues includes producing and laying down new connective tissue and collagen, and vitamin C is a critical factor in collagen formation. In fact, most symptoms of scurvy, the classic deficiency syndrome associated with vitamin C, relate to the vitamin's role in collagen production. Small dotlike bruises under the skin, called petechial hemorrhages, swollen and bleeding gums, slow wound healing, poorly formed scars that break open, scaly skin, and tender joints are symptoms of vitamin C deficiency. Despite the ease in meeting even Recommended Dietary Allowance levels of 60 mg per day, many people consume inadequate amounts of vitamin C, thus potentially interfering with the healing process.

ZINC

A common symptom of zinc deficiency is poor wound healing, probably caused by the defective production of collagen. In addition, trauma such as burns or surgery increases zinc loss in the urine, thus increasing the possibility of poor wound healing. Marginal zinc intake during healthy times has been reported in children, teenagers, pregnant women, seniors, vegetarians, athletes, and people following low-calorie diets. In addition, zinc deficiency is common during sickness and hospitalization.

Although increased intake of zinc either through dietary or supplemental sources is recommended to improve healing and recovery from injury, caution should be used in overdosing. Intakes in excess of 50 mg could result in secondary deficiencies of other trace minerals, such as copper, or possibly in lower HDL-cholesterol, thus placing a person at increased risk of developing heart disease.

OTHER DIETARY FACTORS

Many other substances help in wound healing. For example, garlic has antifungal and antibacterial properties that help combat infection. The juice of the aloe vera plant, when applied topically, is also effective in speeding the healing of cuts, burns, and other minor injuries.

Putting It All Together: Dietary Recommendations

Dietary treatment of severe burns, surgical incisions, and other major wounds requires medical management, including supervision by a dietitian and a physician. Minor cuts, burns, and bruises are most likely to heal quickly and completely if the dietary guidelines outlined in chapter 1 are followed. In addition you should do the following:

1. Consume two to three servings daily of high-quality protein. The typical American diet supplies two to three times normal dietary protein needs and would be more than adequate to meet the extra temporary demands during recovery and repair of damaged tissues. Protein supplements are not needed unless you are recovering from major burns or surgery.
2. Consume two to three servings daily of vitamin C–rich foods and dark green leafy vegetables; beta carotene–rich foods such as orange vegetables; and vitamin E–rich foods such as wheat germ.
3. Consume several servings daily of zinc-rich foods. A supplement containing zinc in doses less than 30 mg might be necessary if dietary intake falls short of recommended amounts. Although zinc is best absorbed from lean meat, supplemental zinc is also well absorbed.

Other life-style habits that encourage optimal immune and circulatory function—effective stress management, regular sleep patterns, daily exercise, avoidance of tobacco, and limited intake of alcohol—also will help in the healing process.

Diabetes

There are two types of diabetes: Type I, also called insulin dependent (IDDM) or juvenile-onset diabetes, and Type II, also called non–insulin dependent (NIDDM) or adult-onset diabetes. IDDM usually begins in childhood, starts suddenly, develops severe symptoms, and requires insulin. NIDDM begins in the adult years. The progression of the disease is slow, with its symptoms mild at first, and it often progresses undetected. It is frequently controlled with a weight-loss diet and life-style modification.

Diabetics are unable to use and metabolize dietary carbohydrates. Consequently, blood sugar levels are elevated (hyperglycemia), and there is an abnormal amount of sugar in the urine. In the diabetic, blood sugar cannot enter the cells at the normal rate. The body cells are starved for energy while blood sugar levels reach abnormally high levels and sugar spills into the urine through the kidneys. Diabetics are at increased risk of other life-threatening diseases—heart disease, blindness, stroke, and gangrene.

Nutrition and Diabetes

Diet is essential in the prevention, treatment, and control of diabetes. Optimal nutrition can help improve overall health, maintain a desirable body weight, stabilize blood sugar levels, and prevent or delay the development of cardiovascular disease, kidney disease, and eye and nerve disorders. The most important aspects of the diet plan are the control of carbohydrate, protein, and fat intake and the maintenance of a balanced calorie intake. Maintaining a desirable weight on the high-fiber, low-fat Healthy Woman's Diet can reduce the need for medication and the risk of secondary diseases in patients with either NIDDM or IDDM. Vitamin and mineral intakes also contribute to the prevention of the disease and provide a second line of defense.

BODY WEIGHT

Being overweight is a primary contributor to the development of NIDDM. More than three out of four diabetics are overweight. In many cases blood sugar stabilizes or returns to normal when a woman loses weight without any other dietary change.

CARBOHYDRATES, PROTEIN, AND FAT

A high complex carbohydrate diet, including whole grain breads and cereals, vegetables, cooked dried beans and peas, potatoes, and other unrefined starches, with moderate amounts of protein and low amounts of fat, is beneficial in the control of diabetes. Complex carbohydrates help maintain optimal insulin use so that blood sugar is easily moved from the blood into the cells. This produces a gradual rise in blood sugar as opposed to refined carbohydrates and sugars that produce a rapid rise in blood sugar levels.

In addition, certain starchy foods produce different blood sugar responses. This effect is called the "glycemic index" of food. The index was developed by comparing the rise in blood sugar after a specific food was eaten. Pure sugar received a score of 100, and other sugary or starchy foods are compared to that. Cooked dried beans and peas produced some of the lowest scores (that is, the smallest rise in blood sugar).

Since most people do not consume one food at a time but instead eat meals containing a variety of foods, the usefulness of the glycemic index has been questioned. In all probability, most important to diabetic control is consuming a variety of complex carbohydrate foods in conjunction with some protein and fat. (See table on page 309.)

Certain forms of fiber also slow the rise in blood sugar after a meal, aid in the maintenance of normal blood sugar levels, and reduce the amount of sugar excreted in the urine. Oat bran, the fiber in cooked dried beans and peas, guar gum, and pectin in fruits are especially effective in the control of blood sugar levels; however, consumption of all fiber foods, including the fiber in whole grain breads and cereals and in vegetables, is encouraged.

Fish oils and monounsaturated fats, such as olive oil, are two types of fat that might help to prevent or control diabetes. Increased supplemental or dietary intake of fish oils increases the concentration of these fats in the pancreas, blood, and muscles, helps regulate blood sugar levels, and reduces the risk of developing heart disease and high blood pressure. Within one month of replacing meat and dairy fats (saturated fats) with monounsaturated fats in their diets, diabetics at

A Partial List of the Glycemic Index

A high score on the glycemic index reflects a rapid rise in blood sugar when a food is consumed. A low score reflects a modest rise in blood sugar.

PERCENT	FOOD
100	Sugar
80 to 90	Carrots, corn flakes, honey, parsnips, potatoes
70 to 79	Whole wheat bread, white rice
60 to 69	Bananas, white bread, raisins, brown rice
50 to 59	Oatmeal muffins, frozen peas, spaghetti, corn, yams, potato chips
40 to 49	Navy beans, oranges, orange juice, dried peas
30 to 39	Apples, chick-peas, milk, tomato soup, yogurt, ice cream
20 to 29	Kidney beans, lentils, fructose
10 to 19	Soybeans, peanuts

Texas Southwestern Medical Center in Dallas showed increased HDL-cholesterol levels, lower blood sugar levels, reduced insulin requirements, and decreased triglyceride levels.

VITAMIN C
Adequate intake of vitamin C might help regulate blood sugar levels and aid in the prevention of diabetes. Diabetics show altered vitamin C metabolism and low tissue levels of the vitamin. This might partially explain why some immune functions are suppressed in diabetics. Caution must be used when diabetics supplement with vitamin C, however, since vitamin C even in moderate doses of 250 mg might interfere with the urinary test for glucose.

VITAMIN E
Inadequate dietary intake of vitamin E alters blood sugar levels, whereas increased intake of vitamin E lowers elevated blood sugar levels in some diabetics. Diabetics and those at risk for developing diabetes often have low blood vitamin E levels, which suggests that the disease alters how the body uses vitamin E. There is limited evidence that the progression of atherosclerosis in diabetics might be slowed when vitamin E is increased in the diet.

NIACIN

Diabetics with IDDM might benefit from niacin supplementation, according to researchers at the University Hospital in Marseilles, France. Their study showed that supplementing the diets of newly diagnosed diabetics with niacin (as nicotin-amide) reduced the amount of insulin needed to control blood sugar; some patients discontinued insulin and remained in remission for at least one year. Niacin therapy should always be monitored closely by a physician since in large amounts this vitamin causes liver damage.

CHROMIUM

The trace mineral chromium is a component of glucose tolerance factor, a compound made in the body that works with the hormone insulin to move sugar out of the blood and into the body's cells. Chromium is, therefore, essential for blood sugar regulation, while a deficiency of this trace mineral results in insulin insensitivity and elevated blood sugar levels. In fact, a chromium deficiency resembles diabetes, including elevated insulin in the blood, numbness in the toes and fingers, increased blood sugar, glucose intolerance, and reduced muscle strength and coordination. These symptoms disappear with chromium supplementation in some people.

Increasing chromium intake sometimes produces dramatic effects on blood sugar regulation in chromium-deficient diabetics; however, increasing intake has no effect on someone who already consumes a chromium-rich diet. More than 90 percent of diets in the United States are low in chromium, according to Dr. Richard Anderson at the U.S.D.A. Human Nutrition Research Center in Beltsville, Maryland. You may be particularly susceptible to marginal chromium intake if your diet is high in fat, refined carbohydrates such as white bread and ready-to-eat cereals, and sugar.

MAGNESIUM

Magnesium metabolism is altered in diabetics and might contribute to the development and progression of the disease. Not only is magnesium deficiency one of the most common disturbances in mineral metabolism observed in diabetics, but low blood magnesium levels are associated with many complications of diabetes, including heart disease and high blood pressure.

Magnesium functions in more than three hundred processes related to carbohydrate, protein, and fat metabolism and is involved in the regulation of insulin and blood sugar regulation. Magnesium supplementation restores low blood and tissue levels, helps correct glucose intolerance, produces a protective effect against heart disease, and might aid in the prevention of eye disorders associated with diabetes and possibly even the progression of the disease.

OTHER MINERALS

Even marginal deficiencies of copper, manganese, and zinc might contribute to abnormal blood sugar regulation and the development or progression of diabetes and its health complications. In addition, deficiencies of these mineral have been identified in diabetics. Urinary losses are often increased, and blood levels are low in uncontrolled diabetes. Zinc is a component of insulin and might aid in insulin regulation. A zinc deficiency also impairs immune function, which would contribute to increased infection, leg ulcers, and other problems in diabetics. Copper and manganese deficiencies are associated with abnormal blood sugar regulation, which is reversed when dietary or supplemental intake of these minerals is increased.

Putting It All Together: Dietary Recommendations

Inconsistency of responses to nutritional therapy among diabetics is probably caused by the individual nature of the disease and each woman's unique nutritional status. For example, it is likely that only those women who are deficient in a mineral will respond to its addition to the diet. On the other hand, the prevalence of marginal nutrient intakes warrants consideration of many dietary factors in the control and prevention of diabetes.

The primary goal in the dietary management of diabetes, both IDDM and NIDDM, is control of blood sugar levels within the narrow range of 60 mg to 160 mg of sugar per deciliter of blood at least 80 percent of the time. Work closely with a physician and dietitian to establish a high-fiber, low-fat diet and exercise program that balances blood sugar and food intake with exercise and body weight. The Healthy Woman's Diet can form the foundation of this individualized nutrition program.

Vitamin and mineral deficiencies are common in NIDDM diabetics. If the calorie intake is below 2,000 calories, a multiple vitamin-mineral supplement that contains all the vitamins and most of the minerals, especially chromium, copper, magnesium, manganese, and zinc, in amounts approaching 100 percent of the U.S. RDA should provide adequate intake of these nutrients. Cooking in stainless-steel cookware also increases the chromium content of the diet; however, if the cookware also contains nickel, this toxic metal can leach into foods.

THE EXCHANGE LISTS

The Diabetic Exchange Lists developed by the American Diabetes Association and the American Dietetic Association are the most widely used system for menu planning. They group foods into seven lists according to calorie, protein, carbohydrate, and fat content.

The term "exchange" refers to a serving of food that can be exchanged for any other food within the same list. The total calorie content of the diet, based on the number of servings from each list, depends on preferences, metabolic needs, and physical activity. The glycemic index was not considered when these lists were developed; however, you can combine the exchange lists with the Glycemic Index and choose those foods within each list that have a score of 50 percent or less. (See table below.)

The American Diabetes Association recommends the following percentages based on total calories: 50 percent to 60 percent carbohydrates, 15 percent to 20 percent protein, and 25 percent to 30 percent fat. For example, a diet that supplies

The Diabetic Exchange Lists

LIST	CARBOHYDRATE (GM)	PROTEIN (GM)	FAT (GM)	CALORIES
1. Milk, nonfat	12	8	Trace	90
low-fat	12	8	5	120
whole	12	8	10	165
2. Vegetable	5	2	0	25
3. Fruit	15	0	0	60
4. Bread/starch	15	3	Trace	80
5. Meat /protein				
low-fat	0	7	3	55
medium-fat	0	7	5	75
high-fat	0	7	8	100
6. Fat	0	0	5	45
7. Free foods	0	0	0	0

2,500 calories would contain no more than 83 grams of fat (2,500 times .30 divided by 9 calories per gram of fat equals 83 grams of fat). Once the calories and grams of carbohydrate, protein, and fat are determined, then the exchange lists are used to make food selections and plan menus. Meal and snack intake must coordinate with insulin administration to guarantee the optimal balance between insulin and blood sugar levels. Vegetarian diets are also effective in the treatment of diabetes and can be designed using the same dietary guidelines and exchange lists.

"DIABETIC" FOODS

Special foods are not necessary since the diabetic can enjoy the same wide variety of foods that are available to the nondiabetic. However, sugary foods prepared with table sugar, dextrose, corn syrup, "natural" sugars, turbinado, or brown sugar should be limited or avoided. Xylitol is a well tolerated sweetener for diabetics, but it must be limited to less than 60 grams per day since it can be converted to glucose (sugar).

No sugar substitute is risk free, and none is an effective aid for weight loss. Aspartame (NutraSweet or Equal) produces a variety of symptoms from headaches to seizures in some sensitive people but is considered relatively safe when consumed in moderation.

LIFE-STYLE AND DIABETES

Aerobic exercise, such as brisk walking, aerobic dance, jumping rope, swimming, jogging, or stationary or outdoor bicycling, performed three to four times a week for twenty minutes or more under the supervision of a physician and a trained exercise physiologist, lowers blood sugar, body weight, and body fat, and reduces the diabetic's risk of developing heart disease.

Endometriosis

Endometriosis is a condition in which fragments of the lining of the uterus (endometrium) develop in other areas, such as the ovaries, the fallopian tubes, the intestine, or the vagina. Each month these fragments bleed like the lining of the uterus, but because they are attached to other tissues, the blood cannot escape. As a result, blood blisters and cysts form that can irritate and scar the surrounding tissue.

Endometriosis is most commonly seen in women between the ages of twenty-five and forty, especially those who have not had children.

Symptoms vary and usually go unnoticed, making diagnosis difficult. When symptoms do occur, they might include abdominal, pelvic, or back pain during menstruation; heavy menstrual flow; aggravated symptoms of Premenstrual syndrome; or painful intercourse. Although most cases are not serious, in some women the condition can progress and result in infertility and reproductive dysfunction.

The causes of endometriosis are poorly understood. The condition might be partly inherited. Women with a short cycle length (less than twenty-seven days), long flow length (more than seven days), fluctuating menstrual cycle lengths, and/or early onset of the menstrual cycle are more prone to developing endometriosis. Endometriosis and another disorder called pelvic inflammatory disease are also more common in women who have used intrauterine devices. This condition also has been linked to immunity since abnormalities in immune responses have been noted in women with endometriosis.

Nutrition and Endometriosis

Little is known about how diet affects the development or progression of endometriosis. One study on rabbits showed that fish oil supplements altered the activity of hormonelike substances called prostaglandins and reduced the growth and spread of endometriosis. No studies have been conducted on humans.

The link between endometriosis risk and suppression of the immune system suggests that a strong immune system might help defend the body against the abnormal cell growth. If this were the case, then all nutrients related to a well-functioning immune system would be involved indirectly in the prevention and control of endometriosis. (See pages 244–49 for more information on nutrition and the immune system.)

Putting It All Together: Dietary Recommendations

Surgical or hormonal therapies are often used to remove the abnormal growths and control future spread of the endometrial fragments. In addition, the Healthy Woman's Diet supplies all the nutrients associated with a strong immune defense and will help strengthen a woman's resistance to disease and infection.

Women who exercise are also at reduced risk of developing endometriosis, possibly because of lower amounts of the female hormone estrogen. Protection is greatest when regular exercise is started at a young age and is continued throughout life.

Eyes and Vision

The link between diet and the development and progression of eye disease has been the subject of numerous studies. For example, a vitamin B1 deficiency results in abnormal eye movements that could interfere with vision. A deficiency of vitamin B2 causes teary or bloodshot eyes, blurred vision, and burning or itching of the eyes. Poor vision is also a symptom of vitamin B12 deficiency and is reversible when dietary intake improves. Finally, the omega-3 fatty acids in fish oils are suspected of being essential nutrients in the formation of healthy eye tissue. A strong and consistent association has recently been found between antioxidant status and the incidence and severity of cataracts, and possibly macular degeneration.

Cataracts: An Overview

The lens of the eye must remain clear to focus light on the retina. As a person ages, an opaque, cloudy area can occur on the lens. This opacification, or cataract, blocks or distorts light entering the eye and progressively reduces vision. The main symptom of cataracts is a slow deterioration of vision in the affected eye(s), with the lens becoming visibly opaque or white in the latter stages.

The primary cause of cataracts was thought to be old age since the majority of people over the age of seventy-five develop cataracts, and many age-related injuries or debilities are associated with damage and accumulation of proteins that cloud the lens. However, many young people also develop the condition. Interestingly, in lesser-developed nations, cataracts occur more frequently in younger segments of the population, suggesting that factors other than age might play a critical role in the genesis and progression.

FREE RADICALS, ANTIOXIDANTS, AND CATARACTS

The formation of cataracts probably involves a number of physiological factors. However, a high correlation between cataract incidence and solar radiation, as well as the known cataract-producing effects of oxygen, suggests that free radical exposure results in a cascade of toxic reactions leading to cataract. (See pages 240–44 for more information on free radicals and antioxidants.)

It is well accepted that exposure to free radicals causes many of the changes in lens proteins throughout life. Proteins within the lens are damaged, probably by repeated exposure to ultraviolet (UV) light and oxygen. These modifications might lead to the formation of protein "clumps" that scatter light and contribute to the development of cataracts. The lens takes the brunt of this exposure since one of its prime functions is to serve as an optical filter so that the amount of UV light received by the retina is greatly minimized. However, this filtering process also subjects the lens to constant exposure to free radicals and potential free radical damage.

Diets rich in antioxidant nutrients might reduce the risk of certain types of cataracts by counteracting the harmful effects of free radicals. For example, studies of the effect of vitamin C on light-induced cataracts and of vitamin E and beta carotene on cataracts induced by various toxic agents repeatedly show a protective effect on either the formation or the progression of cataracts.

People with cataracts consume significantly less beta carotene and vitamin C, less vitamin E, and/or less than four servings a day of fresh fruits and vegetables compared to healthy people. A 50 percent to 70 percent reduction in risk of developing cataracts has been reported when people consume diets rich in carotenoids (the beta carotene–like compounds in dark green and orange vegetables) and vitamins C and E.

VITAMIN C

Some of the highest concentrations of vitamin C in the body are found in various fluids and tissues of the eyes. In humans, the vitamin C content of the eye is twenty times greater than the blood. Interestingly, nocturnal animals with little exposure to UV light have very low concentrations of vitamin C in eye tissue, while diurnal animals have up to thirty-five times the vitamin C in ocular tissues. This phenomenon suggests that a high vitamin C concentration protects the eyes against solar radiation.

Women with cataracts have lower levels of this antioxidant nutrient in eye tissue than women who are cataract-free. Higher vitamin C status, especially among women who have supplemented their diets for years, diminishes the risk of developing various forms of cataracts. But does dietary intake raise vitamin C levels in the eye?

Antioxidant nutrients are found in eye tissue in relation to levels consumed in the diet. A study conducted at the U.S.D.A. Human Nutrition Research Center on Aging at Tufts University reported that supplementation with vitamin C raised eye concentrations of the vitamin. Subjects scheduled for cataract surgery were given either 2 grams of vitamin C or a placebo daily for at least two weeks. At the time of the operations, samples revealed that vitamin C concentrations in blood and lens tissues of the supplemented group were significantly higher than the placebo group even though the placebo group consumed more than twice the RDA of 60 mg of vitamin C in their daily diets. The results of this study suggested that dietary intake of vitamin C might not be adequate to prevent cataract formation, while supplementation might raise eye concentrations to higher levels.

VITAMIN E

Studies show that people with high blood levels of at least two of the three antioxidant vitamins (such as vitamin C, vitamin E, and beta carotene) were at reduced risk of developing cataracts compared with those whose diets were low in two or more of these nutrients. Cataract risk is reduced by as much as 56 percent when people supplement their diets with vitamin E. It appears that vitamin E cannot prevent cataracts, but optimal intake of the vitamin might delay the onset and slow the progression of lens damage associated with them.

Macular Degeneration

Macular degeneration is a disease affecting the retina, the light-sensitive area at the back of the eye that transmits visual impressions from the lens to the brain. Older persons with light-colored eyes are particularly susceptible, as are people who smoke or are frequently exposed to harsh sunlight. However, anyone can develop macular degeneration.

The antioxidant nutrients might counteract some of the harmful processes associated with macular degeneration, thus helping to prevent damage to the retina. The eye has one of the richest stores of selenium. This trace mineral, along with zinc and iron, maintains optimal eye function and protects the eyes from free radical damage. However, the research is preliminary, and additional studies on the role of the antioxidants in the prevention of macular degeneration must be conducted before dietary recommendations can be made.

Zinc has also been linked to the prevention of macular degeneration. A zinc-dependent enzyme that is necessary for normal eye function slows down with age.

Zinc supplements help maintain normal enzyme function and slow the rate of vision loss in people with age-related macular degeneration.

Vision and Nutrition

The best defined function of vitamin A and its building block, beta carotene, is in vision. Vitamin A maintains the cornea—the outer covering of the eye—and enhances night vision. A deficiency of vitamin A results in inflammation of the eye (called xerophthalmia) and night blindness, a condition in which the eye does not adapt quickly to a change from brightness to darkness and the person is "blinded" for several moments after exposure to bright lights.

Putting It All Together: Dietary Recommendations

In short, prolonged exposure to free radicals, not aging per se, is likely to be a primary cause of cataracts. Although the research is in the early stages, optimal intake of zinc and the antioxidant nutrients, especially vitamins C and E, beta carotene, and selenium, might help prevent or slow the progress of eye disorders such as cataracts and macular degeneration.

In some studies a vitamin-rich diet containing four or more servings daily of fresh fruits and vegetables was sufficient to reduce cataract risk. However, other studies show that supplemental doses of vitamin C (500 mg to 1,000 mg) and vitamin E (200 IU to 400 IU) might be necessary to provide maximum protection. Selenium and zinc produce adverse effects when consumed in large doses, so limit daily intake to no more than 200 mcg and 30 mg, respectively, unless monitored by a physician.

In addition to the antioxidant nutrients, optimal intake of the B vitamins, vitamin A or beta carotene, and several servings weekly of fish might help in the prevention and/or treatment of some eye disorders. Limiting or avoiding exposure to free radicals in tobacco smoke, air pollution, and sunlight might also help in the prevention of cataracts.

Fatigue

Fatigue, tiredness, and lethargy are common symptoms of numerous emotional, mental, and physical problems. Stress, poor sleeping habits, overwork, infection, and disease are only a few of the causes of fatigue. A person also may feel "not up to par" because of marginal nutrient deficiencies. (Also see Chronic Fatigue Syndrome on pages 299–301.)

Nutrition and Fatigue

Inadequate intake of any nutrient can cause fatigue. Protein and/or calorie malnutrition results in a number of symptoms, including lethargy and apathy. This condition is rare in the United States but is seen in women with eating disorders, hospitalized patients, and the elderly. A compromised immune system resulting from marginal deficiencies of one or more nutrients also lowers a person's energy level and increases the risk of fatigue, infection, and disease. (See pages 244–49 for more information on nutrition and immunity.)

In addition, poor dietary choices such as grabbing a candy bar for quick energy can affect your energy level. The jolt of energy from a high-sugar food is a temporary high, but within ninety minutes the elevated blood sugar levels are countered by insulin and often fall to below normal levels, leaving you feeling more tired than before the snack.

The combined effect of coffee and doughnuts (or any sugary food) escalates blood sugar problems since caffeine also stimulates the flow of insulin. In contrast, alcohol has a numbing effect on the nervous system, causing drowsiness and apathy. Alcohol and caffeine also interfere with a good night's sleep, resulting in fatigue. Mild dehydration can also cause fatigue and weakness.

VITAMINS

Deficiencies in vitamins E, B2, B6, B12, and C, folic acid, or biotin result in anemia with symptoms of fatigue, poor concentration, apathy, and being out of breath after minor exertion. Many of the B vitamins are vital contributors to the production of energy in the body. It is not surprising that even a marginal deficiency of one or more of these nutrients results in general fatigue, muscle fatigue, and weakness.

MINERALS

A deficiency of one or more minerals results in fatigue because a malnourished body has less energy to complete normal daily tasks and because of direct effects on metabolism and nerve function. A magnesium deficiency causes muscle weakness and fatigue, possibly because of the mineral's roles in converting carbohydrates, protein, and fats into energy; removing toxic substances from the body; nerve transmission; and muscle contraction and relaxation.

Overt magnesium deficiencies are rare in this country; however, many Americans consume less than the RDA levels and are at risk for marginal deficiencies. Life-style factors, such as physical or emotional stress, that are also associated with fatigue, increase urinary loss of magnesium and further increase the need for this mineral.

Although very rare, a sodium deficiency caused by starvation, severe fasting, vomiting, or chronic diarrhea results in weakness, dehydration, and fatigue. Inadequate intake of potassium, chloride, and manganese also causes fatigue and muscle weakness. Deficiencies of cobalt, copper, or selenium result in anemia, which is associated with fatigue, poor concentration, and general weakness. As a component of the thyroid hormones, iodine helps regulate metabolism. Inadequate intake of this mineral results in goiter, with symptoms of lethargy.

Iron gives red blood cells their ability to transport oxygen to all the body's tissues, including the muscles, brain, nervous system, and organs. Inadequate iron intake results in reduced oxygen supply to the tissues, which causes fatigue, weakness, breathlessness after minor physical effort, and poor concentration.

Anemia is the final stage of iron deficiency. You do not have to be anemic, with low hemoglobin or hematocrit blood levels, to experience fatigue. Iron depletion in the tissues prior to any symptoms of anemia also affects energy levels.

Finally, zinc is an essential component of numerous enzymes and functions in the metabolism of protein and the conversion of calorie-containing nutrients to energy. Zinc helps regulate insulin metabolism and blood sugar levels, strengthen the immune system, and maintain normal red blood cell levels. A deficiency of this trace mineral results in anemia and general weakness.

Excessive intake of several essential minerals and toxic metals is also associated with weakness and fatigue. Weakness and lethargy have been associated with cadmium, lead, and aluminum intake. Cadmium enters the food supply when soft water dissolves and washes away the metal from pipes and from cigarette smoke and air pollution. Lead causes nerve damage and is ingested in a variety of sources, including water, lead-based paint, plants grown in lead-contaminated soil, lead-glazed pottery, and air pollution.

Aluminum is toxic to the nervous system and produces nerve damage, of which fatigue is one of the symptoms. Sources of aluminum include antacids and other medications (always read the label), food additives, table salt that contains aluminum additives, and white flour with potassium alum. Even vaginal douches and lipsticks contain aluminum. Cooking in aluminum cookware and coffee pots also contributes to dietary intake; the metal leaches from the pot into the food or beverage. The newer the pot and the longer the cooking time, the higher the aluminum content of the food.

Putting It All Together: Dietary Recommendations

The Healthy Woman's Diet with low-fat, nutrient-dense foods to total at least 2,000 calories is the best protection against diet-induced fatigue. In addition, consume at least six to eight glasses of water daily, even when not thirsty. Since thirst is a poor indicator of water needs, a general guideline for water intake is to drink twice as much water as quenches thirst.

Limit caffeine intake to two cups or less each day, and do not drink caffeinated beverages after midday. Avoid alcohol and sugary foods, and divide the total food intake into four or more small meals throughout the day to maintain normal blood sugar levels.

Make sure to eat breakfast even if not hungry. Not eating in the morning can result in reduced blood sugar levels (and fatigue), which do not return to normal even after eating later in the day. Avoid large or high-fat meals that can leave you drowsy. Finally, include moderate daily aerobic exercise (such as brisk walking, jogging, swimming, and aerobic dance), relaxation, and stress management in the daily routine. Often, energy levels improve with exercise.

Poor dietary habits is one of many causes of fatigue. If the fatigue lingers despite improvements in diet, exercise, and stress management, consult a physician to rule out other causes of chronic tiredness. (Also see Hypoglycemia on pages 344–47, Insomnia on pages 347–49, and Stress on pages 378–81.)

Fertility

Your ability to maintain a regular menstrual cycle, become pregnant, and carry a healthy baby to term is directly and indirectly related to your nutritional status and body weight. Overeating results in obesity, which interferes with ovulation and menstruation and reduces the chances of pregnancy. Even moderate weight loss in the obese woman often restores ovulation and fertility.

The onset and maintenance of menstruation depends on maintaining a desirable weight and a certain amount of essential body fat. Overconcern with being thin, fit, and lean can result in severe calorie restriction and abnormal eating habits, including bingeing, bulimia, and anorexia, which can interfere with normal menstruation and fertility.

Poor nutrition shortens a woman's reproductive life span by producing a late menses and an early menopause. Even if the poorly nourished woman becomes pregnant, she has a high risk of miscarriage or stillbirth. While the pencil-thin body of a model might be attractive for a fashion magazine, it is dangerous for the woman who wishes to maintain her health and fertility or desires a healthy, well-developed baby and a low-risk pregnancy.

Nutrition and Fertility

All aspects of nutrition relate to fertility since optimal health is essential for reproductive function.

PROTEIN, FAT AND CALORIES

Inadequate intake of any of the major nutrients adversely affects reproductive function. For example, inadequate intake of linoleic acid, the essential fatty acid found in safflower oil and other vegetable oils, results in infertility.

VITAMINS

All the vitamins are essential for optimal health and the normal functioning of all body systems, including the reproductive system. For example, vitamin A maintains healthy epithelial tissue that lines all the external and internal surfaces of the body, including the lining of the vagina and uterus. In contrast, vitamin A toxicity from high-dose supplementation results in amenorrhea. One study reported that excessive intake of beta carotene might aggravate menstrual disorders and increase the risk of amenorrhea, which is reversed when beta carotene intake returns to normal. This link between beta carotene and menstrual dysfunction has not been consistently confirmed by other studies.

Vitamin D performs an indirect role in fertility by its effect on the formation of the pelvic bones in women. In fact, the misconception that women should restrict weight gain during pregnancy originated from the days when vitamin D–deficient women with poorly formed pelvises often died giving birth to full-sized babies, while low-birth-weight babies were easier for these malnourished women to deliver.

Although vitamin E does improve fertility in some animals, it has no direct effect on fertility in humans. However, this antioxidant vitamin does affect the production and activity of hormone-like substances in the body called prostaglandins that in turn influence reproduction.

Deficiencies in any of the B vitamins result in lethargy, loss of appetite, and altered hormone metabolism that might indirectly affect reproductive function. For example, folic acid deficiency might result in infertility. In several case studies, women who consumed folic acid–poor diets and who had been unable to get pregnant became pregnant within months of increasing folic acid intake. Supplementation with folic acid prior to conception might also reduce the risk of giving birth to babies with birth defects, including neural tube defects and spina bifida.

Optimal intake of vitamin C might aid in fertility, while excessive vitamin C intake might reduce fertility. In testimonials of vitamin C intake, some women reported that their chances of conceiving were improved by the consumption of up to 1,000 mg of vitamin C. In contrast, some women reported that taking amounts greater than this for long periods resulted in fertility problems. These reports are more "hearsay" than research, and it should be emphasized that the periods prior to conception and during pregnancy are not times to experiment with large supplemental doses of vitamins or minerals or to follow restrictive diets.

MINERALS

Several mineral deficiencies are associated with impaired fertility. Inadequate intake of manganese-rich foods such as spinach, whole grain breads and cereals, and cooked dried beans and peas results in infertility, as does a potassium deficiency. Poor dietary intake of zinc-rich foods, such as oysters, turkey, lean meats, and wheat germ, also increases the risk of sterility, birth defects, delayed sexual maturation, and other reproductive disorders. And while little is known about the trace element vanadium, a deficiency does cause infertility in animals. Dietary sources of this element include whole grain breads and cereals, nuts, root vegetables, fish, and liver.

Putting It All Together: Dietary Recommendations

The best dietary advice for maintaining fertility and maximizing the chances of becoming pregnant is to follow the Healthy Woman's Diet. Maintain a desirable weight with at least 15 percent body fat but not more than 30 percent if possible. Obese women who are infertile or are experiencing amenorrhea should consult their physicians and dietitians about slowly and safely losing a moderate amount of weight. (See chapter 7 for weight-management guidelines.)

The diet should contain at least 100 percent, but not more than 300 percent, of the RDA for all vitamins and minerals and a reliable source of linoleic acid, such as one to two tablespoons daily of safflower oil. Well-balanced vegetarian diets can provide adequate nutrients and calories, but if poorly planned, they can alter female hormone levels and might cause decreased ovulation and infertility.

Avoid excessive exercise that places extreme physical stress on the body and lowers body fat to levels below what is needed to maintain normal menstrual function. Menstrual disorders are frequently reported in athletic women. Even some recreational exercisers have reduced levels of the female hormone progesterone, although the consequences of this are unknown.

Also, avoid alcohol and cigarette smoke, and combine relaxation and effective stress management in the daily routine.

Fibrocystic Breast Disease

Characterized by painful, lumpy breasts, fibrocystic breast disease (FBD) is the most frequent disorder of the breast experienced by premenopausal women. More than 50 percent of all women have obvious signs of FBD; 90 percent have at least the cellular changes associated with the condition. Peak incidence is in women in their forties.

There are three stages of FBD: In the first, which usually develops between the late teens and early thirties, a few lumps are present, and the breasts are tender and full for approximately one week prior to menstruation. In the second stage, which usually develops in the mid-thirties to early forties, the pain intensifies and continues longer. The breasts also might develop a granular or nodular consistency. A woman at this stage often consults a physician for fear the lumps might be cancer. In the third stage, which develops during the late forties and fifties, the discomfort is more diffuse and pain often develops suddenly. Lumps may cluster, and even the slightest touch can be painful.

More than twenty-seven names are used for FBD, including benign breast disease, mammary dysplasia, and cystic mastalgia. FBD is actually an umbrella term for any condition characterized by cyclical changes in the breasts accompanied by lumps, cysts, and pain. Specific names for the condition are based on the type of breast tissue involved, such as the milk ducts, the glands, or other tissue. FBD is such a vague diagnosis, with consequences ranging from none to breast cancer, that the American Cancer Society's National Task Force on Breast Cancer Control discourages the word "disease" and recommends the terms "fibrocystic changes" and "fibrocystic condition."

The cause of FBD is unknown, although an association with hormones is suspected. This theory is supported by findings that oral contraceptives relieve the symptoms of FBD in as many as 85 percent of women. It is unknown, however, whether the association between hormones and FBD is caused by abnormal production of hormones or by exaggerated responses in breast tissue to the hormones. The pain experienced is probably caused by nerve irritation secondary to fluid accumulation (edema). Nerve pinching, the accumulation of tough fibrous tissue (fibrosis), and an associated inflammatory response to the fibrocystic changes also could produce pain and tenderness.

FBD AND BREAST CANCER: IS THERE A LINK?

Since the 1940s, numerous research studies have reported a link between FBD and breast cancer. Both diseases are associated with abnormal hormone metabolism, especially estrogen and progesterone. In addition, the two frequently coexist, which supports a relationship. This relationship is partially explained, however, by the difficulty in detecting a suspicious mass among the background lumps of FBD, consequently delaying or confusing the diagnosis of cancer. Recently, more refined research methods show this link is dependent on the woman's family history of breast disease and the type of cysts, their content, and possibly the number and frequency of development.

In reality, FBD precedes the development of breast cancer by about ten to fifteen years, and only one in every eleven women with FBD develops breast cancer. However, a woman with the wrong type of FBD has a five to nine times greater risk than does a woman with other types of FBD.

The Cancer Committee of the College of American Pathologists has stated that the type of fibrocystic changes must be specified by a biopsy. Women with tissue changes called atypical hyperplasia with borderline lesions (that is, cancerlike cells are observed under a microscope but there are not enough to make a diagnosis of cancer) have a five times greater risk of developing breast cancer. Women with tissue changes called hyperplasia (increased numbers of cells) derived from a specialized cell type in the breast called epithelial cells are one and a half to two times more likely to develop breast cancer, especially if those cells are located in the milk ducts. (A family history of breast cancer raises the risk even higher.) All other types of cysts have little or no association with breast cancer.

Nutrition and Fibrocystic Breast Disease

How and even if diet affects FBD is uncertain. Other life-style factors, such as lean body weight, high socioeconomic status, and advanced education, show a slight positive correlation with the risk of developing FBD. These life-style factors are also related to increased consumption of saturated fats and other harmful dietary substances; however, a direct association between diet and FBD has not been found.

Diets differ between women with FBD and women with breast cancer. Breast cancer patients consume more calories and are heavier; they consume significantly less milk, raw vegetables, pasta, sugar, and butter, and include more poultry, pastry, and margarine in their daily diets. Both FBD and breast cancer patients consume more alcohol and less water than women with no symptoms of breast disorders.

CAFFEINE

In the early 1980s, a researcher at Ohio State University published findings that the consumption of caffeine (or, more specifically, methylxanthines, of which caffeine is an example) was linked to a woman's risk of developing FBD. In these preliminary studies as many as 65 percent of women experienced total disappearance of FBD symptoms when they completely eliminated coffee, tea, chocolate, and other caffeine-containing substances from their diets. However, this research has not been widely accepted because more recent studies have shown little or no association between caffeine consumption and FBD.

VITAMIN E

Early research on vitamin E and FBD produced promising results. However, subsequent studies that were better designed found no consistent association between vitamin E intake and the alleviation of FBD symptoms. Some people apparently do respond favorably to supplemental doses of vitamin E, with improvement in pain, congestion, and tenderness. Interestingly, women in those studies who took a placebo (an inactive pill thought by the subject to be vitamin E) also reported improvement in symptoms, suggesting a possible psychosomatic component to the disorder.

DIETARY FAT

A reduction in dietary fat might help prevent or treat FBD. FBD risk is elevated with increased intake of all fats; however, saturated fats show the strongest association with risk and are dose-related (that is, as saturated fat intake increases, so does FBD risk). When dietary fat is reduced to 20 percent of total calories, some women report a reduction in breast pain, and blood levels of the female hormones estrogen and prolactin decrease. Although a reduction in these hormones is associated with a reduced risk of developing cancer, the link to FBD remains unclear.

Putting It All Together: Dietary Recommendations

To be safe, every woman who notices a solid mass after her menstrual cycle, regardless of what a mammogram shows, should have the tissue biopsied. As many as 15 percent of all palpable breast cancers are not evident on a mammogram, so a biopsy is the only way to determine whether a lump or cyst is cancerous.

Hormone and medication therapy is the most common treatment. Stress also worsens symptoms, so effective stress management is advised.

Until more is known about the link between breast lumps and diet, it is wise to consume the low-fat, nutrient-dense Healthy Woman's Diet that includes fresh fruits and vegetables, cooked dried beans and peas, and whole grain breads and cereals, with a moderate intake of nonfat milk and milk products, fish, and poultry. Avoid or limit saturated fat to no more than 10 percent of calories. Eliminate or limit alcohol consumption as well.

Some women respond favorably to increasing vitamin E intake and eliminating methylxanthine-containing foods such as coffee, cola drinks, and tea. Since there is no harm in testing these dietary changes, a four- to six-month trial might be useful.

Fluid Retention

Fluid retention can result from simple temporary fluctuations in hormones, from excessive intake of salty foods, from malnutrition, or from serious disorders such as congestive heart failure or kidney disease.

Nutrition and Fluid Retention

Edema, or abnormal fluid retention, is a consequence of several severe nutrient deficiencies, including protein and vitamin C. For example, the long-term poor intake of vitamin C results in inadequate production and maintenance of the connective tissue that holds all cells and tissues together. Consequently, the blood vessels, cell membranes, and other barriers that hold fluids in their appropriate spaces become porous, allowing fluids to leak into surrounding tissues and cause swelling. In contrast, excessive intake of some nutrients might also cause fluid retention in some people.

SALT

Do you wake with puffy eyes in the morning? Do your shoes fit too tightly at certain times of the day? Must you wait until afternoon before your rings are loose enough to remove? It is likely your water retention results from eating too much salt. When the diet is high in salt, the body retains fluids in an effort to maintain a constant ratio of water to sodium. Once the sodium dilution becomes normal, then the kidneys excrete the accumulated water along with the sodium. Consequently, the best way to prevent salt-induced fluid retention is to eat a low-salt diet. The best way to treat this condition is to drink more water, which will flush out the sodium.

VITAMIN B6, VITAMIN E, AND GLA

Fluid retention is a common problem in Premenstrual syndrome (PMS). Some studies have reported improvement in PMS-induced swelling with supplements of vitamin B6 or evening primrose oil (a source of the fatty acid GLA), but vitamin E supplements might worsen the condition. In addition, nutrients related to converting GLA to its metabolically active form include magnesium, vitamin B6, zinc, niacin, and vitamin C. However, there is no evidence to indicate that these nutrients decrease fluid retention.

Putting It All Together: Dietary Recommendations

Temporary fluid retention most likely results from excessive salt intake. Eliminating or limiting the intake of salty foods, removing the salt shaker from the table, reducing the amount of salt in recipes, and monitoring other sources of sodium-containing foods and additives will quickly remedy this form of fluid retention.

In addition, you should drink six to eight glasses of water each day. Caffeinated beverages, alcohol, and other "diuretics" could dehydrate the body and interfere with normal sodium excretion; you should therefore use them sparingly and not consider them part of the total fluid intake.

Edema results from protein malnutrition; this condition is rare in the United States, however, because the majority of people eat too much rather than not enough protein. People on very low calorie diets or poorly planned vegetarian diets, hospital patients, and the elderly are at risk for protein malnutrition and are at increased risk of developing a variety of diet-related disorders.

Food Intolerance

One in every three people avoids a food because of related adverse reactions. Considering the millions of known and unknown compounds in foods, both natural and those added during processing and packaging, it is amazing that more people are not affected by food intolerance. It is likely that many symptoms are mild and go unnoticed or the reaction is vague or delayed and is not associated with a particular food.

Reactions to a food are classified as a variety of disorders, including allergies, sensitivities, intolerance, pseudo-intolerance, and idiosyncrasies. Food allergies are rare and result from an immune system response to a food component. Reactions occur within minutes to several hours after consumption of the offending food or may take up to five days to develop. In any case, the symptoms reflect a release of histamine or other physiologically active compounds in the body.

Food sensitivities are a type of allergic response that occur within six to twenty-four hours following ingestion of a food. The reaction may include sweating, faintness, nausea, rapid pulse rate, low blood pressure, confusion, and/or loss of consciousness.

People more commonly misdiagnose a food intolerance as a food allergy. An intolerance to a food results from a genetic defect in a digestive enzyme or other metabolic process that interferes with the digestion or use of a food component.

For example, people with inadequate amounts of the enzyme lactase cannot digest milk sugar, lactose, and are called lactose intolerant. The intestinal gas, bloating, diarrhea, or discomfort that results from drinking milk is not an allergic reaction but the result of undigested sugars that are fermented by intestinal bacteria to form gas. Celiac disease results when a person is unable to digest a protein in wheat flour called gluten. Sensitivities to gluten are also associated with dermatitis and lung disorders.

A pseudo-intolerance or idiosyncrasy is when a food "does not agree" with a person but no physiological reason can be found. In some cases this type of food reaction is psychologically based.

Symptoms of food allergies are restricted to the respiratory tract, the digestive tract, and the skin. Symptoms can be mild to severe, ranging from mild skin redness to anaphylactic reactions. The diagnosis is complicated and requires a diet history, a complete review of a person's medical and symptoms history, and multiple tests conducted by a trained health professional. Self-tests and tests conducted by a nonmedical person, including cytotoxic tests, sublingual tests, and symptom-provocation tests, are not reliable. (See table below.) Although a few studies have shown that vitamin C and fish oils might provide some protection against abnormal inflammatory or allergic responses, the evidence is currently inconclusive.

Symptoms of Food Allergy

RESPIRATORY TRACT		OTHER POSSIBLE SYMPTOMS
Asthma	Cramping and pain	
Rhinitis (inflammation of nasal mucous membranes)	Abdominal discomfort	Anaphylaxis (hypersensitivity)
	Vomiting	Behavioral disorders
	Diarrhea	Epilepsy
	Blood loss in the stool	Arthritis
GASTROINTESTINAL TRACT	SKIN	Ear infections
Swelling or sores of the lips, mouth, tongue	Hives	
Swelling of the throat	Eczema or dermatitis	
Nausea		

Nutrition and Food Intolerance

Any food can cause allergic or adverse reactions; however the most common causes of food allergies are milk, wheat, corn, and eggs. Other common foods include citrus fruits, tomato-based products, shellfish, nuts, fish, and chocolate. Salicylates found in a variety of foods, including grapes, oranges, peanuts, melons, tomatoes, pineapple, apples, pears, nuts, and apricots, also produce allergic-like responses in some people.

ADDITIVES

Most food additives are not associated with food allergies, intolerance, or sensitivities. However, a few additives, such as the sulfiting agents sodium and potassium metasulfite used to keep produce fresh, monosodium glutamate (MSG) used to enhance the flavor of cooked foods, and yellow azo food dyes, produce symptoms in some people. Headaches associated with food sensitivities were reduced by 50 percent in one study when people eliminated all foods containing MSG, yellow dye, yeasts, nitrites, and salicylates from the diet. This suggests that multiple sensitivities might exist in some people.

Sulfites or "whitening agents" have been banned by the Food and Drug Administration for use on fruits and vegetables, and food labels must contain a notice if even "detectable amounts" of this additive are present. Currently, some wine, beer, frozen and dried potatoes, vinegar, cider, maraschino cherries, dried fruits and vegetables, canned seafood soups, baking mixes, seafood such as shrimp, fruit drinks, and colas contain sulfites.

Tartazine or FD&C yellow dye #5 causes allergic reactions in some people. The coloring is difficult to avoid since it is found in a variety of foods, including cake mixes, orange drinks, instant puddings, gelatin, macaroni and cheese dinners, cheese-flavored snacks, and lemon-flavored candy.

Putting It All Together: Dietary Recommendations

Diagnosing food reactions is a complicated process. Allergies are diagnosed differently from intolerances, and different tests are used to identify different food intolerances. For example, lactose intolerance is usually diagnosed by giving a fasting person 50 grams of lactose and measuring blood glucose levels. Celiac disease is often diagnosed by intestinal biopsy and the results of elimination-challenge tests, whereby the gluten-containing foods are first removed from the diet and then are reinstated to observe any adverse effects.

THE FOOD DIARY

Keeping a food and symptom diary is very important. Write down everything you eat and observe any symptoms that develop within the next hour, including tiredness, cramping, stuffy nose, irritability, nausea, sneezing, headaches, or frequent urination. Once the offending food has been identified, the simplest treatment is to avoid that food and use a substitute, such as soy milk for dairy products when it comes to lactose intolerance and gluten-free flour for wheat flour when it comes to celiac disease.

COMBINATION FOODS

Combination foods present another problem since the offending ingredient is not always obvious. If you have lactose intolerance, you should be aware of foods that contain milk products, including breads, biscuits, bologna, some salad dressings, cream sauces and soups, and pancakes. If you are allergic to eggs, you must avoid cream pies, custards, puddings, egg noodles, French toast, many convenience mixes such as pancakes and cookies, Hollandaise sauce, and dumplings.

If you have an intolerance, you must become an avid label reader and familiarize yourself with the composition of all standard foods, such as ketchup, mayonnaise, peanut butter, and ice cream. In addition, you must also consider cross-reactivity. For example, if you are allergic to peanuts, you must be aware of possible reactions to other legumes such as soybeans.

The sensitivity is often not severe, and you may be able to tolerate small amounts of the offending food when combined in a normal diet. For example, if you have lactose intolerance, you may be able to drink small amounts of milk with a meal or eat yogurt or fresh cheese such as cottage cheese and mozzarella. Cooking sometimes deactivates the offending ingredient; raw strawberries may produce symptoms while cooked strawberries do not. Finally, food intolerances often disappear spontaneously, so an offending food might be reintroduced into the diet at a later date without a problem. (See table on page 333.)

THE ELIMINATION DIET

In an avoidance or elimination diet, which is most effective in diagnosing and treating food intolerances and allergies, all suspected foods are excluded. After several days one food is reintroduced, and at intervals foods are reintroduced one

Food Intolerance Symptoms

OFFENDING FOOD	SYMPTOMS
Chocolate, aged cheese, Brewer's yeast, canned fish, red wine	Migraine headaches
Coffee, tea, cola	Nerve disorders
Fermented cheese or foods, pork sausage, sardines, canned tuna	Migraine headaches, skin rash, itching
Food additives	Asthma, headaches, digestive tract problems, itching
Legumes (peanuts, beans)	Flatulence, diarrhea
Monosodium glutamate (MSG)	Asthma, flushing, dizziness, headaches, restless sleep
Strawberries, shellfish, alcohol, pineapple, tomatoes	Eczema, itching, sores on the mouth or tongue
Sulfiting agents	Asthma, fluid retention, nasal congestion, itching

at a time while signs of adverse reactions are noted. A diary of food intake and symptoms is kept, monitoring for changes in energy level, bowel function, headaches, sneezing, watery eyes, gas or abdominal pain, or bloatedness. The final diet is based on all foods that do not cause a reaction.

Designing the diet for food intolerance and allergies is a very individualized process that requires the help of a physician and a dietitian. In contrast, self-diagnosis and designing a restrictive diet is seldom accurate and may result in unnecessary avoidance of nutritious foods.

Hair

Hair, skin, and nails are outer reflections of inner health. Flexible, shiny, vibrant hair is a sign of a healthy, well-nourished body, while dry, dull, lifeless hair is

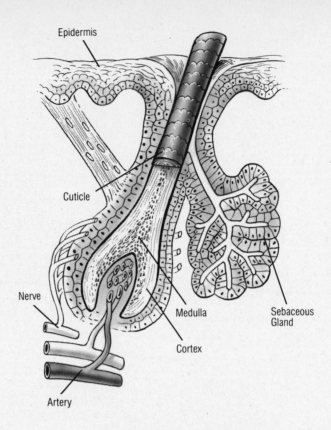

Epidermis

Cuticle

Nerve

Medulla

Sebaceous
Gland

Cortex

Artery

The Hair Shaft and Follicle

a signal of poor nutrition and poor overall health. In fact, hair analysis even uncovers associations between mineral status and physical and emotional disorders.

The hair shaft is composed of three layers: the outer cuticle; the middle, protein-rich cortex; and the inner medulla. Hair color depends on the pigments inside the cortex; an absence of pigments results in white hair. The hair shaft is embedded in a cavity called the follicle, which is surrounded by tiny blood vessels called capillaries that nourish the hair shaft and supply it with oxygen, water, and nutrients. Waste products are also removed via these blood vessels. Oil-secreting glands (called sebaceous glands) also attach to the follicle and secrete "sebum," an oily substance that nourishes and moistens the hair shaft. (See figure above.)

Nutrition and Hair

Almost all of the more than fifty nutrients in the diet are associated with healthy hair, including protein, fat, vitamins, minerals, and water. Nutrients act directly on the growth and maintenance of healthy hair or function indirectly to build a healthy bloodstream that nourishes the hair shaft and follicle.

PROTEIN AND CALORIES

Inadequate intake of either protein or calories results in hair loss and dry, brittle hair. For example, hair loss has been observed in young women with anorexia and in dieters on very low calorie diets that supply insufficient protein or calories to meet minimal daily needs. Protein needs are easily met by following the dietary guidelines outlined in the Healthy Woman's Diet. In fact, Americans in general consume two to three times their protein requirements. Extra protein will not stop hair loss or speed the growth of hair. Instead, it is broken down and either used for energy or stored as body fat.

FAT

The essential dietary fat, linoleic acid, is found in vegetable oils such as safflower oil. Although very rare, a deficiency of this fat or consumption of a fat-free diet can result in reduced oil secretion from the sebaceous glands, causing dry, dull hair. Using oils externally on the hair will not compensate for a poor diet.

VITAMIN A AND BETA CAROTENE

Vitamin A is essential for healthy hair. This fat-soluble vitamin is necessary for normal oil production in the skin and scalp, and optimal intake of either vitamin A or beta carotene helps maintain healthy, shiny hair and scalp. In contrast, a deficiency results in a reddened and sore scalp and hair that is dry and dull. Hair loss and dandruff are common symptoms of vitamin A deficiency. However, vitamin A deficiency is only one of many potential causes of dandruff.

B VITAMINS

The B vitamins associated with healthy hair include B6, B12, folic acid, pantothenic acid, and biotin. For example, certain forms of seborrhea (chronic inflammation of the sebaceous glands that causes overproduction of oil) respond well to vitamin B6. In addition to folic acid and vitamin B12, this B vitamin is essential for optimal red blood cell formation, thus maintaining the oxygen and nutrient supply to the hair. Folic acid and vitamin B12 are also essential for the growth of new hair cells. Consequently, hair growth depends on a constant supply of these B vitamins.

Pantothenic acid is important in the normal growth and color of hair. Limited evidence shows that a deficiency of this B vitamin might result in premature graying of hair. Biotin deficiency, although rare, results in hair loss and dry, dull hair. A protein in raw egg whites called avidin binds to biotin in the intestines and prevents its absorption. A biotin deficiency might develop if several raw eggs were consumed daily. Other causes of biotin or pantothenic acid deficiencies include chronic diarrhea, long-term use of antibiotics, and alcohol abuse.

VITAMIN C

The oil-producing capability of the sebaceous glands depends on adequate vitamin C intake. Inadequate vitamin C results in hair that easily breaks and splits. If the hair breaks just below the surface of the skin, the new hair growing in the follicle will kink and either coil into an abnormal circular pattern or form imperfectly. These hairs are dry, kinky, tangled, and split.

MINERALS

Several minerals are related to the maintenance of healthy hair, including copper, iron, selenium, and zinc. A copper deficiency causes changes or color loss, iron is necessary for optimal blood and oxygen flow to the hair, and hair loss and baldness are signs of either a selenium or a zinc deficiency.

WATER

The most commonly forgotten nutrient necessary for healthy hair is water. Water, the main component of perspiration, is important for keeping skin moisturized and for stimulating the sebaceous glands of the hair follicles to secrete oils that nourish the hair.

Putting It All Together: Dietary Recommendations

Hair problems can result from poor nutrition, although more often the most common problems are caused by other factors such as genetics and the adverse side effects of medications.

In some case, however, hair problems do stem from dietary deficiencies and respond quickly when these deficiencies are remedied. Follow the guidelines for the Healthy Woman's Diet, making sure that your diet contains at least one tablespoon of safflower oil (a source of linoleic acid) and several glasses of water daily. Limit the intake of coffee, tea, alcohol, and other fluids that increase water loss. Consume at least 1,600 to 2,000 calories. Finally, exercise, effective stress management, and regular washing with a mild shampoo help reduce the risk of unnecessary hair problems.

Headaches

Although some headaches are symptoms of other disorders, most headaches occur independently of any other physical problems, develop gradually, and clear up in a few hours with no aftereffects. In other words, most headaches are temporary and are usually brought on by tension, depression, and stress that strains the muscular tissues or blood vessels in the head or neck. Lack of sleep, overeating or overdrinking, noisy or stuffy environments, and strenuous work can also cause temporary headaches.

Migraine headaches are severe, throbbing headaches that are often accompanied by nausea, vomiting, or disturbed vision. Women are more susceptible to migraines than men. Migraines are disabling, intermittent, and last for a few hours to several days. Bright lights may be unbearable, so the person remains in a darkened room or in bed. Migraine headaches tend to occur within families, suggesting there might be a genetic factor to the disorder. In addition, certain foods can cause migraines in some people.

Cluster headaches are a variation on migraines and are more common in men than women. They are characterized by sporadic bouts of extreme pain on one side of the head, typically occurring suddenly during the night. The affected eye is red and watery, and the nostril on the headache side is runny. The headache lasts for several hours and then disappears, only to return within hours. After several days the repeated headaches vanish and may not recur for months or years.

Nutrition and Headaches

Both deficiencies and excesses of certain nutrients can cause headaches. In addition, some food substances can trigger migraine headaches.

VITAMIN A

Large supplemental doses of vitamin A can cause headaches. Signs of toxicity usually develop only after long-term daily intakes exceeding 50,000 IU in adults. Beta carotene, even in large supplemental doses consumed for long periods of time, is not associated with headaches.

B VITAMINS

Marginal deficiencies of many of the B vitamins, such as niacin, folic acid, and pantothenic acid, can produce headaches. A vitamin B1 deficiency is associated with reduced tolerance to pain and heightened pain response. In one study it was found that women who suffered from stress-induced headaches consumed suboptimal amounts of vitamin B1, vitamin B2, and folic acid. In many cases headache symptoms improved with increased intake of these nutrients. (See pages 378–81 for more information on stress and nutrition.)

The use of vitamin B6 in the treatment of migraines is based on the vitamin's role in producing the nerve chemical (called a neurotransmitter) serotonin. If serotonin is involved in migraines, vitamin B6 might increase the pain. In contrast, if migraines are caused by a depletion of serotonin, then vitamin B6 supplementation would help raise serotonin levels and prevent or modify the pain. To date, vitamin B6 has not proven to be consistently effective in causing, preventing, or treating migraines. However, vitamin B6 might benefit women who suffer from tension headaches.

Vitamin B6 was successful in treating headaches associated with Premenstrual syndrome (PMS) in some cases. The treatment appears most effective if taken for five days prior to the onset of PMS. In addition, estrogen-related headaches that occur during the early stages of pregnancy, with the use of postmenopausal estrogen, or with the birth control pill appear to be responsive to vitamin B6 supplementation.

CHOLINE

Choline is a dietary substance found in eggs, liver, meat, wheat germ, and green peas. It is a building block for another neurotransmitter called acetylcholine, which regulates numerous nerve functions. One study reported that choline levels are low in patients who suffer from cluster headaches. Increasing the body's choline content alleviated headache symptoms.

MINERALS

Marginal intake of several minerals, including iron and copper, is associated with increased incidence of headaches.

FOOD COMPONENTS

Several substances in foods trigger headaches and migraines. For example, a compound called tyramine might produce migraines. Tyramine-containing foods include herring, organ meats, aged cheeses, peanuts and peanut butter, fermented sausages such as bologna and pepperoni, chocolate, sauerkraut, and alcoholic beverages. Other foods associated with headaches include milk and cheese, wheat, grapes and raisins, and shellfish.

Phenylethylamine, a compound in chocolate, affects the blood vessels and might produce migraine headaches. Chocolate is more likely to cause headaches than carob, a chocolate-like replacement.

Some food additives, such as monosodium glutamate (MSG) used as a flavor enhancer in Chinese foods and many processed foods, also cause headaches in susceptible people. Nitrites found naturally in foods and used as preservatives in hot dogs and other processed meats have been reported to cause headaches. Finally, some people report increased frequency of headaches when they consume the noncaloric sweetener aspartame (NutraSweet).

Coffee, and possibly tea, is linked to headaches. Some people develop allergiclike symptoms to coffee and tea, including irritability, heart irregularities, and headache. In addition, coffee withdrawal results in headaches that may linger for several days.

FISH OILS

The oils in fish and fish oil capsules might help prevent or treat migraine headaches. Several studies have reported improvements in headache symptoms even in patients unresponsive to medication when fish oil was included in the diet. Although poorly understood, researchers have speculated that fish oils reduce spasms of the cerebral arteries and possibly alter serotonin levels.

Putting it All Together: Dietary Recommendations

Eliminating tyramine-containing foods is the first line of treatment for migraine headaches. If headaches persist after following a tyramine-free diet, then other foods thought to aggravate the condition should be eliminated one at a time to determine the source of the problem. This type of elimination diet should be monitored closely by a physician and/or a dietitian.

For other headaches, you should avoid caffeine-containing beverages, alcohol, and tobacco smoke; eat frequent, small, nutrient-dense meals throughout the day; and obtain regular and adequate sleep. Finally, effective coping skills are also helpful to reduce the stress associated with headaches. Make sure your diet contains at least Recommended Dietary Allowance levels of all vitamins and minerals. Chronic trouble with headaches should be reviewed by a physician.

Additional information on services and educational materials can be obtained from the National Headache Foundation at 800-843-2256 and the American Council for Headache Education at 800-255-ACHE.

Hypertension

More than 61 million Americans have hypertension (high blood pressure). Many of them are unaware they even have the disorder, and only a small percentage have their blood pressure under control through medication and/or diet.

A blood pressure reading contains two figures: the top and higher number (systolic blood pressure) reflects the maximum amount of blood pressure in the arteries when the heart contracts; the bottom and lower number (diastolic blood pressure) is the lowest amount of pressure in the arteries when the heart relaxes between beats. Although hypertension is not a disease, it is an indication of cardiovascular problems and is a major risk factor in the development of atherosclerosis, stroke, and other cardiovascular diseases, as well as kidney failure and hemorrhages in the eye. (See table on page 341.)

Nutrition and Hypertension

In most cases blood pressure drops and even normalizes with changes in diet, exercise, and body weight. In fact, the National Institutes of Health in 1984 released a statement recommending that physicians have their patients try a three- to six-month trial of dietary and behavioral change before they prescribe medication to control hypertension. Antihypertensive medications are a last resort, especially since some of their side effects, such as elevated blood fats and lowered magnesium levels, increase a person's risk of developing heart disease.

Blood Pressure Readings

	SYSTOLIC/DIASTOLIC
Normal	120/80 or less
Mild or borderline hypertension	140/90 to 160/95
Hypertension	160/95 or higher

WEIGHT CONTROL

Some researchers have reported that weight loss has the greatest effect on lowering blood pressure of any nonmedical treatment. Even small amounts of weight loss result in significant reductions in blood pressure. The benefits are directly proportional to the amount of weight lost, while blood pressure tends to increase as a person gains weight.

SODIUM, POTASSIUM, MAGNESIUM, AND CALCIUM

At one time the effect of diet on hypertension was thought to be a simple matter of restricting salt intake. Current understanding of the mechanisms that control blood pressure is that it is much more complex than previously thought, with several minerals (called electrolytes) working as a team.

It is well known that populations that consume salty diets, such as the Japanese and Americans, have a higher incidence of hypertension than societies where salt intake is low. Approximately one-half of all hypertensives are "salt sensitive" and respond favorably when salt (that is, sodium) is restricted.

The average American consumes ten to twenty times the recommended amount of sodium, which would be considered a "megadose" of any other nutrient. The kidneys cannot always keep up with the excessive influx of sodium, so the body tries to minimize the toxic excess by diluting it with water in the blood and cells of the body. A person may be carrying five to ten pounds of excess fluid in the body just to keep the accumulated salt diluted. The expanded blood volume places pressure on the cardiovascular system, and hypertension develops. Diuretic medications force the kidneys to excrete water and sodium at a faster rate, thus reducing blood pressure in some people.

The ratio of potassium to sodium in the diet may be as, or even more, important than sodium alone. The American diet is low in potassium relative to sodium. The body appears to retain sodium and water when potassium intake is low. An increased intake of potassium combined with salt restriction increases sodium excretion, reduces the risk of developing hypertension, lowers blood pressure, and reduces medication requirements.

Low magnesium intake, although not a cause of hypertension, contributes to its development by its direct effect on the blood vessels and by indirectly affecting potassium balance in the body. Approximately 30 percent of those with hypertension consume inadequate amounts of magnesium. In addition, many diuretic medications increase urinary loss of this essential mineral. Low magnesium status results in low potassium levels, which in turn alters sodium and increases blood pressure. In contrast, consumption of magnesium-rich foods or magnesium supplementation often aids in the prevention and treatment of hypertension and other cardiovascular disorders.

Calcium also has an integral role in blood pressure, in part by interacting with sodium, potassium, and magnesium. Increased calcium intake can offset some of the hypertensive effects of sodium, possibly by increasing urinary excretion of sodium. In one study, calcium supplementation (1,000 mg per day for twelve weeks) increased urinary excretion of sodium and consequently reduced both systolic and diastolic blood pressures in women over the age of forty. In contrast, a high-sodium diet increased urinary calcium loss and increased the risk of developing hypertension. Replacing table salt (sodium chloride) with potassium salt halts calcium loss and lowers hypertension risk in women.

Calcium even lowers blood pressure in healthy women with normal blood pressures. Interestingly, low-fat, calcium-rich foods and calcium supplements lower blood pressure, while calcium sources with a higher fat content, such as cheese, do not. In addition, studies on animals have shown that a pregnant mother who consumes ample calcium during pregnancy is less likely to have children who suffer from hypertension. Potassium might also play a role in maintaining normal calcium balance in the body, further showing the interrelationship between these minerals.

VITAMINS

Both a vitamin C–rich diet and vitamin C supplementation are associated with a reduced risk of developing hypertension. In contrast, the diet and blood of hypertensives are often low in vitamin C. Although more research is needed, researchers at the U.S.D.A. Human Nutrition Research Center in Beltsville, Maryland, have recommended vitamin C supplements as a companion to other therapies in the treatment of hypertension.

Limited evidence has shown a link between low dietary intake of vitamin D and an increased risk of hypertension in women. One study of more than three hundred women ages twenty to eighty showed that as vitamin D intake decreased, blood pressure increased, especially in younger women. It is likely that vitamin D has a secondary effect on hypertension by altering calcium absorption and metabolism.

FIBER, FAT, AND SUGAR

A low-fat, low-sugar, high-fiber diet also helps prevent and treat hypertension. A high-fat diet increases the risk of developing hypertension, while a reduction in saturated fat primarily from foods of animal sources and a moderate increase in polyunsaturated fats from vegetable oils, nuts, and seeds reduces blood pressure. Researchers have speculated that polyunsaturated fats are converted to hormone-like substances called prostaglandins that help regulate blood pressure. For the same reason, frequent inclusion of fish in the diet or supplementing with fish oils lowers blood pressure, especially when consumed in conjunction with a low-salt, high-calcium diet.

Fiber helps lower blood pressure, especially when combined with a low-fat diet. In contrast, high-sugar diets raise blood pressure, probably because these diets are low in potassium and other blood pressure–lowering minerals.

Putting It All Together: Dietary Recommendations

Researchers have stated that if fat is reduced to 25 percent or less of total calories, salt is restricted, and a desirable body weight is maintained, hypertension would be controlled or eliminated in 85 percent of all hypertensives without the use of medication.

To restrict salt intake, you should eliminate or curb the use of salt in cooking or at the table. Purchase low-salt foods, avoid processed foods high in salt, and gradually reduce salt in recipes to wean yourself from the salty taste. (See below for more information on reducing salt in the diet.)

The diet should also be high in potassium, magnesium, calcium, vitamin C, and fiber, preferably from dietary sources such as fresh fruits and vegetables, whole grain breads and cereals, cooked dried beans and peas, and low-fat or nonfat milk products. Consuming small amounts or eliminating meat and chicken also helps lower blood pressure. Include two or more servings of fish each week. If the diet is inadequate in calcium and/or magnesium, consider a supplement that supplies these two minerals in a ratio of 2 parts calcium for every 1 to 1.5 parts magnesium (for example, 800 mg calcium and 400 to 500 mg magnesium).

Coffee and tea should be eliminated or consumed in moderation. A few studies have shown an association between tea or coffee intake and increased risk of developing hypertension, possibly because these beverages increase urinary excretion of calcium or contain substances that directly affect blood pressure.

A word of caution about eliminating all salt from the diet: Preliminary evidence has shown that totally eliminating salt from the diet of those without hypertension might alter blood fat and sugar levels and increase the risk of developing heart disease. Thus, the old adage "everything in moderation" holds true even for salt.

Other life-style habits associated with a reduced risk of developing hypertension include reducing alcohol intake to five or fewer drinks a week, reducing stress and competitive behaviors, exercising aerobically (a brisk walk, jog, or swim) four to five days a week, avoiding oral contraceptives, and not smoking. Also, if you are one of those people who have normal blood pressure at home but are hypertensive at the doctor's office, you might learn how to take your blood pressure routinely at home or at work. You can also ask the physician to take several blood pressure readings at different times and average the results. Finally, you should comply with medication and physician instructions if you have been diagnosed as having hypertension.

Hypoglycemia

Hypoglycemia or low blood sugar is not a disease but a symptom of abnormal blood sugar regulation. It is common in diabetes and in other conditions, and is typically characterized by blood sugar levels below 50 mg per 100 deciliters of blood with associated symptoms, including pallor, fatigue, irritability, inability to concentrate, headaches, palpitations, perspiration, anxiety, hunger, and shakiness or internal trembling.

Hypoglycemia has traditionally been divided into two basic categories: reactive hypoglycemia, which develops within three to four hours after a meal, and fasting or organic hypoglycemia, which is characterized by symptoms that develop eight hours or more after a meal. Reactive hypoglycemia results from food intake, especially sugary foods in sensitive people. This condition is sometimes

---

CUT THE SALT

To reduce dietary intake of salt (sodium), use the following foods in moderation:

    Lightly salted seasonings

    Tomato puree and sauce

    Grain products made with small amounts of salt, baking powder, and baking soda

    Packaged mixes for biscuits and muffins

    Lightly salted vegetables

    Canned vegetables

    Fresh shellfish

Use the following foods sparingly:

    Salt

    Soy sauce

    Highly salted seasonings

    Highly salted grain products

    Pretzels, potato chips, corn chips, and other commercial snack foods

    Crackers

    Salted popcorn

    Highly salted vegetables

    Pickled vegetables

    Olives and pickles

    Sauerkraut

    Smoked, cured, or pickled products

    Bacon or other processed meats

    American cheese

    Processed cheese product

---

associated with an increased risk of developing diabetes and reflects a delay in the secretion of insulin, the hormone that regulates blood sugar levels. Fasting hypoglycemia is rare and usually results from other serious conditions such as diabetes, a tumor on the pancreas (the organ that secretes insulin), liver damage, starvation, or cancer.

Many more people complain of hypoglycemiclike symptoms than actually show specific low blood sugar levels on a glucose tolerance test (GTT). In fact, hypoglycemia became a fad in the 1970s when popular books attributed everything from behavior problems and crime to heart disease and allergies to this condition. None of these associations have been verified by well-designed studies. However, although many cases of hypoglycemia are more psychological than physiological, there is more to low blood sugar than was previously thought.

Low blood sugar syndromes develop on a continuum, with very healthy people who occasionally experience a slight decrease in blood sugar with no or mild symptoms at one end and the rare case of fasting hypoglycemia at the other end. In between there are as many variations on blood sugar levels and symptoms as there are people who complain of hypoglycemia.

The GTT should be the definitive test for monitoring blood sugar levels; however, it is inconclusive in the diagnosis of hypoglycemia. For this test a person consumes a sugary drink on an empty stomach, and then blood sugar levels are monitored every half hour. The GTT can produce false positive results since it creates an unrealistic situation—people seldom consume only sugar.

Another test, the meal tolerance test (MTT), provides a more reliable estimate of blood sugar levels and reflects blood sugar response to normal dietary intake. Even in the MTT, however, one person showing low blood sugar levels may exhibit no symptoms, while another person with normal blood sugar levels will report numerous symptoms.

Thus, the traditional definition of "normal" or "low" blood sugar is likely to be arbitrary, with low blood sugar levels affecting different people differently. What is clear is that self-diagnosis and using inadequate procedures such as questionnaires to identify hypoglycemia are unreliable.

Putting It All Together: Dietary Recommendations

The diet for hypoglycemics is similar to that for diabetics. (See pages 311–13.) The low-fat, high-fiber, nutrient-dense Healthy Woman's Diet should be consumed with no more than 30 percent fat calories, no more than 20 percent protein calories, and the rest complex carbohydrates, such as breads, cereals, starchy vegetables, fruits and vegetables, and cooked dried beans and peas.

The soluble fibers found in fruits, vegetables, cooked dried beans and peas, and oats, and in guar gum supplements are especially effective in helping to regulate blood sugar levels. Sugar, sugary foods, caffeine, and alcohol should be avoided. The diet should be divided into six or more mini-meals and snacks throughout the day, with each meal containing some protein, starch, and fiber. This will slow the rate of absorption of dietary sugar and help regulate blood sugar levels.

Supplementation with 200 mcg of chromium has proved beneficial in some cases of hypoglycemia since this trace mineral is essential in insulin metabolism and blood sugar regulation. In addition to consuming chromium-rich foods, cooking in stainless-steel cookware increases the chromium content of food because the mineral leaches from the pot into the food during preparation.

Maintenance of a desirable body weight and daily exercise lasting from at least twenty to forty minutes are also associated with a reduced risk of developing hypoglycemia. Finally, you should avoid overeating in response to hypoglycemic symptoms since this may aggravate blood sugar irregularities.

Insomnia

Insomnia—having difficulty falling or staying asleep or waking too early—is the most common sleep disturbance. Sleep problems usually result from or accompany other life events such as stress, depression, physical discomfort, or medication use. In some cases, however, nutrition might aggravate or cause insomnia.

Nutrition and Insomnia

Deficiencies and excesses of certain vitamins and minerals are associated with insomnia. For example, an inadequate intake of niacin, pantothenic acid, and magnesium have been associated with sleep problems. Vitamin B6 assists in the formation of the neurotransmitter serotonin, which helps regulate sleep. Marginal dietary intake of this B vitamin is associated with insomnia, irritability, and depression. These symptoms disappear when vitamin B6 intake increases. Large doses of vitamin B12 administered with physician supervision have also proven successful in several case studies of people with long-standing sleep disturbances.

Inadequate trace mineral intake might also increase the risk of insomnia. For example, poor copper intake is linked to difficulty falling asleep, longer total sleep time, and feeling less rested after waking. Low iron intake might contribute to increased nighttime wakings and longer total sleep time, possibly because of iron's role in serotonin metabolism. Optimal magnesium intake and avoidance of aluminum-containing foods were associated with high-quality sleep time and few nighttime wakings in one study on women with sleep disorders.

Tryptophan, an amino acid found in protein-rich foods, improves sleep patterns in people suffering from insomnia. Tryptophan is the building block for the neurotransmitter serotonin, which regulates sleep. Increased dietary intake of tryptophan increases blood and brain levels of serotonin, which in turn lowers the time needed to fall asleep by as much as 50 percent and improves the quality and length of time asleep.

For maximum effectiveness, tryptophan must be consumed just prior to bedtime, preferably with a carbohydrate-rich snack such as crackers or a bagel. Although milk and turkey are good sources of tryptophan, they also contain other amino acids that compete with tryptophan for absorption, thus reducing tryptophan's entry into the brain and its conversion to serotonin.

Tryptophan supplements were banned by the Food and Drug Administration (FDA) in 1989 because of reports that they caused a rare disorder called eosinophilia-myalgia syndrome. Although the harmful effects were traced to contaminants in supplements made by the Japanese firm Showa Denko, the FDA ban is still in force.

Putting It All Together: Dietary Recommendations

Several dietary habits might cause or aggravate insomnia. Late-night meals cause the digestive system to work overtime and might result in difficulty falling asleep or staying asleep. Women on very low calorie diets sometimes complain of sleep disorders; eating a light snack prior to bedtime might help alleviate these sleep problems. Spicy, gas-forming, or MSG-laden foods can cause heartburn, digestive tract upsets, or nervous system disturbances that can keep you awake or cause restless sleep. Food allergies can trigger sleep problems, but the only true way to identify allergies is testing by a physician.

No specific dietary recommendations have been identified for sleep disorders. The Healthy Woman's Diet will ensure adequate intake of all vitamins and minerals. In addition, although alcohol might help a person fall asleep, it often results in troubled or restless sleep and should be limited or avoided.

Finally, caffeine might contribute to sleep disorders. You might have trouble getting to sleep and staying asleep even if your last cup of coffee was several hours prior to bedtime. Avoid coffee, tea, colas, and other caffeinated beverages or medications for two weeks to see if sleep habits improve.

Effective stress management and daily exercise also help prevent and treat sleep disorders. Prolonged insomnia should be treated by a physician and might require medication or psychological counseling.

Mood and Emotions

Since the dawn of civilization, people have used food to alter mood. Until recently, however, scientists thought the brain was relatively impermeable to diet and dietary changes. A "blood brain barrier" supposedly shielded the brain from changes in the chemical composition of the blood caused by diet, drugs, or other substances. Science now recognizes that this view was incomplete and concedes what people have known all along: What you eat affects how you feel, think, and act.

Nutrition, Emotions, and Mood

Poor dietary habits are common in people who suffer from depression and other mental disorders. Even marginal nutrient deficiencies are associated with changes in mood and altered brain waves recorded on an EEG. Memory loss, confusion, depression, and other mental disorders, once attributed to aging, can be consequences of poor diet.

NEUROTRANSMITTERS: A REVIEW

Nerves are the fundamental unit of the nervous system. Nerve cells transmit signals throughout the body and are responsible for everything a person thinks, feels, or does. Nerves communicate by releasing different chemicals called neurotransmitters. Some neurotransmitters stimulate nerves and are responsible for increased mental processes. Other neurotransmitters inhibit nerve function and result in relaxation and other calming mental processes. Diet affects the formation and activity of these neurotransmitters by regulating how much of them the body makes.

CARBOHYDRATES, PROTEIN, AND MEAL COMPOSITION

It is no coincidence that women turn to pasta, desserts, and other carbohydrate-rich foods when they feel down in the dumps. Carbohydrates have a profound effect on numerous body chemicals that regulate how a person feels and acts.

Carbohydrate-rich foods increase brain concentrations of an amino acid called tryptophan, which is the building block for the neurotransmitter serotonin. Consequently, increased tryptophan means higher levels of serotonin in the brain, which in turn relieves depression, insomnia, and irritability.

Interestingly, people with Seasonal Affective Disorder (SAD)—an illness characterized by depression, lethargy, and an inability to concentrate combined with episodic bouts of overeating and excessive weight gain—crave carbohydrates during the depressive phase (usually winter) of this illness. Like patients with SAD, many people report increased desire to snack on sweets when they feel depressed or emotionally vulnerable. The"craving" for carbohydrates is often described as "I just need something to calm myself." A more relaxed and clear-headed feeling results from the snack.

In contrast, a high-protein meal such as a ham sandwich or a steak reduces tryptophan and serotonin levels in the brain. Consequently, a woman who eats a high-protein meal for breakfast may crave a carbohydrate-rich mid-morning snack. (See pages 152–55 for more information on food cravings.)

SUGAR HIGHS AND LOWS

Sugar, although a carbohydrate, might affect mood and behavior for other reasons than its effect on serotonin production. It provides an energy boost followed by an energy lull as the hormone insulin reacts to the elevated blood sugar levels and transfers the sugar from the blood into the cells, resulting in fatigue, depression, confusion, or an increase in appetite.

Using sugar to self-regulate mood is a temporary fix. In the long run it could create a vicious cycle: You may relieve the fatigue and feel better for a short while, but the depression and fatigue will return.

A researcher at Texas A&M University reported that some depressed individuals unresponsive to normal psychiatric or medication therapy showed changes in brain waves corresponding to improvements in mood when sugar (and caffeine) were eliminated from the diet. The depression returned when sugar was added back to the diet. As opposed to the temporary sugar high, eliminating sugar and caffeine from the diet is a permanent solution.

In contrast, a researcher at Johns Hopkins University in Baltimore has researched the calming effects of sugar on distressed newborns. These infants quickly stop crying when given small amounts of a diluted sugar solution and the calming effect persists over time, even when the sugar is removed.

This research suggests that sugar affects natural, morphine-like chemicals in the brain called endorphins that ease stress and discomfort. In essence, the sweet taste might stimulate the release of these endorphins and result in a calming effect.

The sugar-endorphin theory has not been tested in adults, but it does provide

The Sugar Content of Selected Foods

FOOD	QUANTITY	SUGAR (TEASPOON)	FOOD	QUANTITY	SUGAR (TEASPOON)
Applesauce	½ cup	2	Ice cream	½ cup	5–6
Apricots, canned	4 halves	3½	Jam, strawberry	1 tablespoon	4
Brownie	2 inches by 2 inches by ¾ inch	3	Jell-O	⅓ cup	4½
			Jelly	1 tablespoon	4–5
			Marmalade	1 tablespoon	4–5
Cake	1 piece	4 to 15	Milk drink, chocolate	1 cup	6
Catsup	2 tablespoons	1½	Milk drink, eggnog	1 cup	4½
Cereals:			Orange drink	6-ounce glass	5½
Instant oatmeal with cinnamon spice	1 serving	4	Peaches, canned in syrup	2 halves	3½
Sugar frosted flakes	1 cup	4	Peanut butter, with sugar added	2 tablespoons	⅓
Lucky Charms	1 cup	3+	Pie, apple	⅙ medium pie	12
Chewing gum	1 stick	½	Pie, pumpkin	⅙ medium pie	10
Cookies, chocolate chip	1	2–3	Pop Tart	1	4
Cool Whip	1 tablespoon	0.23	Salad dressing, blue cheese	1 tablespoon	¼
Cranberry sauce	½ cup	12			
Doughnut, glazed	1	6			
Doughnut, plain	3-inch diameter	4	Sherbet	½ cup	6–8
			Soft drinks, cola	12-ounce can	9
Fruit cocktail	½ cup	5	Sweet roll, plain	1	4
Graham crackers	2	0.9	Syrup, maple	1 tablespoon	2½
Grape drink	6-ounce glass	4	Yogurt, frozen	1 cup	5⅓
Grape juice	6-ounce glass	1	Yogurt, fruited	1 cup	7½
Honey	1 tablespoon	3			

an interesting link among the cravings for sweets in Premenstrual syndrome (PMS), people quitting alcohol or tobacco, and bulimia, the attraction to chocolate during times of stress, and the almost immediate relief from depression, tension, or fatigue. In essence, the craving for sweets might be a craving for the endorphin "high" that calms these people and gives them a sense of well-being. (See table on page 351.)

When to Eat and How Much

Researchers at Texas Technical University studied the effects of different meal compositions on alertness and work performance. The results showed that women who were not carbohydrate cravers were less alert, had trouble concentrating, and felt sleepier after a carbohydrate-rich meal. Carbohydrate-rich meals or snacks produced the opposite effects in carbohydrate cravers, leaving them more alert and less sleepy.

The size of a meal might also affect mood. A big lunch that supplies 1,000 calories or more interferes with mental alertness, especially if you are not accustomed to eating a large midday meal. In contrast, small, low-fat midday meals and snacks improve mental alertness and work performance.

Coffee and Caffeine

Caffeinated beverages are central nervous system stimulants that affect a woman's mood. One to two cups of coffee increase alertness, combat fatigue, and improve performance of work tasks that require detailed attention. Higher doses result in agitation, headaches, nervousness, and decreased ability to concentrate.

In women who do not regularly consume caffeine, even a small dose of caffeine results in irritability, nervousness, and insomnia. In contrast, regular coffee drinkers develop similar symptoms when they are deprived of coffee. Some individuals who suffer from depression and other distress symptoms respond favorably to the removal of caffeine (and sugar) from the diet.

VITAMINS

B vitamin deficiencies, including B1, B2, B6, B12, niacin, and folic acid, and Vitamin C deficiencies are often found in psychiatric patients. In some cases these deficiencies result from poor dietary habits. However, vitamin deficiencies often produce a cycle of depression, uninterest in food or poor eating habits, progressive malnutrition, and increasing mental or emotional disorders, which respond best to a combination of diet and moderate supplementation. Vitamin deficiencies seldom occur alone and are almost always accompanied by inadequate intake of other vitamins, protein, iron, and/or trace minerals.

Even marginal deficiencies of vitamins B1, B2, B6, and niacin are associated with irritability, nervousness, fatigue, mental confusion, depression, memory loss, and emotional instability. Other symptoms include personality changes, dramatic mood changes, insomnia, abnormal EEG readings, and aggressiveness. These deficiencies are common in people who suffer from depression and negative mood patterns. For example, vitamin B6–deficient mothers are less responsive to their newborns and are more apt to have older siblings care for them than mothers who consume optimal amounts of the vitamin. (The babies born to vitamin B6–deficient mothers are more irritable, easily upset, and less consolable than other babies.) Increased dietary intake or supplements often improve depression and stabilize mood, which suggests that B vitamin deficiencies might be the cause of certain forms of depression or mood changes.

Vitamin B12 is essential for the formation and maintenance of the insulation around nerve cells. A long-term deficiency of this B vitamin results in moodiness, confusion, agitation, delusions, dizziness, disorientation, and, in severe cases, permanent nerve damage. A folic acid deficiency is also directly linked to depression and mood changes. Mental illness in the elderly is often attributed not to aging but to poor dietary intake or absorption of one or both of these B vitamins.

In addition, vitamin B12 and folic acid are essential for the formation of all body cells. A deficiency of folic acid or vitamin B12 results in anemia, lethargy, depression, and fatigue, which is treatable with improved diet.

Mental changes associated with vitamin C deficiency include depression and lethargy. Vitamin C is involved in the production of several essential nerve chemicals, which might explain the vitamin's role in mood and behavior.

MINERALS

Both calcium and magnesium are essential for normal nerve function and in neurotransmitter production. Although no association between calcium and behavior has been noted, even marginal magnesium deficiency results in confusion, personality changes, depression, lack of coordination, weakness, and poor concentration.

Poor dietary intake of iron causes anemia and altered brain and nervous system chemistry, which results in mood disorders, lethargy, depression, poor concentration, impaired reasoning and judgment skills, irritability, decreased attention span, apathy, personality changes, and a reduced desire to learn. Iron-deficient children and iron-deficient college students have reduced verbal ability, perform poorly on intelligence tests, and exhibit impaired concentration and memory skills. Even iron-deficient infants who later consume adequate amounts of iron score lower on mental and physical tests than iron-adequate children when they enter school. These findings are consistent with studies on adults, which show that work performance, mood, and memory are impaired when iron intake is suboptimal. (See pages 254–57 for more information on iron.)

In a study conducted at the University College in Wales, people taking selenium supplements (100 mcg per day) showed improved mood and reduced anxiety, fatigue, and depression. As dietary intake of selenium was reduced, reports of anxiety, depression, and fatigue increased. How selenium affects the brain and nervous system is unknown.

While some dietary minerals and metals might play a beneficial role in maintaining healthy emotions and attitudes, other minerals consumed in excess are harmful. For example, excess copper and manganese impair brain function. Lead and mercury poisoning also have profound effects on the nervous system.

Putting It All Together: Dietary Recommendations

Depression and other mood disorders are common symptoms of many physical, emotional, and situational problems unrelated to diet or nutritional studies. In some cases, however, improving dietary habits or choosing a well-balanced vitamin-mineral supplement might improve or even cure a troublesome condition.

Any drastic change in normal eating patterns can alter brain chemistry. Severe dieting, bingeing on sweets, skipping meals such as breakfast, or other abnormal eating habits affect neurotransmitter levels and, consequently, mood and behavior.

The Healthy Woman's Diet is the foundation of dietary management of moods. Consume several small meals or snacks throughout the day rather than

THE "FEELING GOOD" DIET

How a carbohydrate craver plans her daily food intake is slightly different from how other women plan theirs. Carbohydrates give cravers a "boost," but they make other women drowsy. These foods should be included in the day's meal pattern in a way that will enhance energy and work performance.

Meal	Cravers	Noncravers
Breakfast	Cereal and milk, fruit	Egg beaters, toast, fruit
Snack	Cinnamon-raisin bagel and fruit	Peanut butter on bagel, yogurt
Lunch	Linguine and clam sauce, salad, milk	Turkey sandwich, coleslaw, milk
Snack	Pretzels, vegetables, other carbohydrate-rich snacks	Nonfat cheese and crackers, vegetables
Dinner		
If you want to relax:	Meat, vegetable, potato, milk	Spaghetti, bread, salad, fruit juice
If you want to exercise or work:	Same	A light meal with protein and a small amount of carbohydrate

two or three big meals to avoid wide fluctuations in blood sugar and neurotransmitter levels.

Carbohydrate cravers cannot "will away" their cravings, so they should work with them instead. Make sure every meal contains some complex carbohydrate. In addition, plan a carbohydrate-rich snack during that time of the day when most vulnerable to snack attacks, and choose whole grain breads and cereals rather than sugary foods. (See pages 152–55 for more information on food cravings and how to manage them.)

When the diet is not optimal, consider choosing a well-balanced vitamin-mineral supplement. (See chapter 5 for more information on choosing a supplement.) Emphasize tryptophan-enhancing foods such as complex carbohydrates.

You should include regular exercise, coping skills, and a strong social support system in your daily life. Limit or avoid alcohol, cigarettes, and medications that compound emotional problems. Finally, consult a physician if emotional problems persist or interfere long-term with the quality of your life and health.

Muscle Cramps

A cramp is an involuntary, violent, and painful spasm of a muscle. Especially during pregnancy and performing intense exercise, women are likely to experience cramps mostly in the calf muscles, hamstrings, quadriceps, and small muscles of the feet and hands.

Clarifying the type of cramp provides the first clue to the underlying physiological causes and subsequent treatment. A true cramp, or "charley horse," is most common. These cramps are most frequent in people with well-developed muscles. Heat cramps develop when a person performs intense muscular work in a hot environment and perspires profusely. During heat exposure, electrolytes (sodium, potassium, chloride, and other minerals) are lost in perspiration. Muscle pain and spasms may occur, especially in the calves, if these electrolytes are not replaced. Intermittent, painful spasms of the muscles, called tetany, are usually attributed to low calcium levels, but low potassium levels have also produced tetanylike symptoms in individuals. Low blood magnesium levels have also resulted in tremors and seizures.

Until the 1950s cramps were commonly thought to be psychosomatic, occurring primarily in people who were tense, anxious, and insecure, and who fought feelings of anger and guilt. Today, with these wives' tales behind us, researchers suspect that cramps result from overactivity of the nerves sending messages to specific muscle groups. In addition, changes in the fluid outside the cells, such as occurs in dehydration and electrolyte imbalances, or alteration of intracellular metabolites, such as enzymes, can initiate and terminate muscle cramps.

Nutrition and Muscle Cramps

Alterations in tissue mineral levels are linked to all forms of muscle cramps. The minerals and electrolytes that are most likely to affect the muscles are calcium, magnesium, potassium, and some trace minerals. The physiological functions of these minerals are interdependent. For example, low blood magnesium levels often develop when a person is deficient in potassium and/or calcium. In addition, vitamin E shows moderate usefulness in the treatment and prevention of muscle fatigue and cramping.

CALCIUM

Regulation of muscle contraction depends on the presence of calcium, which is stored within the muscle cells. Low calcium levels increase the irritability of the nerves and result in muscle spasms. The condition is called tetany. Increased calcium intake might help alleviate this condition, but the research is inconclusive at this time.

MAGNESIUM

The balance between calcium and magnesium is critical to normal muscle function: Calcium stimulates muscle contraction, while magnesium stimulates muscle relaxation. The two minerals also help regulate nerve transmission and the heartbeat. Inadequate magnesium intake affects all tissues, especially the muscles. Even a marginal deficiency of magnesium can result in tremors, spasms, and weakness of the muscles.

Strenuous exercise alters magnesium concentrations in the muscles and blood, which might affect muscle relaxation and contraction. Blood levels of magnesium are low after endurance exercise, and blood levels remain below preexercise values for as long as several months after a strenuous exercise session. A temporary increase in blood magnesium values following exercise probably reflects magnesium loss from damaged muscle cells. Levels of hormones, such as norepinephrine and epinephrine (adrenaline), rise in response to strenuous exercise, and these hormones also increase urinary loss of magnesium. In addition, muscle concentrations of magnesium can be low despite normal blood concentrations of the mineral. Low blood levels reflect potentially serious tissue depletion of magnesium.

Dietary surveys have shown that self-selected diets often contain less than the RDA levels of magnesium. In addition, current research on magnesium and muscle physiology suggests that RDA levels for magnesium might not be optimal for most people, especially those who exercise. The physical stress of sports training, exercising in the heat, and even the psychological stress of competition increase magnesium losses. High calcium intake with even RDA intakes of magnesium also results in negative magnesium balance.

Dr. Mildred Seelig of the American College of Nutrition in New York states that optimal magnesium intake might be as much as 500 mg per day for a 135-pound woman (current adult RDA is 280 mg), especially if daily calcium intake is less than 1,400 mg. An intake that ranges between 350 mg and 450 mg is probably adequate for nonexercising women who suffer from leg cramps.

POTASSIUM

Potassium is the main electrolyte inside the muscle cells. It maintains nerve and muscle function and normal contraction of the muscles and heart. Muscle spasms, tremors, tetany, heart arrhythmias, and muscle weakness are caused by increased nerve excitability associated with inadequate intake of potassium. Chronic low intake of potassium combined with frequent exercise or work in hot climates could increase a woman's need for potassium.

ZINC

Several cellular components associated with muscle cramping could be susceptible to the harmful effects of free radicals. (See page 240 for an explanation of free radicals and antioxidants.) Free radical activity is higher in zinc-depleted tissues than in tissues with adequate levels of this trace mineral, which places these tissues at risk for damage, cramps, and generalized weakness. Zinc intake is often low, and the physiological demands of both exercise and pregnancy increase the risk of poor zinc status.

Putting It All Together: Dietary Recommendations

Although the exact cause of muscle cramps is unknown, it is likely that cramps result from a variety of factors working independently or in combination. Regardless of the type of muscle cramp, several minerals including calcium, magnesium, potassium, and zinc apparently perform combined roles in the prevention of muscle injury and cramps. You should include several servings daily of foods rich in these minerals. (See chapter 6 for dietary sources of these nutrients.)

General recommendations for preventing muscle cramps include drinking plenty of water and fluids, consuming a high-carbohydrate, nutrient-dense diet, maintaining optimal mineral and electrolyte intake, and frequently and gently stretching the troublesome muscles and/or warming up and cooling down before and after exercise.

Osteoporosis

Osteoporosis is a condition, not a disease, in which the calcium content of the bones is depleted over time to the extent that the bones become brittle, porous, and are likely to fracture with even minimal trauma. In advanced osteoporosis the bones of the spine collapse, giving a woman a stooped posture called "dowager's hump." There are no symptoms of osteoporosis until a fracture occurs, indicating the condition is in the advanced stages with little likelihood of successful treatment.

More than 20 million people are affected by osteoporosis, mostly women over the age of forty-five. Women are especially susceptible to osteoporosis because their bones are smaller than men's, so less calcium can be lost before obvious problems occur. In addition, women are more likely to follow low-calorie diets that supply inadequate amounts of dietary calcium and other nutrients essential for bone maintenance. Women also engage in fewer weight-bearing exercises, which place stress on the bones and help maintain their density.

Nutrition and Osteoporosis

CALCIUM

Calcium plays the primary role in the prevention and treatment of osteoporosis. A woman's greatest bone mass and density (called "peak" bone mass) is reached when she is thirty to forty years old. Prior to this time the best prevention is consuming a calcium- and nutrient-rich diet, plus exercise to maximize bone density.

Shortly after peak bone mass is reached, age-related bone loss begins at a rate of 1 percent per year in women and continues until menopause. Optimal calcium and nutrient intake plus exercise during the childbearing years slows this natural bone loss process. After menopause the loss accelerates and can reach 6 percent per year in the spine. High calcium intake (1,500 mg per day), exercise, and hormone replacement therapy can slow or halt the postmenopausal acceleration of bone loss.

In contrast, osteoporosis is most common in women who consume calcium-poor diets during their early years so that their bones do not reach their maximum density and/or they continue to consume inadequate amounts of calcium during their adult years. For example, calcium is readily lost from the bones when women consume diets that contain 50 percent to 75 percent of the Recommended Dietary Allowances (RDAs), which is typical in the United States. In addition, there is controversy as to whether the RDA levels for calcium are adequate to prevent or treat osteoporosis.

It is never too late to correct a calcium-poor diet, although the more progressed the disease, the longer it may take to strengthen the bones. Unfortunately, nothing can mend the damage caused when osteoporosis is allowed to progress unchecked to advanced stages.

CALCIUM AND POSTMENOPAUSAL WOMEN

The bone density of women after menopause is directly related to their calcium intake. However, the issue is more complicated than just calcium intake and bone strength. The rate of bone loss increases during the first two to five years following the onset of menopause, so the responsiveness of early postmenopausal women to calcium supplementation is different from that of younger or older women.

In studies on early postmenopausal women, calcium supplementation improved bone mineral content and slowed bone loss in some bones but did not entirely prevent the condition. Women who have consumed calcium-poor diets show the greatest improvement in reducing bone loss, whereas women whose diets were optimal in calcium do not show additional benefits when they increase calcium intake. The rate of bone loss in later postmenopausal women is approximately half that of early postmenopausal women; however, optimal calcium intake is still effective in slowing bone loss in these women.

In short, calcium provides a protective effect in the development of bone loss and osteoporosis. Hip fracture risk is reduced by as much as 75 percent in those who consume high-calcium diets, whereas those who consume lowcalcium diets throughout their lives are at high risk of developing bone disorders. In addition, other life-style factors such as alcohol abuse, multiple pregnancies, and avoidance of weight-bearing activity contribute to the development of osteoporosis.

Previous concerns that calcium supplementation might increase a woman's risk of developing kidney stones are unfounded. A recent study found no increases in urinary calcium levels or risk of developing kidney stones in women who consumed 1,100 mg or more of calcium from dietary and supplemental sources.

EXERCISE AND CALCIUM

A sedentary life-style results in substantial bone loss, while weight-bearing and possibly resistance or weight-training exercise increases bone mass and prevents osteoporosis. In fact, the combination of weight-bearing exercise, such as walking and jogging, and calcium supplementation is more effective than calcium alone. Although one study reported that a combination of hormone replacement therapy (HRT) and exercise was most effective in preventing bone loss, the researchers also warned that HRT also produced more side effects.

SALT AND CALCIUM

A salty diet might interfere with calcium retention and increase the risk of developing osteoporosis. Researchers at the National Institute of Health and Nutrition in Tokyo have reported that a high-salt diet increases calcium loss in the urine, which could reduce bone density if prolonged. In contrast, other dietary factors, such as lactose in milk, increase calcium absorption and help prevent osteoporosis.

WHICH CALCIUM SOURCE IS BEST?

Calcium from low-fat and nonfat milk and milk products is the best absorbed source of calcium. Dark green leafy vegetables are excellent sources of calcium, but the mineral is not as well absorbed as it is from milk. Calcium supplements also are best absorbed if taken with milk.

The form of supplemental calcium that is best absorbed and most available for bone metabolism is currently under investigation. Most studies on osteoporosis have used calcium carbonate because it is inexpensive, has a high calcium content, and is well tolerated.

Several studies have shown, however, that people with low stomach acid (a condition called achlorhydria) absorb calcium better from calcium citrate or calcium citrate/malate than from calcium carbonate. Calcium citrate/malate was better absorbed and produced a 44 percent to 47 percent greater increase in bone than calcium carbonate. Calcium citrate is apparently most effective when taken on an empty stomach, whereas carbonate or other forms of supplemental calcium taken with food are well absorbed in most people.

VITAMIN D AND CALCIUM

Vitamin D is essential for maintaining healthy bone tissue. Prior to the overt symptoms of a vitamin D deficiency, such as the bone-crippling disease of osteomalacia, bone fractures increase as much as 40 percent. Vitamin D is also directly related to the prevention and/or development of osteoporosis and is recommended in the treatment of osteoporosis in postmenopausal women.

Vitamin D deficiency might be more common than previously recognized. Sunlight on the skin and diet are two sources of vitamin D, but the relative importance of each is poorly understood. In white postmenopausal women, the population at highest risk for osteoporosis, vitamin D deficiency might result from reduced exposure to sunlight, reduced ability to manufacture vitamin D in the body, and low dietary intake of the vitamin.

For many women, diet fails to provide enough vitamin D to compensate for inadequate sunlight exposure or reduced ability to manufacture vitamin D. Consequently, the use of a supplemental form of the vitamin, in conjunction with calcium and magnesium, might be necessary.

MAGNESIUM

Approximately 60 percent of the body's magnesium is in the bones. Research shows that magnesium affects bone status from conception, and inadequate intake might contribute to the development of osteoporosis. In addition, magnesium and calcium absorption and metabolism are interrelated; consequently, increasing calcium intake without a concurrent increase in magnesium intake can reduce magnesium levels in bone and other tissues.

Women on average consume approximately 200 mg of magnesium each day, or slightly more than half the 1980 Recommended Dietary Allowance (RDA). The adequacy of the 1989 RDAs is also controversial, and Dr. Mildred Seelig of the American College of Nutrition has reported that the RDA of 280 mg for women should be increased to 6 to 8 mg per kilogram of body weight per day or 368 to 490 mg for a 135-pound woman.

OTHER MINERALS: COPPER, FLUORIDE, MANGANESE, AND ZINC

Calcium and magnesium work as a team with other minerals in the maintenance of healthy bones. Inadequate copper intake is associated with calcium loss from the bones, reduced bone formation, and bone deformities.

Fluoride supplementation has produced contradictory results. Fluoride strengthens the crystalline structure of bones and teeth, and women who live in areas where the water is fluoridated have a lower incidence of developing osteoporosis. However, other studies have reported that 80 mg of fluoride daily increases the risk of hairline fractures in the spine of postmenopausal women with osteoporosis.

Manganese is also important in bone growth and metabolism. A deficiency of this trace mineral increases calcium loss from the bone and the risk of fractures. Finally, zinc intake is directly related to bone density; as zinc intake increases (up to RDA levels), bone loss decreases in women of all ages.

Putting It All Together: Dietary Recommendations

The Healthy Woman's Diet forms the foundation for preventing and treating osteoporosis. Consuming this low-fat, nutrient-dense diet with moderate amounts of protein will increase calcium absorption or reduce calcium loss in the urine, thus maximizing calcium availability for bone growth and maintenance.

Calcium intake should be maintained at least at RDA levels of 800 mg to 1,200 mg a day (the Healthy Woman's Diet supplies this amount of calcium) and increased to 1,500 mg during adolescence, when breast-feeding, and after the onset of menopause. (See chapter 6 for other dietary sources of calcium.)

A supplement that contains calcium is recommended for people who are lactose intolerant and do not consume dairy products, and for people who do not routinely consume the recommended three or more servings daily of calcium-rich foods in the Healthy Woman's Diet. As long as the supplement is taken with food there is little difference in the types of supplemental calcium. However, calcium citrate is best for older women with low stomach acid or people who take supplements on an empty stomach.

Researchers at the U.S. Department of Agriculture Human Nutrition Center at Tufts University recommend consuming at least 500 IU of vitamin D daily to reduce bone loss and improve bone density, especially during the winter months when sunlight exposure is limited. Magnesium intake also should be at or above RDA levels and increased if a calcium supplement is taken.

Caffeine, coffee, tea, and alcohol have been suspected of increasing the risk of developing osteoporosis, probably because they increase calcium excretion. A recent investigation of the effects of caffeine on osteoporosis risk showed that moderate caffeine consumption—two cups of coffee or less each day—did not increase the risk of developing osteoporosis. However, high caffeine intake might increase bone loss in elderly women who are already deficient in calcium and might increase their risk of developing osteoporosis.

UP WITH CALCIUM

You can increase your dietary intake of calcium by doing the following:

1. Consume daily two or more servings of calcium-rich vegetables such as collard greens, spinach, broccoli, and kale.
2. Drink three or more glasses of nonfat milk or the equivalent (1 cup of nonfat yogurt, 2 cups of cottage cheese).
3. Add nonfat milk powder to casseroles, soups, cheese sauces, milk shakes, and meatloaf.
4. Cook rice, noodles, oatmeal, and other grains in nonfat milk.
5. Add nonfat milk powder to recipes such as French toast, muffins, breads, mashed potatoes, creamed pies, and dips.
6. Use nonfat condensed milk for cream sauces, gravies, and soup bases.
7. Use nonfat yogurt as a replacement for sour cream.
8. Add nonfat milk powder to nonfat milk.

In addition to diet, avoiding tobacco and increasing weight-bearing exercises such as walking, jogging, and jumping rope are essential for the prevention and treatment of osteoporosis. Since stress increases the loss of magnesium and other minerals in the urine, effective coping skills and relaxation might also be useful in preventing bone deterioration.

Hormone replacement therapy (HRT) is the only therapy that reduces fractures in both the spine and the femur (thigh bone) and is thus likely to remain the therapy of choice for the prevention and treatment of osteoporosis. There is some debate about how long this protection lasts after discontinuation of HRT since a rapid increase in bone loss without HRT could mean treatment must be continued for life. Careful consideration before initiating HRT is essential because this therapy has serious adverse side effects. (See pages 207–8 for more information on HRT.)

Premenstrual Syndrome

Premenstrual syndrome (PMS) is a complex of symptoms that occurs one to fourteen days prior to the onset of menstruation. Symptoms improve once menstruation begins, and there is a symptom-free phase once the period is over. The symptoms vary and include emotional, behavioral, and physical changes.

More than 150 different symptoms have been documented. A woman may have any one or a combination of symptoms, and the symptoms might vary each month depending on life-style changes or stress. For example, stress, a sedentary life-style, and a diet that is high in sugar and refined carbohydrates, salt, fat, and caffeine have an effect on PMS sufferers.

Several researchers have attempted to identify patterns in symptoms. For example, one researcher created eight groupings:

1. Pain: headache, backache, fatigue
2. Poor concentration: forgetfulness, poor motor coordination, confusion
3. Behavioral changes: poor work or school performance, avoidance of social activities
4. Nervous system reactions: dizziness, nausea, cold sweats
5. Water retention: weight gain, swelling, breast tenderness
6. Negative emotions: crying, anxiety, irritability, depression, mood swings, tension
7. Arousal: bursts of energy, excitation
8. Miscellaneous: heart pounding, blurred vision

Another researcher, Dr. Guy Abraham, grouped symptoms into four clusters. These groupings are the basis for the Menstrual Symptom Diary (MSD) used to

Premenstrual Syndrome Clusters

CLUSTER	SYMPTOMS	INCIDENCE (PERCENT)
PMT-A	Nervous tension, irritability, mood swings, anxiety	66
PMT-H	Weight gain, swelling of extremities, breast tenderness, abdominal bloating	65
PMT-C	Headache, sweets cravings, increased appetite, heart pounding, fainting, fatigue, dizziness	24
PMT-D	Depression, forgetfulness, confusion, crying, insomnia	23

The Menstrual Symptoms Diary

Grading of Menses: 0 = none, 1 = slight, 2 = moderate, 3 = heavy, 4 = very heavy

Grading of symptoms: 0 = none, 1 = mild and does not interfere with activities, 2 = moderate but not disabling, 3 = severe and disabling

Day of cycle	1	2	3	4	5	6	7	8	9	10	11	12	13	14	15	16	17	18	19	20	21	22	23	24	25	26	27	28	29	30	31	32	33	34	35	36
Date																																				
Menses																																				

PMT-A

Nervous tension																																				
Mood swings																																				
Irritability																																				
Anxiety																																				

PMT-H

Weight gain																																				
Swelling of extremities																																				
Breast tenderness																																				
Abdominal bloating																																				

PMT-C

Headaches																																				
Craving for sweets																																				
Increased appetite																																				
Heart pounding																																				
Fatigue																																				
Dizziness or fainting																																				

PMT-D

Depression																																				
Forgetfulness																																				
Crying																																				
Confusion																																				
Insomnia																																				

DYSMENORRHEA PAIN

Cramps (low abdominal)																																				
Backache																																				
General aches and pains																																				

Reprinted with the permission of Guy E. Abraham, M.D.

monitor the occurrence and severity of PMS symptoms. Maintaining a diary of body and mood changes is the best way to determine if the symptoms occur during the two weeks prior to menstruation and are associated with PMS. (See table on page 365 and chart on page 366.)

Between 40 percent and 90 percent of women experience PMS on a regular basis, with the greatest percentage occurring during the thirties and forties. For years women were told that these difficulties were "all in their heads." Current research shows, however, that there is a physiological basis for PMS. It is likely that PMS results from a complex of factors, including hormone imbalances, fluid and sodium retention, alterations in neurotransmitters and prostaglandins (hormonelike substances that affect the nervous system and numerous metabolic functions), low blood sugar, and nutritional inadequacies or excesses.

Nutrition and PMS

Numerous dietary factors might contribute to the development or severity of the symptoms of PMS. These include calories, fat, sugar, fiber, and salt intake; food cravings; several vitamins and minerals.

For example, studies have shown that women with PMS consume fewer B vitamins, half as much zinc and iron, one-quarter as much manganese, and more dairy products, salt, sugar, protein, and fat and protein from foods of animal origin. Some women respond to vitamin-mineral supplementation despite normal blood levels of these nutrients. Therefore, higher than RDA levels of certain nutrients might act like a drug rather than a nutrient that corrects simple nutrient deficiencies.

CALORIE INTAKE

Approximately a quarter of women report increased appetite during the premenstrual phase. During this phase women consume as much as 87 percent more calories than at any other time during the month. Hormonal changes coincide with the increased appetite and might be partially responsible. For example, estrogen and progesterone levels are highest when women experience the greatest increase in hunger. In addition, energy expenditure often increases by as much as 11.5 percent during the same phase, which is attributed to the metabolic-stimulating effect of the female hormone progesterone and might explain why some women feel warm and get overheated during the premenstrual phase.

Often accompanying the increase in calories are food cravings, including cravings for carbohydrates, sweets, and/or chocolate. Women with PMS consume as much as twenty teaspoons of sugar daily. PMS-induced depression is linked to fluid retention and increased cravings for sweets and chocolate, and women who do not suffer from depression are also less likely to crave sweets. A high-carbohydrate, low-sugar, low-protein diet during the premenstrual phase sometimes improves the symptoms of depression—anxiety, anger, fatigue, and confusion—while it increases alertness and tranquillity, possibly by increasing the levels of the neurotransmitter serotonin. (See pages 349–56 for more information on food and mood.)

Some researchers have suggested that the craving for chocolate is actually a craving for a compound called phenylethylamine, a substance that stimulates the release of a hormone-like substance called dopamine, which helps regulate mood. (See pages 152–55 and pages 350–52 for more information on food cravings.)

VITAMIN B6

Some women respond favorably to vitamin B6 supplementation during the premenstrual phase. While on the supplement, some women reported significantly less depression, irritability, dizziness, vomiting, headaches, swelling, acne, and fatigue. Interestingly, many women experienced no improvements while in some cases 70 percent of the women taking placebos also reported improvements in symptoms. This suggests a possible psychosomatic component to some women's PMS symptoms that is responsive to any type of therapy the woman believes will work.

VITAMIN E

Vitamin E supplementation (100 IU to 300 IU per day) might improve the PMS symptoms associated with PMT-A, PMT-C, and PMT-D in some women. In contrast, doses greater than 600 IU might aggravate some symptoms of PMS. However, the research linking vitamin E with PMS is conflicting, and prevention or treatment of PMS with this vitamin is considered experimental.

MAGNESIUM

Red blood cell concentrations of magnesium are low in women with PMS, although other blood indices of magnesium are normal. Symptoms of magnesium deficiency resemble those of PMS, including muscle spasms, appetite changes, nausea, personality changes, and apathy. Some researchers have speculated that stress promotes magnesium excretion, which in turn leads to fluid and sodium retention. A magnesium deficiency also reduces brain dopamine levels, which could cause or aggravate PMT-A symptoms.

FIBER, PROTEIN, AND FAT

Elevated estrogen levels might contribute to the symptoms of PMT-A. Dietary fiber helps remove excess estrogen from the body and might help alleviate some of these symptoms.

Reducing the consumption of meat and limiting protein is recommended for some symptoms of PMS. Vegetarian diets are associated with reduced estrogen and progesterone levels during the premenstrual phase and consequently might be helpful in reducing PMS symptoms. (See chapter 3 for information on how to plan a vegetarian diet.)

Some research has shown that limiting dietary fat, especially animal fats, and emphasizing vegetable oils might aid in the regulation of PMS symptoms. Animal fat directly influences blood estrogen levels, and since excess blood estrogen might contribute to PMT-A symptoms, avoiding saturated animal fats might help. Evening primrose oil, which contains vitamin E and a fatty acid called gamma linolenic acid (GLA), might help regulate the production of hormonelike compounds called prostaglandins that affect PMS symptoms such as breast tenderness, irritability, and depression.

Putting It All Together: Dietary Recommendations

PMS is so common and so intertwined with normal fluctuations in a woman's hormones that the condition is more a natural biological and emotional experience than a disease or even a disorder. Dr. Joyce Mills has emphasized that Native Americans view women's cycles as "a source of growth and empowerment" rather than a "curse," which therefore should be appreciated. However, for those women whose lives are seriously affected by PMS or who have developed symptoms because of unhealthful life-style habits, then diet, exercise, or other changes are recommended to curb PMS suffering and improve overall health.

The following dietary recommendations might help reduce PMS symptoms:

- Consume a high-complex carbohydrate diet.
- Limit sugar to less than 10 percent of total calories.

- Limit protein to 15 percent of total calories and limit or avoid protein from animal sources.
- For chocolate cravers, choose moderate amounts of low-fat chocolate foods such as cocoa made with nonfat milk and chocolate cake with no frosting.
- Reduce fat intake to no more than 30 percent of calories.
- Reduce saturated fat to less than 10 percent of calories.
- Include one to two tablespoons of safflower oil in the daily diet.
- Limit salt to minimize fluid retention and swelling.
- Consume several servings daily of fiber-rich foods to ensure a fiber intake ranging between 20 grams and 40 grams.
- Avoid caffeine, especially when anxiety and breast tenderness are problems.
- Consume at least RDA levels of magnesium, iron, and the B-complex vitamins, and no more than 300 IU of vitamin E (RDA is 12 IU).
- Vitamin B6 supplementation (50 to 150 mg per day) started on day ten of the menstrual cycle and continued through day three of the next cycle has produced positive results in some women. The RDA for vitamin B6 is 1.6 mg per day. Vitamin B6 in doses greater than 100 mg a day should be taken only with the supervision of a physician since the vitamin can produce toxic symptoms, including irreversible nerve damage, when consumed in large amounts for extended periods of time.
- Include physical activity in the daily routine.
- Practice effective stress-management techniques.

A physician should be consulted if symptoms intensify or persist since hormone and/or drug therapy might be indicated.

Sexually Transmitted Diseases (STD)

Sexually transmitted diseases, also called venereal diseases, are infections transmitted from one person to another through sexual contact. Examples of STDs include gonorrhea, nonspecific urethritis (NSU), syphilis, herpes genitalis, and genital warts. The vaginal infections trichomoniasis and yeast infection can be transmitted through sexual conduct but are more frequently contracted through nonsexual means. (See pages 382–86 for more information on yeast infections and pages 250–53 for more information on AIDS.)

Nutrition and STDs

The literature is sketchy on how diet affects a woman's risk of contracting an STD. Since maintaining a strong immune system is a primary defense against all forms of infection and disease, it is wise to consume a diet high in the nutrients known to aid in immunity, including the antioxidant nutrients (vitamin C, vitamin E, beta carotene, and selenium), the B vitamins, and the minerals iron, magnesium, and zinc.

One study from the Centers for Disease Control in Atlanta reported that vitamin C inactivated the herpes virus within days of exposure. This study concluded that vitamin C might be an effective antiviral agent in the treatment of both oral and genital herpes. (See pages 244–49 for more information on nutrition and immunity.)

LYSINE AND HERPES

In the 1970s, researchers reported that supplemental doses of the amino acid lysine were effective in reducing the severity and frequency of herpes infections; however, lysine had no effect on preventing the infection. Some people reported that the pain subsided within hours and the herpes sores did not spread when supplements containing between 800 mg and 2 grams of lysine were consumed. In addition, healing normally took six to fifteen days, but with lysine, as many as 83 percent of patients reported their lesions healed in five days or less. Some studies have shown that if the maintenance dose is too small (less than 750 mg per day) or is discontinued, herpes lesions reappear within one to four weeks.

L-lysine is thought to be the only effective form of lysine. Failures with lysine therapy might result from an inadequate dose of the amino acid or using D-lysine, which has no effect on viral growth. Normal dietary intake of lysine is not sufficient to produce the beneficial effects observed in some patients taking supplements.

The theory is that the herpes virus cannot grow in a lysine-rich environment, while another amino acid, arginine, triggers the growth of this virus. Consequently, an arginine-poor diet combined with lysine supplements is recommended for the treatment of herpes infections. Some studies have shown improvements in herpes symptoms in both the lysine-supplemented and the placebo groups, suggesting that a psychological factor exists and a person might be able to "will away" some infections.

Putting It All Together: Dietary Recommendations

The only dietary advice for the prevention and treatment of STDs is to consume a low-fat, nutrient-dense diet such as the Healthy Woman's Diet. This diet supplies ample amounts of all the nutrients known to strengthen the immune system. In addition, supplementation with L-lysine (in doses of 750 mg or higher) combined with avoidance of arginine-containing foods such as nuts, seeds, and chocolate might reduce the frequency or severity of recurrent infections.

Good sleeping habits, relaxation, and effective stress management are important since physical and emotional stress suppress the immune system, which in turn increases a person's susceptibility to infection. Other items that should be avoided include tobacco smoke, alcohol, and caffeinated beverages.

The use of condoms is one way of reducing the risk of contracting an STD (other than abstinence). Inspecting the partner's genitals, routine medical evaluations, as well the use of birth control foams, jellies, or creams might also reduce STD risk. In addition, the more sexual partners a woman has, the higher her risk of contracting an STD.

In all cases, diet plays a minor role in the prevention and treatment of STDs. More important, a physician should be consulted at the first suspicion of infection, and diagnostic tests and medical treatment should be initiated immediately.

Skin

The skin is an outer reflection of a woman's inner health. The skin's cells have a short life span and are replaced every few days; consequently, signs of nutritional deficiencies develop quickly. In contrast, clear, moist, glowing skin is a sign of internal health and optimal nutritional status.

The skin is composed of three layers. The subcutaneous layer is the deepest layer and is primarily fat and a protein called collagen. The corium, or middle layer, shields underlying layers from injury and repairs surrounding layers when they are damaged. The upper portion of this layer has an abundant supply of blood vessels and nerve endings; it is here that wrinkles originate. The epidermis, or top layer, is the thinnest layer of skin. The nails and hair grow from the epidermis.

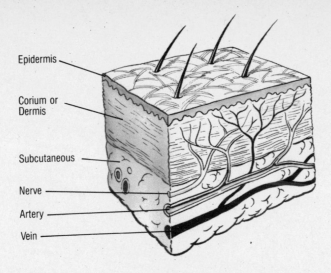

Epidermis

Corium or Dermis

Subcutaneous

Nerve

Artery

Vein

The Layers of the Skin

The skin consists of three layers: the subcutaneous, the corium or dermis (middle layer), and the epidermis (outer layer).

Covering all the layers of the skin is a layer of dead "keratinized" cells that swell in response to moisture and are shed daily. (See figure above.)

Nutrition and the Skin

All nutrients, including calories, protein, fat, vitamins, minerals, and water, play important roles in maintaining healthy skin and in treating many skin disorders. For example, inadequate intake of any nutrient or calories results in reduced blood and oxygen flow to the skin, altered oil secretions within the skin, diminished maintenance and repair of injured tissue, dry skin, alterations in skin color, and limited ability to fight off infections.

ACNE

The primary aid in the prevention and treatment of acne is to keep the skin clean and oil-free. Poor diet suppresses the immune system and increases the risk of skin infections; however, no one dietary component, from chocolate to greasy foods, has been shown to cause acne. Allergic reactions to some foods might cause skin eruptions that resemble acne, and elimination of the aggravating foods will produce immediate results. Sometimes the food can be reintroduced in small doses after several months of abstinence.

A synthetic form of vitamin A called retinoic acid, or 13-cis-retinoic acid, a prescription medication, helps in the treatment of acne but produces some side effects. Unfortunately, dietary vitamin A and beta carotene are not effective in the prevention or treatment of acne. A zinc deficiency might aggravate a preexisting acne condition, and some people report fewer skin sores and reduced oiliness after supplementation with zinc.

The Healthy Woman's Diet plus regular exercise, effective stress management, avoidance of tobacco and alcohol, and moderate exposure to sunlight also help in the prevention and treatment of acne.

AGING

The skin is a blueprint for aging. In youth the skin is soft and smooth. Collagen gives skin its strength and firmness, while elastin in the middle layer of the skin provides resilience. Wrinkles and sagging gradually develop as the skin's elastin and collagen fibers start to deteriorate. The process begins in the thirties, progresses slowly throughout the rest of life, and is escalated by sun damage.

The antioxidant nutrients show promise in slowing the rate of both natural and sun-induced aging of the skin. The antioxidants protect the skin and other tissues from the aging effects of free radicals found in air pollution and tobacco smoke, generated by ultraviolet radiation in sunlight, and produced naturally in the body. Vitamin E helps prevent liver spots and protects the polyunsaturated fats in cell membranes from damage. Consequently, the skin remains more youthful longer. However, the antiaging effects of any dietary substance, if any, are not as potent as the aging effects of sun exposure!

Repeated bouts of weight loss and weight gain also take a toll on the skin, resulting in sagging, stretch marks, and wrinkling. Avoid the yo-yo dieting cycle and "crash diets" by following the guidelines in chapters 1 and 7 for designing a low-fat, nutrient-dense diet that helps maintain a desirable weight.

In addition, regular aerobic exercise improves blood flow and helps nourish the skin, while drinking six to eight glasses of water daily helps to remove cellular waste products and to moisten the skin from within. The use of sunscreens combined with topical application of vitamin C or vitamin E throughout life will have the greatest impact on the prevention of premature aging of the skin.

Finally, you should read the labels on all creams and lotions before using them on your skin. Some products, especially creams sold as "freckle removers," contain mercury, which can penetrate the skin, raise blood levels of this toxic metal, and produce nerve damage.

DERMATITIS

Dermatitis is an umbrella term for any inflammation of the skin and includes symptoms such as rash, itching, burning, dryness, blemishes. Treatment will depend on the cause of the dermatitis; however, many nutrient deficiencies produce dermatitislike symptoms.

A vitamin A deficiency produces bumpy, scaly, rough skin resembling "goose flesh" or "alligator skin." Several B vitamin deficiencies, including vitamin B2, niacin, vitamin B6, vitamin B12, biotin, and pantothenic acid, affect the skin and produce redness, soreness, dryness or excessive oiliness, scaliness, changes in pigmentation, and burning sensations or numbing and tingling of the hands and feet. Small pinpoint bruises under the skin can reflect a vitamin C deficiency, while dry, scaly skin is also a result of inadequate dietary intake of linoleic acid, the essential fatty acid in safflower oil. In all cases these skin abnormalities heal quickly when the deficient nutrient is added back to the diet.

Sometimes dermatitis results from an intolerance to certain food components, such as a protein in wheat called gluten. A physician can assess the foods that might be causing a reaction, and a dietitian can tailor a diet to remove any offending foods.

ECZEMA

Eczema is another skin disorder that includes chronic inflammation and irritation. Eczema is often the result of allergic reactions to pollen, cosmetics, dust, dry air, chemical irritants, or sunburn. Stress and lack of sleep often aggravate the condition. Several nutrient deficiencies produce eczemalike symptoms, including vitamin A, the B vitamins, vitamin C, and linoleic acid. In addition, symptoms sometimes improve when dairy products and eggs are removed from the diet and are replaced with soy-based milk.

ITCHING

Itching is a common symptom of many diseases and other disorders of the body as well as a common side effect of many medications. Chemical irritants, stress, and even exposure to wind and other elements can cause itching. Nutrient deficiencies that might result in skin disorders include vitamin A, vitamin B2, niacin, vitamin B6, vitamin B12, biotin, pantothenic acid, vitamin C, iron, zinc, protein, and the essential fatty acid linoleic acid. In addition, excessive intake of vitamin A, vitamin D, and niacin might also cause itching. Avoiding anything that is drying to the skin, including tobacco smoke, alcohol and caffeine intake, stress, inadequate intake of water, or a dry climate, might help alleviate itching.

PSORIASIS

Psoriasis is a chronic, inflammatory skin condition characterized by dry, red skin patches covered with silvery white scales and with bleeding spots under the sores. The condition might come and go but is usually chronic and is often triggered by stress. Although few dietary practices will effectively alleviate psoriasis in everyone, research studies have reported improvement in symptoms when dietary intake of vitamin D, zinc, or linoleic acid is increased.

Fish oils also show some success in treating psoriasis. Fish oils suppress a group of hormonelike substances called leukotrienes that otherwise trigger inflammation. Increased intake of fish or fish oils lowers blood levels of leukotrienes and halts the inflammatory processes associated with psoriasis. These dietary changes are in addition to following a low-fat, nutrient-dense diet.

SKIN CANCER

One in every four people will develop skin cancer, with women at higher risk than men. Most cases, if caught early, are highly treatable; however, melanoma, the most serious form of skin cancer, and other skin cancers caused approximately nine thousand deaths in 1992. Melanoma was once rare in this country, but its rate is now increasing faster than any other form of cancer. By the year 2000, one in every ninety persons will develop melanoma.

The antioxidant nutrients show promise in the prevention of skin cancer. Applied topically to the skin prior to sun exposure, the antioxidants might help reduce the risk of developing skin cancer.

The greatest risk factors are exposure to the sun and a fair complexion; consequently, the best prevention is avoidance of sun exposure through the use of sunscreens, hats, sunglasses, and clothing. Treatment is most effective if begun early, so watch for the warning signals, including any unusual skin condition and especially a change in the size or color of a mole or other darkly pigmented growth or spot. Scaling, oozing, bleeding, or a change in the appearance of a bump or nodule or a change in sensation, itchiness, tenderness, or pain are also warning signals that you should be checked immediately by a physician.

SUN DAMAGE

The sun does more damage to the skin than anything else. The ultraviolet rays of the sun increase premature aging, wrinkling and sagging, varicose veins, dry skin, liver spots and other pigmentation changes, and the risk of developing skin cancer. The best way to avoid this damage is to limit your exposure to direct sunlight, that is, minimize exposure during the hours of 10 A.M. to 3 P.M.; liberally use a #15 SPF (sun protective factor) or higher sunscreen; and wear hats with large brims, long-sleeved shirts with a tightly woven fabric, long pants, and sunglasses. Use sunscreens even on cloudy or overcast days. (Remember to increase dietary or supplemental vitamin D when avoiding sunlight or using sunscreens.)

The antioxidant nutrients might help avoid some of the harmful effects of sun exposure. Results of several studies have shown that both dietary and topical application of vitamins E and C might be effective in protecting the epidermis against the sun's ultraviolet radiation. Dr. Helen Gunsler at the University of Arizona also reported that vitamin E is an effective sunblock and should be added to sunscreen lotions.

Repeated exposure to sunlight also increases a woman's requirements for beta carotene, according to researchers at Cornell University. In addition, both dietary and topical application of vitamin A and some of its derivatives enhance skin repair after ultraviolet damage and have been used in combination with conventional therapies for the treatment of ultraviolet-damaged skin, skin cancer, and precancerous skin damage.

Putting It All Together: Dietary Recommendations

Skin disorders are as diverse as the factors that cause them. In general, the Healthy Woman's Diet is the best dietary advice for aiding in the prevention and treatment of most skin disorders. Increased fish consumption, because of the fish oils, might help inflammatory skin disorders. The antioxidant nutrients also show promise in helping to prevent excessive damage from the sun, although by far the best recommendation is to avoid sun exposure.

If general skin problems such as itching, dryness, scaly or oily skin, and rashes reflect an underlying nutrient deficiency, then increased intake of the nutrient will produce immediate improvement in symptoms. Any skin condition should be checked by a physician, especially if changes suggest possible skin cancer.

Stress

Stress is integrally related to a woman's mental, emotional, physical, and nutritional well-being. For example, stress and depression suppress the immune system and increase urinary loss of several nutrients that are also essential for optimal immune function. A woman's health and nutritional status has a primary effect on how she handles stress and, consequently, what impact stress has on her health today and in the future. A positive outlook on life, enhanced immunity, effective coping skills, optimal nutrition, and increased resistance to disease are also related. In many cases, stress-related disease is preventable when effective coping skills and guidelines for a low-fat, nutrient-dense diet are followed.

Nutrition and Stress

Nutritional status and stress are closely related. Nutrient deficiencies are stressful to the body, and the nutritional status of the body determines how well it defends itself against the stress of disease. Stress also reduces the absorption and increases the urinary excretion of certain nutrients, potentially producing a nutrient deficiency or aggravating a preexisting one. Stress alters the nervous and hormonal systems of the body, which in turn influence metabolism and dietary requirements for nutrients. Nutrition is also a critical component in the body's immune system. (See pages 244–49 for more information on nutrition and immunity.)

The body's response to stress suppresses the immune system. Nutrient stores are less likely to be depleted and the immune system is less likely to be jeopardized if nutrient intake is optimal prior to, during, and following times of stress. Stress also affects eating habits; some women eat less and some eat more of the wrong types of food, with the result being either malnutrition or obesity. In short, a well-nourished woman is better able to cope than a poorly nourished one.

Stress is an elusive term. No two people respond to the same event or situation in the same way. What is stressful to one person is not stressful to another. Since it is difficult to measure the effects of stress on nutrition, research has focused primarily on definable and observable physical stress, such as intensive exercise and illness. However, preliminary studies have also shown that emotional or psychological stress has a similar impact on nutritional status, with reduced blood levels, increased urinary excretion, and greater than "normal" requirements of certain nutrients.

Researchers at the U.S. Department of Agriculture measured blood mineral levels in people during a five-day period of severe psychological stress. Results showed that despite adequate dietary intake, blood levels of several minerals dropped as much as 33 percent, and there was evidence of tissue depletion of nutrients.

CALORIES AND PROTEIN

Severe physical stress, such as burns, trauma, fever, or surgery, increases the metabolic rate by as much as 55 percent, which increases the need for calories and protein. These requirements remain elevated until the repair process is completed. Calorie and protein needs do not appear to be affected by moderate physical or emotional stress.

VITAMIN C

Both emotional and physical stress affect the status of vitamin C, increasing the amount of dietary vitamin C needed to maintain normal blood levels. In addition, the vitamin C content of stress-related tissues such as the adrenal and pituitary glands is depleted during times of stress. On the other hand, vitamin C is essential for maintaining the immune system.

Consequently, a cycle develops whereby stress depletes vitamin C levels in the body, which in turn reduces the body's resistance to infection and disease and increases the likelihood of further stress. The self-perpetuating spiral continues until the person intervenes and improves her diet. When vitamin C intake is increased, the harmful effects of the stress hormones are reduced, and the body's ability to cope with the stress response improves.

B VITAMINS

Most of the B vitamins function in the development or maintenance of the nervous system. The requirements for B vitamins are based on calorie intake. A marginal deficiency can therefore result from either a vitamin-poor diet or an excessive intake of high-calorie, nutrient-poor foods such as sweets and refined/highly processed foods. The harmful effects of vitamin deficiencies on the nervous system might increase the risk of developing stress-related symptoms such as irritability, lethargy, and depression.

VITAMIN E

Some environmental stressors such as air pollution might increase a person's need for the antioxidant nutrient vitamin E. Ozone reacts with the body's tissues to form highly reactive free radicals. Vitamin E protects lung tissue from free radical damage, thus potentially increasing resistance to disease and possibly cancer. In contrast, inadequate vitamin E levels are associated with increased tissue damage from ozone.

Numerous studies have shown that supplementation with vitamin E above the recommended dietary amounts might be necessary to provide a strong defense against ozone exposure, especially in athletes and people who live in large cities and inhale greater amounts of this damaging compound. (See pages 240–44 for more information on free radicals and antioxidants.)

MAGNESIUM

Stress and magnesium are interrelated. Both physical and psychological stress stimulate the stress hormones, which in turn increase magnesium loss from the cells (especially from the heart and other vital organs), stimulate urinary excretion of magnesium, and increase dietary requirements for the mineral. A magnesium deficiency, on the other hand, increases secretion of the stress hormones, aggravates the stress response, and results in depression and irritability. For example, magnesium-deficient animals are overly sensitive to noise and crowding, while animals that consume more magnesium are better able to cope.

In studies on people, subjects with "type A" personalities (overachievers and those highly stressed) have higher blood levels of the stress hormones and lower magnesium levels than people who are generally more relaxed. Finally, women who cope with stress by eating more sweets also increase their risk of magnesium deficiency since sugar triggers urinary loss of magnesium. Researchers at the American College of Nutrition have recommended magnesium supplementation during times of stress because of increased magnesium loss and elevated requirements.

TRACE MINERALS

Physical stress such as illness, hospitalization, or strenuous exercise increases urinary and/or perspiration loss of many trace minerals, including chromium, copper, iron, and zinc. In addition, blood levels of these minerals are often low in physically stressed individuals. Many of these minerals help regulate the immune function, and even a marginal deficiency could increase the risk of stress-related illness or disease.

Putting It All Together: Dietary Recommendations

People in general are better able to cope with stress when their diets are low in refined carbohydrates (sugar and white breads and cereals) and fat, and high in nutrient-dense foods, such as whole grain breads and cereals, fruits and vegetables, cooked dried beans and peas, and lean or nonfat foods of animal origin.

Caffeine in coffee, colas, tea, and some over-the-counter medications should be eliminated during stressful times. Caffeine increases the secretion of the stress hormones and produces symptoms of anxiety, including nervousness, restlessness, and insomnia, that only aggravate the stress response. You should use decaffeinated beverages, all-roasted grain beverages, fruit juice, or herbal teas. Drink six or more glasses of water daily, and avoid alcohol or consume it in moderation (less than five drinks a week, with one drink equivalent to one beer, one glass of wine, or one ounce of liquor).

A multiple vitamin-mineral supplement that supplies no more than 300 percent of the U.S. RDA for all vitamins and minerals, including the B vitamins, vitamin C, magnesium, and the trace minerals, might also be useful nutritional "insurance." Vitamin E is safe in doses up to 200 IU. A supplement taken in small, multiple doses does increase the absorption and usefulness of the vitamins and minerals, as compared to a one-pill-per-day supplement. For example, magnesium absorption is best at doses of 100 mg or less per meal. Large doses of magnesium have a laxative effect, while frequent small doses are less likely to cause diarrhea. (Magnesium is the active ingredient in Milk of Magnesia!)

Avoid "stress" supplements that contain randomly formulated megadoses of some nutrients and little or none of the others. At best you are wasting your money. At worst, excessive intake of a nutrient could produce toxic effects or result in a secondary deficiency of another nutrient, which might affect the immune function and the body's ability to cope with stress.

Urinary Tract Infections

Urinary tract infections (UTI) or bladder infections are the most common kidney-related disorder. Bladder infections can be caused by congenital obstruction, kidney stones, injury to the urinary tract, or chronic inflammation by bacteria. In the latter, bacteria migrate from the outside of the body, up the urethra, and into the bladder. They can also travel to the kidneys from another part of the body through the bloodstream. Once in the urinary tract, the bacteria multiply and spread, which disrupts normal function and causes inflammation and swelling. If allowed to go untreated, bladder infections can lead to chronic pyelonephritis, a condition in which the kidneys become increasingly damaged by repeated infections.

Symptoms of a bladder infection include pain when urinating, frequent need to urinate, and sometimes blood in the urine. Urethritis is inflammation of the urethra (the tube that leads from the bladder to the outside of the body). The symptoms are similar to a bladder infection, but urethritis usually occurs in women as a result of bruising during sexual intercourse.

Putting It All Together: Dietary Recommendations

The common nutritional therapy for bladder infections is to force fluids—three to four quarts of water daily—and an "acid-ash" diet, which consists of high-protein foods such as meats, fish, eggs, and gelatin products; cranberries, plums, and prunes; and vitamin C supplements. This produces an acidic urine that helps limit bacterial growth.

Vitamin C might also have a direct effect on reducing the growth of bacteria in the urinary tract. Women who have suffered repeated bladder infections say that large amounts of cranberry juice and avoidance of coffee and tea is sometimes an effective treatment.

Although vitamin A is essential for the development and maintenance of a healthy urinary tract, there is no evidence that this vitamin is effective in the prevention or treatment of bladder infections. In addition, large doses of vitamin D can irritate the urinary tract, and there is preliminary evidence that excessive vitamin D intake is linked to kidney stones in people who are susceptible to stone formation.

Always seek immediate medical advice for the treatment of bladder infections and comply with medication use. To prevent bladder infections, you should drink 6 to 8 glasses of fluid daily, wear cotton underwear, urinate regularly, empty the urinary bladder after intercourse, avoid bath salts or bubble bath, and wipe front to back.

Yeast Infections

Candida albicans is a common organism found on the skin; in the mouth, digestive tract, or vagina; and on other areas of the body. Under normal conditions this fungus causes no problems; the numbers are small, are kept in check by harmless bacteria, and do not cause symptoms. The "yeasts" proliferate, and symptoms develop, when conditions change to favor their growth. The result is a yeast infection that causes numerous problems, including vaginitis.

For example, antibiotic medications or feminine hygiene sprays destroy helpful bacteria and allow uncontrolled growth of Candida in the vagina. Pregnancy, diabetes, douching, sexual activity, and taking birth control pills also alter the vaginal environment and favor the growth of yeast, as does a compromised immune system.

Symptoms of Candida albicans growth include itching, a thick white discharge, irritation of the vagina, and swelling or redness of the vulva. Pain or soreness during intercourse and a need to urinate more frequently might also develop. Candida also might trigger nonspecific "allergic" reactions, including histamine release.

Nutrition and Yeast Infections

SUGAR AND FIBER

The role of diet in the development and progression of yeast infections is unclear. A study at the University of Michigan stated that consuming a diet high in concentrated sweets or alcohol increased the urinary loss of sugar and elevated the risk of vaginal Candida infection. Reducing your intake of sugar and dairy products lowers the amount of sugar loss in the urine and results in fewer complaints of yeast infection.

According to the University of Michigan study, a high-fiber diet, in particular insoluble fibers found in whole grains and wheat bran, also increases the risk of Candida infection. Soluble fibers in fruits, vegetables, cooked dried beans and peas, and oats did not affect infection risk.

FISH OILS

Preliminary research has also shown a possible association between fish oils and Candida albicans infection. A fatty acid in fish oils called EPA (eicosapentaenoic acid) reduces inflammation and enhances the body's immune response to counteract the growth of Candida infection.

YOGURT

The old wives' tale that yogurt is useful in the treatment of Candida infections might have merit. In a recent study there was a threefold decrease in Candida infections and a significant reduction in the amount of Candida albicans numbers in the vaginas of women who daily consumed one cup of yogurt containing Lactobacillus acidophilus. This culture does not kill the infection but changes the microbial environment of the vagina to encourage the growth of normal, healthy bacteria. In addition, consuming the live, active cultures found in yogurt enhances specific immune processes and might have a secondary benefit in strengthening a woman's defense against future infections.

YEAST-CONTAINING FOODS

Limited research has also shown a possible connection between the dietary intake of yeast-containing foods and Candida albicans infection. People already at risk for developing an infection, such as those on long-term antibiotic therapy, have unusually high antibodies to yeasts found in baker's and Brewer's yeasts. This hypersensitivity to dietary yeast products might contribute to the development of Candida albicans infections. In some cases recurrent yeast infections have been successfully managed with medication and by reducing the intake of yeast-containing foods.

GARLIC

Garlic has shown some effectiveness in the prevention and treatment of Candida albicans. A component in garlic called allicin is a potent fighter against yeast. Garlic supplements must contain allicin to provide a protective effect. An optimal dose is unknown, although daily inclusion of a clove or two in the normal diet is safe, tolerable, and potentially useful.

VITAMINS

Vaginal yeast infections are associated with impaired immunity. The number and activity of specialized immune cells, called monocytes, is reduced in women who are susceptible to repeated infections of Candida albicans, which might be caused by fluctuations in female hormones, especially progesterone, or other factors that suppress the immune system, including marginal nutrient intake.

Limited research has shown a connection between vitamin status and the risk of Candida infections. Vitamin A helps maintain the lining of the vagina and stimulates immune responses that defend against infection. Vitamin A deficiency has been noted in some women with recurrent vaginitis; however, the evidence is inconclusive whether a deficiency causes or is a result of the infection. Other vitamins found to be low in the diet or blood of women suffering from recurrent yeast infections include vitamin B6, vitamin B2, and biotin.

MINERALS

Magnesium deficiency is sometimes noted in women with Candida albicans infection. How magnesium might affect the development and progression of infection is unknown. Dr. Leo Galland, a member of the World Health Medical Group in New York, has speculated that a magnesium deficiency might reduce resistance to Candida infection or stimulate the release of histamine, which suppresses the immune system. A magnesium deficiency might also be secondary to the marginal intake of vitamin B6. Mild zinc deficiency also might increase a woman's susceptibility to, or contribute to, the development and progression of yeast infections.

Putting It All Together: Dietary Recommendations

The connection between diet and yeast infections remains controversial, and specific dietary recommendations are sketchy at best. Until more is known about how diet affects the risk and development of this type of infection, it is best to consume a low-fat, nutrient-dense diet such as the Healthy Woman's Diet, which supplies ample amounts of all the nutrients associated with a strong immune system.

You should avoid foods that contain sugar, including table sugar, honey, "raw" sugar, or corn syrup, and consume fiber-rich foods such as fruits and vegetables, cooked dried beans and peas, whole grain breads and cereals, and nuts. You should avoid processed fiber foods such as bran cereal. (See pages 244–49 for more information on immunity and nutrition.)

Include one or more servings daily of yogurt that contains the L. acidophilus bacteria. Not all yogurt contains L. acidophilus, while many commercial yogurts include cultures of L. bulgaricus, L. lactis, or S. thermophilus. These bacteria do not establish residency in the intestine or migrate as well into the vagina and do not show the same beneficial effects of L. acidophilus.

In addition, some commercial yogurts claim to have L. acidophilus, but actually contain little or none. The effectiveness of L. acidophilus tablets is controversial; some women report they are effective, while other women must rely on yogurt or bottled refrigerated L. acidophilus liquid. You should research the content of any commercial yogurt to make sure it contains the advertised L. acidophilus. Whether L. acidophilus is consumed from dietary or supplemental sources, moderation remains the rule. More is not necessarily better.

Finally, if the above dietary recommendations combined with medication therapy are not effective, you should try to avoid yeast-containing foods, such as yeasted breads, Brewer's yeast, and pastries made with yeast. There is no need to continue this dietary change if no improvements are noted within a few months.

In addition to dietary changes, you should avoid wearing nylon underwear or panty hose; long hours in tight-fitting clothes such as leotards, bathing suits, and garments made from fabrics that do not breathe naturally; and fabrics that irritate. Instead, you should do the following:

- Wear cotton underwear and polypropylene workout clothes.
- Use a hair dryer on a cool setting to dry the pubic area after a workout or shower.
- Sleep in cotton pajamas to allow air to circulate at night.
- Do not use feminine hygiene sprays or powders, or douche the vaginal area more than once a week.

Expanded Glossary

Acetylcholine: A neurotransmitter associated with the regulation of numerous body processes, including memory.

Achlorhydria: Reduced stomach acid.

Acid: A chemical substance that contains hydrogen and usually tastes sour. Hydrochloric acid in the stomach, vinegar, and acetic acid are examples of acids. An acid has a pH (a measure of acidity) of less than 7.

Acid-Base Balance: The equilibrium between acids and bases (alkaline) in the body.

Acute: Sharp and severe onset of disease.

Additive: A chemical substance added to food, either intentionally or unintentionally.

Adrenaline: A hormone secreted by the adrenal glands that aids in the release of stored sugar in the liver, contraction of muscles, and increased blood supply to the muscles, all in response to stress.

Aerobic: In the presence of oxygen. Aerobic exercise is any slow, steady exercise, such as bicycling, jogging, swimming, or walking, that requires constant long-term use of large muscle groups. Aerobic fitness refers to increased ability to transport oxygen to the tissues and is associated with cardiovascular fitness.

Aerobic Capacity: A measurement of athletic ability, especially endurance sports such as running.

Aflatoxin: A potent cancer-causing mold that can grow on peanuts, corn, and some grains.

Alkaline: A chemical substance called a base that will neutralize an acid to form a salt. Baking soda is an example of an alkaline substance. Alkaline compounds have a pH of more than 7.

Allicin: A substance in garlic that is responsible for garlic's odor, inhibits the growth of bacteria, and strengthens the immune system.

Alliin: A compound in garlic that converts to allicin when garlic is chopped or crushed.

Amenorrhea: Cessation of menstruation.

Amino Acid: A building block or precursor of protein. More than twenty-one amino acids are used by the body to manufacture different proteins in hair, skin, blood, and other tissues.

Anaerobic: High-intensity exercise performed without sufficient oxygen to the tissues. Examples include sprinting, volleyball, football, and other stop-and-start sports.

Anemia: A reduction in the size, number, or color of red blood cells that results in the reduced oxygen-carrying capacity of the blood.

Angina: Chest pain usually associated with reduced oxygen to the heart and heart disease.

Anorexia: The lack or loss of appetite for food, associated with weight loss and muscle wastage. Anorexia nervosa is a condition characterized by self-induced starvation.

Anthropometric: Measurements of the body, including weight, height, and circumferences of various body parts.

Antibody: A substance in body fluids that is a component of the immune system and protects the body against disease and infection.

Antioxidant: A compound produced in the body or a nutrient supplied in the diet that neutralizes harmful substances called free radicals. Examples of antioxidants include vitamin C, vitamin E, beta carotene, and selenium.

Apgar: A numerical score that represents an infant's condition sixty seconds after birth, based on heart rate, respiratory effort, muscle tone, reflex irritability, and color.

Apo B: A protein attached to LDL-cholesterol.

Arginine: An amino acid.

Arrhythmia: Irregular heartbeat.

Arteriosclerosis: A general term for hardening and thickening of the arteries.

Artery: A blood vessel that supplies blood, oxygen, and nutrients to the tissues.

Ascorbic Acid: Vitamin C.

Atherosclerosis: A form of arteriosclerosis characterized by the accumulation of fat in the artery wall. It is the underlying cause of cardiovascular disease.

Atrophic Vaginitis: Infection of the vagina causing a decrease in the amount of normally developed tissue.

Balanced Diet: A diet in which all vitamins, minerals, protein, essential fats, fiber, and other nutrients are supplied in optimal amounts. The typical balanced diet supplies a variety of foods from the Basic Four Food Groups: fruits and vegetables, breads and cereals, low-fat milk products, and extra lean meats, chicken, fish, and cooked dried beans and peas.

Basal Metabolism: Energy used for basic body processes, including the heartbeat and the repair and maintenance of tissues. Also called basal metabolic rate, or BMR.

Beriberi: A disease caused by a deficiency of vitamin B1 and characterized by nerve disorders, weakness, mental disturbances, dermatitis, and heart failure.

Beta Carotene: A building block of vitamin A found in dark green or orange fruits and vegetables. Independent of its vitamin A activity, beta carotene also functions as an antioxidant.

Bile: An emulsifying fluid produced from cholesterol in the liver and stored in the gall bladder to be secreted into the intestine as a digestive acid when fats are present in the diet.

Bioflavonoids: More than two hundred substances, including rutin, hesperidin, and quercetin, found in the peel of citrus fruits, leafy vegetables, red onions, and coffee and thought to enhance vitamin C activity and possibly exert some antioxidant capabilities.

Biological Activity: The potency of a vitamin or mineral within the body.

Biotin: One of the B vitamins that is important in the breakdown of fats, proteins, and carbohydrates for energy.

Blood Cholesterol Levels: These are the best indicators of whether a person will have or has developed heart disease. A total blood cholesterol level greater than 200 mg per deciliter of blood is indicative of elevated risk.

Bulimia: An eating disorder characterized by excessive food intake followed by vomiting, laxative use, or fasting.

Caloric Density: Refers to the amount of calories in a food relative to its nutrient content. A calorie-dense food supplies few nutrients for its calorie cost.

Calorie: A measurement of energy in food. Dietary calories are really kilocalories or kcalories and are one thousand times as large as the physicist's calorie. A kcalorie is the amount of heat energy necessary to raise the temperature of 1,000 grams of water 1 degree Centigrade. ("Calor" means heat and "kilo" means one thousand.) In foods, protein and carbohydrates supply 4 calories per gram, fat supplies 9 calories per gram, and alcohol supplies 7+ calories per gram.

Candida: An infection by a fungus called Candida albicans. The infection can occur in the lungs, heart, vagina, gastrointestinal tract, skin, nails, or other tissues. Also called a "yeast" infection.

Carbohydrate: The starches and sugars in the diet.

Carcinogen: A substance that causes cancer.

Cardiomyopathy: A chronic disorder of the heart muscle.

Cardiovascular Disease: A disease of the heart and blood vessels often caused by the accumulation of plaque in the lining of the blood vessels.

Cataract: A milky film that forms over the eye and is one of the most common reasons for loss of eyesight.

Celiac Disease: A digestive tract disease caused by a sensitivity to a protein in wheat called gluten. Other terms for this condition include gluten-sensitive enteropathy, nontropical sprue, and idiopathic steatorrhea.

Cell-Mediated Immunity: The aspect of the immune response inside the cells and tissues that protects these tissues against invasion by bacteria and other microorganisms and from abnormal cell growth. It includes T lymphocytes (or T-cells) and interferon.

Cell Membrane: The outer covering of each cell composed of fats and proteins.

Cellulite: Normal subcutaneous body fat that is irregular or "waffled" in appearance, probably caused by the webwork of connective tissue that binds it to underlying tissues.

Cellulose: One type of fiber in food; a plant-derived carbohydrate composed of glucose, which humans cannot digest.

Cervix: The neck or opening to the uterus.

Chelated: A mineral combined with another compound, such as chromium picolinate.

Chelator: A compound that combines with a mineral to form a weak bond where the mineral is part of a chemical ring structure. Picolinic acid is the chelator in the supplement chromium picolinate.

Cholesterol: Cholesterol is a type of fat, but it supplies no calories and consequently cannot be "burned off" or "sweated out." It is found only in foods of animal origin, such as eggs, organ meats, meat, chicken, fish, dairy products, and in processed foods made with these ingredients. No foods of plant origin contain cholesterol. Increased dietary intake of cholesterol-rich foods is associated with elevated blood levels of cholesterol and an increased risk of developing heart disease.

Cholesterol is an essential component in the body and is needed for the manufacture of certain hormones, bile, and other compounds. The body manufactures all of its needs, however, so dietary intake of this fat only contributes to excesses, not to health.

Cholesterol Oxides: Cholesterol damaged by free radicals.

Choline: A B vitamin–like compound obtained from the diet and manufactured by the body. Whether or not choline is an essential nutrient remains controversial.

Chromic Chloride: The inorganic salt of chromium used in many supplements.

Chronic: Long-term; cardiovascular disease and diabetes are chronic diseases.

Clinical: Pertaining to the observable signs of a disease.

Co-enzyme: A compound required in order for an enzyme to function. Many of the B vitamins are co-enzymes.

Collagen: A protein in connective tissues and the organic substance in teeth and bones.

Complementary Protein: Two or more proteins whose amino acid compositions complement each other so that the essential amino acids missing from one are supplied by the other. An example would be whole wheat bread and cooked split peas.

Complex Carbohydrate: Starches and some fibers in the diet, such as cellulose, containing from ten to more than a thousand glucose units linked much like pearls on a string.

Connective Tissue: A weblike tissue located in every organ that holds together and supports the various tissues within the organ.

Cornea: The exposed and transparent portion of the eyeball.

Coronary Arteries: The blood vessels that supply the heart.

Cortisol: A hormone secreted by the adrenal glands that acts much like cortisone in stimulating the body to manufacture more glucose for energy.

Cruciferous Vegetables: Vegetables in the cabbage family, including broccoli, asparagus, Brussels sprouts, kohlrabi, and cabbage, that contain compounds called "indoles," which are protective against cancer.

Diastolic Blood Pressure: The lower of two readings that make up a blood pressure test. Diastolic blood pressure corresponds to the least amount of pressure in the cardiovascular system at any one time and reflects the pressure inherent in the heart and blood vessels when the heart relaxes between beats (contractions).

Dolomite: A mineral composed of calcium and magnesium.

Duodenal Ulcer: An ulcer in the first or upper part of the small intestine.

Dysplasia: Abnormal cell development.

Eicosapentaenoic Acid (EPA): An omega-3 fatty acid in fish oils that lowers the risk of developing cardiovascular disease.

Electrolyte: A substance or salt that dissolves into positive or negative charged particles and conducts an electrical charge. Sodium, potassium, and chloride are examples of electrolytes.

Electrolyte Balance: The distribution of electrolytes (salts) among the body fluids.

Endocrine Glands: Ductless glands that secrete hormones, which in turn have profound effects on the regulation of body processes. Examples of endocrine glands are the ovaries, thyroid, and pancreas.

Endorphins: A group of neurotransmitter-like substances that produce a calming effect on the brain much like morphine.

Energy: The fuel that powers all body processes. Equivalent to calories. The nutrients that supply energy or calories include protein (4 calories/gram), carbohydrates (4 calories/gram), fat (9 calories/gram), and alcohol (7+ calories/gram). The body stores energy as fat tissue, and to a limited amount as glycogen (sugar) in the muscles and liver.

Enriched: The addition to processed foods of a few nutrients to bring the level back to the original vitamin or mineral content. Only four nutrients are added back in the enrichment process, while many more nutrients are lost.

Enzyme: A compound that acts as a catalyst in starting chemical reactions in the body.

All enzymes are made from protein and often work closely with B vitamins and some minerals.

Epithelial: The tissues that line the internal and external surfaces of the body, including the skin, blood vessels, uterus, urinary bladder, and the outer surface of the eye.

Esophagus: The passageway or tube from the throat to the stomach.

Essential Fatty Acid: A polyunsaturated fat that cannot be manufactured by the body, such as linoleic acid found in safflower oil.

Essential Nutrient: A substance that cannot be manufactured in sufficient amounts in the body and must be obtained regularly from the diet. A nutrient is used in the body to promote growth, maintenance, and repair of tissues.

Estrogen: A family of female hormones that regulates menstruation and possibly protects against heart disease and osteoporosis.

Extracellular: Outside the cells. Extracellular fluid includes the blood, lymph, and fluid between the cells (interstitial fluid).

Fat Burners: People who primarily burn fat for energy during and after exercise, unlike those whose bodies resist mobilizing fat from storage. In many cases a person is genetically programmed to burn more or less fat; however, diet and exercise habits can modify this genetic programming.

Slow, prolonged exercise burns fat as its primary fuel, while short, intense exercise uses primarily sugar or glucose. Low-fat foods combined with daily, prolonged aerobic exercise condition the body through a variety of mechanisms, including alterations in fat-mobilizing enzymes and hormones, to remove fat from storage and burn it for fuel.

Fat Calories: The number of calories that come from fat. The amount of fat in the diet is directly linked to disease, weight gain, body fat percentage, and overall health. Fat in foods is measured by weight (grams). For example, hamburger meat is listed as 9 percent fat, 15 percent fat, or 22 percent fat by weight. In terms of health, however, dietary fat is more accurately represented as a percentage of total calories.

"Fat calories" should not exceed 30 percent of total calorie intake. Less is better. This percentage is calculated by multiplying the total grams of fat in a food or menu by 9 (fat supplies 9 calories per gram), dividing by the total calories in the food or menu, and multiplying by 100.

Fatty Acid: A fat-soluble molecule that consists of a long chain of carbon atoms with hydrogen attached. Three fatty acids linked to a glycerol molecule compose a triglyceride. Eicosapentaenoic acid (EPA) and linoleic acid are examples of fatty acids.

Ferritin: A form of iron in the blood. The serum ferritin test measures iron status, in particular iron deficiency prior to the onset of anemia.

Ferrous: Iron.

Fiber: The indigestible residue of food, composed of the carbohydrates cellulose, pectin, and hemicellulose; vegetable gums; and the noncarbohydrate lignin.

Folacin: Folic acid, a B vitamin.

Food and Drug Administration (FDA): An agency of the U.S. government responsible for monitoring the safety and effectiveness of food, drugs, and cosmetics sold in the United States.

Food Intolerance: The inability to digest a food as a result of individual chemical idiosyncrasies, food contamination, psychological factors, or digestive enzyme deficiencies. Lactose intolerance, for example, results from inadequate amounts of the digestive enzyme lactase.

Fortified: The addition of vitamins or minerals to a processed food. Milk is fortified with vitamin D; salt is fortified with iodine.

Free Radical: Highly reactive substances found in air pollution, tobacco smoke, foods, pesticides, and ultraviolet sunlight, and manufactured during normal body processes. They damage cell membranes and result in tissue damage associated with heart disease, cancer, cataracts, arthritis, premature aging, and many other conditions.

Fructose: A simple sugar or carbohydrate sometimes known as fruit sugar. High fructose corn syrup (HFCS) used in soft drinks contains between 40 percent and 90 percent fructose. Honey is approximately 50 percent fructose.

FSH: Follicle stimulating hormone, which stimulates the release of the ovum (egg) from the ovary.

Gamma Linolenic Acid (GSA): An omega-3 fatty acid.

Gastritis: Inflammation of the stomach lining.

Gastrointestinal Tract: The digestive tract, including the stomach and intestines.

Genetics: The branch of biology that studies heredity and biological variation.

Glucose: Sugar, blood sugar, the building blocks of starch.

Glucose Polymers: Manufactured strings of glucose (sugar) molecules that slow the release of sugar from the digestive tract into the blood. Used in drinks for athletes.

Glucose Tolerance Factor (GTF): A compound containing chromium that aids the hormone insulin in regulating blood sugar levels.

Glucose Tolerance Test: A test that measures blood sugar regulation, in particular the presence of hyperglycemia or diabetes and hypoglycemia. A glucose solution is taken orally on an empty stomach, and then the blood sugar levels are monitored up to four hours.

Glutathione: A nonessential substance in the diet that has antioxidant capabilities.

Glycogen: The storage form of glucose in the body. Glycogen is formed and stored in the liver and muscles, and is converted to glucose when energy is needed.

Goiter: Enlargement of the thyroid gland.

Gram: A unit of weight. Twenty-eight grams equal one ounce.

Growth Hormone: A substance produced by a section of the brain called the anterior pituitary that promotes the increased size of cells and increased development of new cells, resulting in tissue growth.

Gynoid: Pertaining to women.

Hamstrings: The muscles in the back of the thigh.

HDL-Cholesterol: Cholesterol packaged in high-density lipoproteins. HDL is composed of fats and protein, and serves as a transport for fats in the blood. A high level of HDL is associated with a reduced risk of developing cardiovascular disease.

Heart Palpitations: Rapid beating of the heart.

Hematocrit: A test for iron-deficiency anemia. The volume percent of red blood cells in blood.

Heme Iron: Iron associated with hemoglobin in red blood cells. This form of iron, found in meat, chicken, and fish, is well absorbed; up to 30 percent is absorbed compared to only 2 percent to 7 percent absorption in nonheme iron foods such as vegetables, grains, and fruit.

Hemoglobin: The oxygen-carrying protein in red blood cells. Each molecule of hemoglobin contains four atoms of iron. The hemoglobin test is a measure of iron status, in particular iron-deficiency anemia.

Hormone: A substance produced by an organ called an endocrine gland; it is released into the blood and transported to another organ or tissue, where it performs a specific action. Examples of hormones include adrenaline and estrogen.

Hot Flashes: Visible redness in the face, neck, and throat, followed by profuse sweating and lasting for at least two or three minutes. A common symptom of menopause, possibly caused by fluctuation in hormones.

Human Immunodeficiency Virus (HIV): The virus thought to be associated with the development of AIDS.

Hyperglycemia: High blood sugar levels, often associated with diabetes or the risk of developing diabetes.

Hypertension: High blood pressure.

Hypoglycemia: Low blood sugar levels.

Immune System: A complex system of substances, tissues, and organs that protect the body against disease and infection.

Immunity: The body's resistance to disease provided by a complex system of specialized cells, tissues, organs, and chemicals, such as antibodies and interferon.

Indoles: A group of compounds in cruciferous vegetables (vegetables in the cabbage family) associated with a reduced risk of developing cancer.

Inositol: A vitamin-like compound found in food and produced in the body. There are no deficiency or toxicity symptoms of inositol, so it is not considered an essential nutrient.

Insomnia: Inability to sleep, to stay asleep, or to fall asleep.

Insulin: A hormone produced by the pancreas that regulates blood sugar levels.

Interferon: An immune system chemical produced in response to a virus that prevents the virus from multiplying.

Intermittent Claudication: Intermittent lameness caused by obstruction of the blood vessels that supply blood and oxygen to the legs.

International Unit (IU): An arbitrary measurement used for the fat-soluble vitamins A, D, and E. These units standardize the potency of the vitamin rather than measure it by weight. IUs can be converted to weight measurements (for example, 3.33 IU of vitamin A are equivalent to 1 mcg).

Intracellular: Inside the cell.

Intrinsic Factor: A substance secreted in the digestive tract that is essential for vitamin B12 absorption.

Keratin: A tough protein substance that gives hardness or structure to nails, hair, and the skin.

Ketogenic: Producing ketones or by-products of fat metabolism. Ketosis is an acidic condition associated with excessive amounts of ketones in the blood.

Lactation: Breast-feeding.

Lactobacillus acidophilus: A bacteria found in some yogurt that helps maintain a healthy environment in the digestive tract and vagina. Also called L. acidophilus or acidophilus.

Lacto-Ovo Vegetarian Diet: A diet that omits meat, chicken, and fish, and is derived from fruit, vegetables, whole grain breads and cereals, nuts, seeds, eggs, and dairy products.

Lactose: Milk sugar.

LDL-Cholesterol: Low-density lipoprotein; a molecule composed of fats and protein that transports cholesterol in the blood. A high level of LDL is associated with an increased risk of developing cardiovascular disease.

Lecithin: A compound that has fat-soluble and water-soluble sides, thus making it a good emulsifier. Lecithin is a source of choline, is a constituent of cell membranes, is manufactured in the liver, and is found in food. It is used in commercial products, such as salad dressing, to suspend oil in water.

Legume: Dried beans and peas.

Lethargy: Feeling tired or sluggish, lacking energy.

Leukotrienes: A group of hormone-like substances involved in inflammation.

Linoleic Acid: An essential polyunsaturated fatty acid found in safflower oil and to a lesser extent in other vegetable oils.

Lipid: Fat, including triglycerides, phospholipids, and cholesterol.

Lipoprotein: A compound made up of fat and protein that carries fats in the blood. Cholesterol is a fat and therefore cannot travel in the watery medium of the blood without being "packaged" in a lipoprotein, a water-soluble "bubble." In a blood test the total cholesterol reading is actually a sum of all the cholesterol packaged in the various lipoproteins. The more total cholesterol that is packaged in high-density lipoproteins (HDL-cholesterol), the lower a person's risk of developing heart disease. The more total blood cholesterol packaged in low-density lipoproteins (LDL-cholesterol), the higher a person's risk. Consequently, HDL is considered the "good" cholesterol and LDL the "bad" cholesterol. Neither LDL nor HDL cholesterol is found in food; they are found only as carriers of cholesterol in the blood.

Lipoprotein Lipase: An enzyme that functions in converting blood fats into storage fat.

Listeria: A type of bacterial food poisoning that can be deadly.

Lymphocyte: A specialized white blood cell that is a component of the immune system and aids in the protection of the body against disease and infection. There are B lymphocytes and T lymphocytes, or B-cells and T-cells.

Lysine: One of the ten essential amino acids that make up protein.

Macrophage: A large blood cell involved in the immune response and the body's resistance to infection and disease.

Macula: Macula lutea. A pigment area of the retina in the eye.

Magnesium: A mineral essential in bone development, muscle relaxation, nerve transmission, blood sugar regulation, and the prevention of heart disease and high blood pressure.

Manganese: A trace mineral essential in connective tissue formation, fat and cholesterol metabolism, bone development, blood clotting, and protein metabolism. It also might have antioxidant capabilities.

Megadose: Large intake of a nutrient; more than ten times the RDA for a vitamin or mineral.

Megaloblastic Anemia: Anemia characterized by large, misshapen red blood cells that result from a deficiency of folic acid or vitamin B12.

Menopause: The permanent cessation of the menstrual cycle.

Menorrhagia: Heavy blood loss during menstruation.

Menses: Menstruation.

Menstrual: Pertaining to menstruation or the monthly discharge of blood and tissue from the uterus that occurs between puberty and menopause.

Menstruation: The monthly discharge of blood and tissue from the uterus.

Metabolism: The sum of all the chemical processes that convert food and its components to the fundamental chemicals that the body uses for energy or for repair, maintenance, and growth of tissues. Metabolism includes all the building-up processes, such as bone maintenance and nail and hair growth, and all the tearing-down processes, such as the breaking down of fat tissue or carbohydrate for energy. Tissue growth, such as building muscles and gaining weight, indicates that the building processes outweigh the tearing-down processes. In contrast, losing weight is an example of the tearing-down processes (removing fat from storage) outweighing the building-up processes.

Metabolite: Any product of metabolism.

Methionine: One of the ten essential amino acids that make up proteins.

Methylxanthine: A group of related compounds that include caffeine and caffeine-like substances.

Microgram (mcg): A metric unit of weight equivalent to one one-thousandth of a milligram or one millionth of a gram.

Microorganisms: Bacteria, viruses, and other minute life forms that are visible only through a microscope.

Milligram (mg): A metric unit of weight equivalent to one one-thousandth of a gram.

Mineral: An inorganic fundamental substance found naturally in the soil that has specific chemical and structural properties. Many minerals are essential nutrients for growth, maintenance, and repair of tissues.

Molybdenum: A trace mineral essential in the formation of uric acid (a normal breakdown product of metabolism), in the transport of iron out of the tissues, and in normal growth and development.

Monocyte: A specialized white blood cell important in the immune response.

Monounsaturated Fat: A type of fat that has one site on the fatty acid for the addition of a hydrogen atom. An example of a monounsaturated fat is oleic acid in olive oil. Other oils high in monounsaturated fats include canola oil and peanut oil.

Mucus: A thick liquid secreted by the mucous glands.

Myoglobin: The iron-containing storage molecule for oxygen in the tissues, similar to hemoglobin in the blood.

Myristic Acid: A saturated fatty acid found in coconut oil and milk that is four times as potent in raising blood cholesterol levels as other saturated fatty acids.

Neurotoxin: Any chemical or substance that is irritating or damaging to the nerves.

Neurotransmitter: A chemical that serves as a communication link between nerve cells or between a nerve cell and a muscle or organ. Serotonin and acetylcholine are examples of neurotransmitters.

Niacin: A B vitamin important in breaking down carbohydrates, protein, and fat for energy. Also called nicotinic acid or niacinamide.

Nutrient Density: Refers to the amount of vitamins, minerals, and other nutrients in a food relative to its calorie content. A nutrient-dense food is one that supplies ample amounts of nutrients for few calories.

Nutritional Pharmacology: Using nutrients in amounts larger than typical dietary intake for the prevention or treatment of disease.

Nutritious Food: A food that provides a high quantity of one or more essential nutrients, with a small quantity of calories. (See Nutrient Density.)

Obesity: Body fat weight more than 20 percent above ideal body weight. The body weight is excess fat, not muscle or lean tissue.

Omega-3 Fatty Acid: Fatty acids found in fish oils and gamma linolenic acid that might reduce the risk of heart disease, cancer, arthritis, and other disorders, while strengthening the immune system.

Oral: Pertaining to the mouth.

Ovary: A glandular organ in the female reproductive system that produces the ovum (egg) and secretes the female hormones estrogen and progesterone.

Ovulation: The growth, maturation, and release of the egg (ovum) from the ovaries each month.

Oxidative Stress or Oxidative Damage: Free radical damage to tissues and molecules in the body associated with premature aging, disease, and suppressed immune function.

Oxidized LDL-Cholesterol: LDL-cholesterol that has been damaged by free radicals and is suspected of promoting the development of atherosclerosis more than normal LDL-cholesterol.

Ozone: A highly reactive modification of oxygen whereby the two atoms in oxygen (O_2) are increased to three (O_3).

Pancreas: The organ responsible for the production and secretion of numerous digestive enzymes and the hormone insulin.

Pancreatic Amylase: A digestive enzyme secreted by the pancreas that helps break down starches.

Parathyroid Hormone: A substance secreted by the parathyroid gland, which is located by the thyroid gland and regulates phosphorus and blood calcium levels.

Pepsin: A digestive enzyme in the stomach that breaks down proteins.

Perimenopause: The period immediately prior to and following the menopause with hormonal, chemical, and biological symptoms that are associated with menopause.

Peripheral Neuropathy: A condition characterized by tingling and numbness of the hands.

Pernicious Anemia: Anemia caused by an inadequate secretion of an intrinsic factor; consequently, vitamin B12 is not absorbed and anemia develops.

Peroxide: One of a number of highly reactive free radicals.

Petechial Hemorrhages: Pinpoint hemorrhages below the skin associated with vitamin C deficiency.

PKU: Phenylketonuria. Excretion in the urine of excessive amounts of a breakdown product of the amino acid phenylalanine. It results from a genetically determined metabolic disorder and causes mental retardation unless all foods containing phenylalanine are eliminated from the diet.

Placebo: A medicine or pill that has no pharmacologic effect but is given to please or humor a patient. In the "placebo effect," a health condition improves when the patient believes the treatment will work even if the patient is taking a placebo. The patient's belief that a pill or treatment will work can set up metabolic processes in the body that encourage healing. In contrast, negative thoughts such as guilt, hopelessness, and tension might suppress immune responses and aid in the promotion of disease.

Plaque: The accumulation of fat, calcium, and other debris in the artery walls; it is associated with the development of atherosclerosis.

Platelets: Blood cell fragments that aid in blood coagulation. Abnormal clumping of platelets is associated with atherosclerosis.

Polyunsaturated Fat: A triglyceride in which one or more of the three fatty acids is unsaturated, that is, it has room for more than one hydrogen atom. Examples include the fats in vegetable oils and fish oils.

Postmenopause: After the menopause; determined after a period of twelve months of spontaneous amenorrhea has been observed.

Precursor: A substance used as a building block for another substance. Beta carotene is a precursor of vitamin A, and tryptophan is the precursor of serotonin and niacin.

Pre-Eclampsia: Toxemia associated with the latter stages of pregnancy; characterized by high blood pressure, edema, and protein in the urine.

Premenopausal: Prior to the onset of menopause.

Progesterone: A female hormone that induces premenstrual changes of the uterus lining following ovulation and possibly inhibits contractions of the uterus during early pregnancy. Also called progestin.

Prolactin: A female hormone released from a region in the brain called the anterior pituitary, which stimulates milk secretion.

Prostaglandin: A group of hormone-like substances formed from polyunsaturated fatty acids that have a profound effect on the body, including contraction of smooth muscle and dilation or contraction of blood vessels in the regulation of blood pressure.

Quadriceps: The four muscles in the front of the thigh.

Recommended Daily Allowances (RDA): Reference amounts of most vitamins and minerals necessary for health, based on a person's gender, age, and size.

Refined: The process whereby the coarse parts of plants are removed. For example, the refining of whole wheat into white wheat flour involves removing three of the four parts of the kernel—the chaff, the bran, and the germ—leaving only the endosperm or high-carbohydrate inner core.

Retina: The layer of light-sensitive cells lining the back of the inside of the eye.

Retinol: Vitamin A.

Retinol Equivalents (RE): A unit of measurement for vitamin A; 1 RE is equivalent to 1 mcg or 3.33 IU of vitamin A as retinol.

Saponins: A group of substances in seeds, dried beans, and peas that might lower blood cholesterol levels.

Saturated Fat: A triglyceride with the maximum possible number of hydrogen atoms. Saturated fats are solid at room temperature, such as butter, lard, and hydrogenated vegetable oils in margarine and shortening. Exceptions to this rule are coconut and palm oils, which are liquid vegetable oils high in saturated fats. A diet high in saturated fats increases the risk for elevated blood triglyceride and heart disease.

Schilling Test: A test for vitamin B12 status.

Scurvy: A disease caused by a deficiency of vitamin C and characterized by bleeding gums, loose teeth, small hemorrhages below the skin, and weakness.

Sebaceous Glands: Cells in the skin that secrete a greasy lubricating substance called sebum.

Secondary Deficiency: A nutrient deficiency caused by something other than poor dietary intake, including excessive intake of one nutrient that interferes with absorption or utilization of other nutrients.

Selenite: The inorganic salt of selenium used in supplements; also called sodium selenite.

Selenium: A trace mineral required in small amounts for health and that functions as an antioxidant to prevent the development of disease and infections.

Serotonin: A neurotransmitter produced in the brain that regulates mood, sleep, pain, and numerous other body processes.

Simple Carbohydrate: Sugars in the diet, including sucrose (table sugar), glucose, fructose (in fruits and honey), and lactose (in milk).

Sodium: An electrolyte that combined with chloride makes table salt.

Strict Vegetarian Diet: A diet that contains only foods of plant origin, such as whole grain breads and cereals, cooked dried beans and peas, fruits, vegetables, and nuts and seeds. Also called a vegan diet.

Subclinical Deficiency: A nutrient deficiency that does not produce overt physical symptoms. Also called a marginal deficiency.

Synthesize: The process of combining two or more substances into a new compound in the body.

Systolic Blood Pressure: The higher of the two readings that make up a blood pressure test. Systolic blood pressure represents the greatest amount of pressure in the cardiovascular system at any moment and corresponds to the pressure exerted by the heart during a heartbeat (contraction).

Tannin: Tannic acid. A yellowish astringent compound in tea.

Tetany: Muscle twitching, cramps, and convulsions.

Thromboxane: A prostaglandin (a hormone-like substance) that in high concentrations might be associated with the progression of atherosclerosis.

Tocopherol: Vitamin E.

Total Iron Binding Capacity (TIBC): A test to measure iron status, in particular iron deficiency prior to the onset of anemia.

Toxemia: A disorder that sometimes develops in the latter portion of pregnancy characterized by the symptoms of eclampsia, such as high blood pressure, protein in the urine, edema, salt retention, convulsions, and sometimes coma.

Toxicity: The ability of a substance to cause harmful effects. Any substance is toxic if consumed in high enough concentrations.

Trace Mineral: An essential mineral found in the body in amounts less than .0005 percent of body weight.

Trans Fatty Acids: Polyunsaturated fats formed during hydrogenation of vegetable oils to make margarine or shortening. The shape of these fats is different from other polyunsaturated fats, and it is suspected that they act more like saturated fats in the promotion of heart disease.

Triglycerides: The primary fats in food, in a person's fat tissue, and in the blood. Triglycerides can be saturated or unsaturated, and the unsaturated ones can be either monounsaturated or polyunsaturated. Regardless of the type, all triglycerides supply more than 250 calories per ounce (or 9 calories per gram), can contribute to weight gain and elevated body fat, and are associated with numerous diseases, from heart disease to cancer.

Triglycerides are composed of three fatty acids attached to a "backbone" molecule called glycerol. It is the composition of these fatty acids that determines if the fat is saturated or unsaturated. One fatty acid called linoleic acid is found only in polyunsaturated fats and is essential in the diet since it is one of the few fats the body cannot manufacture. The omega-3 fatty acids in fish oil might also be essential fats.

Tryptophan: An amino acid essential for life and converted in the body to the B vitamin niacin.

Unsaturated Fat: A triglyceride that contains one or more fatty acids that could accept more hydrogen atoms. Unsaturated fats are liquid at room temperature. Examples of unsaturated fats include vegetable oils and fish oils.

Urinary: Pertaining to urine.

U.S. RDA: The United States Recommended Daily Allowances are obtained from the

RDA figures for use on labels. In most cases, the highest value for a nutrient suggested in the RDA tables for any age or gender group is used for the U.S. RDA.

Vaginitis: Inflammation of the vagina.

Vanadium: A trace mineral found in whole grains, nuts, root vegetables, liver, fish, and vegetable oils. Whether or not vanadium is essential to humans remains controversial.

Vegan: A strict vegetarian who consumes no foods of animal origin.

Virus: Any of a large group of minute particles that are capable of infecting plants, animals, and humans.

Vitamin: An essential nutrient that must be obtained from the diet and is required by the body in minute amounts.

Vulva: The external genital organs at the opening of the vagina, consisting of the labia minora and the labia majora.

Waist-to-Hip Ratio (WHR): A measurement of regional distribution of body fat. A high WHR reflects excessive fat accumulation above the waist, which is associated with increased risk of heart disease, diabetes, cancer, and other disorders.

Whole Grain: An unrefined grain that retains its edible outside layers (the bran) and the highly nutritious inner germ.

Xerophthalmia: A disease that impairs vision and is caused by a deficiency of vitamin A. This disorder is characterized by a thickening and inflammation of the outer surface of the eye.

Yo-Yo Dieting: Repeated attempts to lose weight, followed by a regain of the lost

References

INTRODUCTION

The American Dietetic Association's nutrition recommendations for women. *J Am Diet A* 1986;86(12):1663–1664.

Anderson R, Kozlovsky A: Chromium intake, absorption and excretion in subjects consuming self-selected diets. *Am J Clin N* 1985;41:1177–1183.

Baker H, Frank O, Zetterman R, et al: Inability of chronic alcoholics with liver disease to use food as a source of folates, thiamin, and vitamin B6. *Am J Clin N* 1975; 28:1377–1380.

Block G, Dresser C, Hartman A, et al: Nutrient sources in the American Diet: Quantitative data from the NHANES II survey. 2. Macronutrients and fats. *Am J Epidem* 1985;122(1):27–40.

Commentary, Oral contraceptives and nutrition. *J Am Diet A* 1976; 68:419–420.

Downing D: Recommended daily allowances—success or failure? *J Nutr Med* 1990; 1:89–92.

Haines P, Hungerford D, Popkin B, et al: Eating patterns and energy nutrient intakes of U.S. women. *J Am Diet A* 1992;92(6):698–707.

Johnson P, Gallaher D, Lykken G, et al: Zinc availability from beef served with various carbohydrates or beverages. *Nutr Res* 1990;10:155–162.

Krebs-Smith S, Cronin F, Haytowitz D: Food sources of energy, macronutrients, cholesterol, and fiber in diets of women. *J Am Diet A* 1992;92:168–174.

Mareschi J, Magliola C, Couzy F, et al: The well-balanced diet and the at-risk micronutrients: A forecasting nutritional index. *Int J Vit N* 1987;57:79–85.

Monti D, Troiano L, Tropea F, et al: Apoptosis: Programmed cell death: A role in the aging process? *Am J Clin N* 1992;55:1208S–1214S.

Munger R, Folsom A, Kushi L, et al: Dietary assessment of older Iowa women with a food frequency questionnaire: Nutrient intake, reproducibility, and comparison with 24-hour dietary recall interviews. *Am J Epidem* 1992;136(2):192–200.

Murphy S, Calloway D: Nutrient intakes of women in NHANES II, emphasizing trace minerals, fiber, and phytate. *J Am Diet A* 1986;86(10):1366–1372.

National Research Council, Food and Nutrition Board: *Recommended Dietary Allowances,* 10th edition. Washington, D.C., National Academy Press, 1989.

Nationwide Food Consumption Survey, Spring 1980. U.S. Department of Agriculture, Science and Education Administration, Beltsville, MD.

Pennington J, Young D: Total Diet Study nutritional elements 1982–1989. *J Am Diet A* 1991;91:179–183.

Pietrzik K: Concept of borderline vitamin deficiencies, in Hanck A, Hornig D (eds): Vitamins: Nutrients and therapeutic agents. *Int J Vit N* 1985;Suppl 27:61–73.

Pryor W: The antioxidant nutrients and disease prevention: What do we know and what do we need to find out? *Am J Clin N* 1991;53:391S–393S.

Recommended Dietary Allowances: Scientific issues and process for the future: A statement of the Food and Nutrition Board. *J Nutr* 1986;116:482–488.

Smith J, Turner J: A perspective on the history and use of the recommended dietary allowances. *Currents* 1986;2(1):1–8.

Somer E: The 1986 RDAs: A step backward. *Nutr Rep* 1986;March:18,24.

———. *The Essential Guide to Vitamins and Minerals.* New York, HarperCollins, 1992.

Wynn V: Vitamins and oral contraceptive use. *Lancet* 1975;I:561–564.

INTRODUCTION TO PART ONE

Kristal A, White E, Shattuck A, et al: Long-term maintenance of a low-fat diet: Durability of fat-related dietary habits in the Women's Health Trial. *J Am Diet A* 1992;92:553–559.

Thompson F, Sowers M, Frongillo E, et al: Sources of fiber and fat in the diets of U.S. women aged 19 to 50: Implications for nutrition education and policy. *Am J Pub He* 1992;82(5):695–702.

CHAPTER ONE

Blundell J: Paradoxical effects of an intense sweetener (aspartame) on appetite. *Lancet* 1986;I:1092.

Burr M, Fehily A, Butland B, et al: Alcohol and high-density lipoprotein cholesterol: A randomized controlled trial. *Br J Nutr* 1986;56:81–86.

Cluette-Brown J, Mulligan J, Igoe F, et al: Dietary ethanol alters plasma sex hormones and lipoprotein cholesterol. *Clin Res* 1986;34:A854.

Council on Scientific Affairs: Aspartame: Review of safety issues. *J Am Med A* 1985; 254:400.

Dews P: Meeting report: Summary report of an international aspartame workshop. *Fd Chem Toxic* 1987;25:549–552.

Ferrence R: Alcohol and the prevention of coronary heart disease. *Nutr Rep* 1987; 5(8):56,64.

Jacobson M: *Eater's Digest: The Consumer's Factbook of Food Additives.* Garden City, New York, Doubleday and Company, 1976.

Maher T: Neurotoxicity of food additives. *Neurotoxico* 1986;7(2):183–196.

Pinner R, Schuchat A, Swaminathan B, et al: Role of foods in sporadic listeriosis. *J Am Med A* 1992;267(15):2046–2050.

Somer E: Trans fatty acids and disease: Fact or fallacy? *Nutr Rep* 1991;June:42.

Stellman S, Garfinkel L: Artificial sweetener use and one-year weight change among women. *Prev Med* 1986;15:195.

Taylor S, Bush R: Sulfites as food ingredients. *Cont Nutr* 1986;11(10):1–2.

Walton R: Seizure and mania after high intake of aspartame. *Psychosomat* 1986; 27:218–219.

Wurtman R: Neurochemical changes following high-dose aspartame with dietary carbohydrates. *N Eng J Med* 1983;389:429–430.

Yokogoshi H, Roberts C, Caballero B, et al: Effects of aspartame and glucose administration on brain and plasma levels of large neutral amino acids and brain 5-hydroxyindoles. *Am J Clin N* 1984;40:1–7.

CHAPTER TWO

Anderson R, Kozlovsky A, Moser P: Effects of diets high in simple sugars on urinary chromium excretion of humans. *Fed Proc* 1985;44:751.

Block G, Dresser C, Hartman A, et al: Nutrient sources in the American Diet: Quantitative data from the NHANES II survey. 2. Macronutrients and fats. *Am J Epidem* 1985;122:27–40.

Blume E: Why oxidized fats are in your food and why you wish they weren't. *Nutr Action Health Letter* 1987;December:1,4–6.

Brewster L, Jacobson M: *The Changing American Diet: A Chronicle of American Eating Habits from 1910–1980.* Washington, DC, Center for Science in the Public Interest, 1983.

The Changing American Diet: Update. Washington, DC, Center for Science in the Public Interest, 1982.

Heaton K: The sweet road to gall stones. *Br Med J* 1984;288:1103–1104.

Katschinski B, Logan R, Edmond M, et al: Dietary fiber, sugar, and the risk of duodenal ulcer. *Gastroenty* 1987;92:1460.

Kavanagh M, Prendiville V, Buxton A, et al: Does sucrose damage kidneys? *Br J Urol* 1986;58:353–357.

Kristal A, White E, Shattuck A, et al: Long-term maintenance of a low-fat diet: Durability of fat-related dietary habits in the Women's Health Trial. *J Am Diet A* 1992;92:553–559.

Kruis W, Forstmaier G, Scheurlen C, et al: Effect of diets low and high in refined sugars on gut transit, bile acid metabolism, and bacterial fermentation. *Gut* 1991; 32(4):367–371.

Pivonka E, Grunewald K: Aspartame- or sugar-sweetened beverages: Effects on mood in young women. *J Am Diet A* 1990;90:250–254.

Sparks J, Sparks C, Kritchevsky D: Hypercholesterolemia and aortic glysosaminoglycans of rabbits fed semi-purified diets containing sucrose and lactose. *Atheroscler* 1986;60:183–196.

Yudkin J, Eisa O, Kang S, et al: Dietary sucrose affects plasma HDL cholesterol concentration in young men. *Ann Nutr M* 1986;30:261–266.

CHAPTER THREE

Freeland-Graves J, Ebangit L, Hendrikson P: Alterations in zinc absorption and salivary sediment zinc after a lacto-ovo vegetarian diet. *Am J Clin N* 1980;33:1757–1766.

Grundy S, Arky R, Bray G, et al: Coronary risk factor statement for the American public. *Arterioscle* 1985;5(6):A678–A682.

Hunt I, Murphy N, Henderson C: Food and nutrient intake of Seventh-Day Adventist women. *Am J Clin N* 1988;48:850–851.

Kjeldsen-Kragh J, Haugen M, Borchgrevink C, et al: Controlled trial of fasting and one-year vegetarian diet in rheumatoid arthritis. *Lancet* 1991;336(8772):899–902.

Margetts B, Beilin L, Vandongen R, et al: Vegetarian diet in mild hypertension: A randomized controlled trial. *Br Med J* 1986;293:1468–1471.

McMurry M, Cerquiera T, Connor S, et al: Changes in lipid and lipoprotein levels and body weight in Tarahumara Indians after consumption of an affluent diet. *N Eng J Med* 1991;325:1704–1708.

National Cholesterol Education Program: Report of the expert panel on population strategies for blood cholesterol reduction: Executive summary. *Arch in Med* 1991;151:1071–1084.

Pronczuk A, Kipervarg Y, Hayes K: Vegetarians have higher plasma alpha-tocopherol relative to cholesterol than do nonvegetarians. *J Am Col N* 1992;11(1):50–55.

Rationale of the diet-heart statement of the American Heart Association: Report of the AHA Nutrition Committee. *Arterioscle* 1982;4:177–191.

Srikumar T, Johansson G, Ockerman P, et al: Trace element status in healthy subjects switching from a mixed to a lactovegetarian diet for 12 months. *Am J Clin N* 1992;55:885–890.

Srikumar T, Ockerman P, Akesson B: Trace element status in vegetarians from southern India. *Nutr Res* 1992;12:187–198.

Willett W, Stampfer M, Colditz G, et al: Dietary fat and the risk of breast cancer. *N Eng J Med* 1987;316(1):22–28.

CHAPTER FOUR

Alper J: Diet sabotage. *Self* 1990;May:232–233,249–251.

Blair A, Lewis V, Booth D: Does emotional eating interfere with success in attempts at weight control? *Appetite* 1990;15:151–157.

Brownell K: When and how to diet. *Psych Today* 1989;June:40–44.

DeCastro J, Brewer E, Elmore D, et al: Social facilitation of the spontaneous meal size of humans occurs regardless of time, place, alcohol, or snacks. *Appetite* 1990; 15:89–101.

Paulsen B, Lutz R, McReynolds W, et al: Behavior therapy for weight control: Long-term results of two programs with nutritionists as therapists. *Am J Clin N* 1976;29:880–888.

Promoting a healthy weight. *Dairy Council Digest* 1991;March–April:7–12.

Stalonas P, Perri M, Kerzner A: Do behavioral treatments of obesity last? A five-year follow-up investigation. *Addict Beha* 1984;175–183.

Wing R: Behavioral treatment of severe obesity. *Am J Clin N* 1992;55:545S–551S.

CHAPTER FIVE

Adler A, Shainkin-Kestenbaum, R, Berlyne, G: Aluminum absorption and intestinal vitamin D dependent Ca binding protein. *Kidney Int* 1990;37:471.

Dietary Intake Source Data: United States 1976–1980. Data from the National Health Survey, Series 11, No. 231, DHHS Publication No (PHS) 83-1681, March 1983.

First Health and Nutrition Examination Survey. Public Health Service, Health Resources Administration, U.S. Department of Health, 1971–1972.

Mareschi J, Magliola C, Couzy F, et al: The well-balanced diet and the "at risk" micronutrients: A forecasting nutritional index. *Int J Vit N* 1987;57:79–85.

Nationwide Food Consumption Survey, Spring 1980. U.S. Department of Agriculture, Science and Education Administration, Beltsville, MD.

Pennington J: Total Diet Study: Nutritional elements. *Nutr Rep* 1992 May;10(5):33,40.

Tamura T: Folic acid. *Nutr MD* 1984;10:1–2.

CHAPTER SIX

Zeisel S: Choline: An important nutrient in brain development, liver function, and carcinogenesis. *J Am Col N* 1992;11(5):473–481.

CHAPTER SEVEN

A critique of low-carbohydrate ketogenic weight reduction regimens. Chicago, IL, AMA Council on Foods and Nutrition, 1973.

Andrews J: Exercise for slimming. *P Nutr Soc* 1991;50:459–471.

Ballor D, Keesey R: A meta-analysis of the factors affecting exercise-induced changes in body mass, fat mass, and fat-free mass in males and females. *Int J Obes* 1991; 15:717–726.

Bjorntorp P: Abdominal fat distribution and disease: An overview of epidemiological data. *Ann Med* 1992;24:15–18.

————: The association between obesity, adipose tissue distribution, and disease. *Act Med Sc* 1991;723 (Suppl):121–134.

Bjorvell H, Rossner S: A ten-year follow-up of weight change in severely obese subjects treated in a combined behavioral modification programme. *Int J Obes* 1992; 16:623–625.

Boeder C, Burrhus K, Svanevik L, et al: The effects of either high-intensity resistance or endurance training on resting metabolic rate. *Am J Clin N* 1992;55:802–810.

Bouchard C: Heredity and the path to overweight and obesity. *Med Sci Spt* 1992; 23(3):285–291.

Bowyer C: A diet for slimming? *P Nutr Soc* 1991;50:433–440.

Bradstock M, Serdula M, Marks J, et al: Evaluation of reactions to food additives: The aspartame experience. *Am J Clin N* 1986;43(3):464–469.

Bryce-Smith D, Simpson R: Case of anorexia nervosa responding to zinc sulphate. *Lancet* 1984;II:350.

Calles-Escandion J, Horton E: The thermogenic role of exercise in the treatment of morbid obesity: A critical evaluation. *Am J Clin N* 1992;55:533S–537S.

Chromium picolinate and bariatric medicine. *Int J Biosoc Med Res* 1991;13(2):152–153.

Chung Y, Daghestani A: Seasonal affective disorder: Shedding light on a dark subject. *Postgr Med* 1989;86(5):309–314.

Dalvit-McPhillips S: A dietary approach to bulimia treatment. *Physl Behav* 1984; 33:769–775.

deZwaan M, Mitchell J: Binge eating in the obese. *Ann Med* 1992;24:303–308.

Fenner L: Cellulite: Hard to budge pudge. *FDA Consumer* 1980;May.

Fernstrom J: Tryptophan, serotonin, and carbohydrate appetite: Will the real carbohydrate craver please stand up! *J Nutr* 1988;118:1417–1419.

Ferraro R, Lillioja S, Fontvielle A, et al: Lower sedentary metabolic rate in women compared to men. *J Clin Inv* 1992;90(3):780–784.

Fisher M, Lachance P: Nutrition evaluation of published weight-reducing diets. *J Am Diet A* 1985;85:451–455.

Foreyt J, Goodrick G: Factors common to successful therapy for the obese patient. *Med Sci Spt* 1991;23(3):292–297.

Grave, R, Bussinello P, Zeni A: Short-term effect of a very low calorie diet on body composition and fat distribution. *Int J Obes* 1989;13 (Supple. 2):177–178.

Griffiths R, Woodson P: Reinforcing effects of caffeine in humans. *J Pharm Exp* 1988; 246(1):21.

Grodner M: "Forever dieting": Chronic dieting syndrome. *J Nutr Ed* 1992;24(4): 207–210.

Hall R, Hoffman R, Beresford T, et al: Refractory hypokalemia secondary to hypomagnesemia in eating-disorder patients. *Psychosomat* 1988;29(4):435–437.

———: Hypomagnesemia in patients with eating disorders. *Psychosomat* 1988; 29(3):264–272.

Hamilton C, Anderson J: Fiber and weight management. *J Florida M A* 1992; 79(6):379–381.

Heaton K: The sweet road to gall stones. *Br Med J* 1984;288:1103–1104.

———: Intestinal carcinogenesis: The role of diet. *Br J Can* 1986;54:138.

Jen K, Almario R, Ilagan J, et al: Long-term exercise training and retirement in genetically obese rats: Effects on food intake, feeding efficiency and carcass composition. *Int J Obes* 1992;16:519–527.

Jenkins D, Ocana A, Jenkins A, et al: Metabolic advantages of spreading the nutrient load: Effects on increased meal frequency in non–insulin dependent diabetes. *Am J Clin N* 1992;55:461–467.

Jenkins D, Wolever T, Vuksan V, et al: Nibbling versus gorging: Metabolic advantages of increased meal frequency. *N Eng J Med* 1989;321:929–934.

Kavanagh M, Prendiville V, Buxton A, et al: Does sucrose damage kidneys? *Br J Urol* 1986;58:353–357.

Keno Y, Matsuzawa Y, Tokunaga K, et al: High sucrose diet increases visceral fat accumulation in VMH-lesioned obese rats. *Int J Obes* 1991;15:205–211.

Kruis W, Forstmaier G, Scheurlen C, et al: Effect of diets low and high in refined sugars on gut transit, bile acid metabolism, and bacterial fermentation. *Gut* 1991; 32(4):367–371.

Kuczmarski R: Prevalence of overweight and weight gain in the United States. *Am J Clin N* 1992;55:495S–502S.

Lissner L, Odell P, D'Aostino R, et al: Variability of body weight and health outcomes in the Framingham Population. *N Eng J Med* 1991;324:1839–1844.

Livingstone M, Strain J, Prentice A, et al: Potential contribution of leisure activity to the energy expenditure patterns of sedentary populations. *Br J Nutr* 1991;65: 145–155.

Miller W: Diet composition, energy intake, and nutritional status in relation to obesity in men and women. *Med Sci Spt* 1991; 23(3):280–284.

Patton G: Eating disorders: Antecedents, evolution and course. *Ann Med* 1992; 24: 281–285.

Pi-Sunyer F: The role of very-low-calorie diets in obesity. *Am J Clin N* 1992;56:240S–243S.

Pivonka E, Grunewald K: Aspartame- or sugar-sweetened beverages: Effects on mood in young women. *J Am Diet A* 1990;90:250–254.

Prewitt T, Schmeisser D, Bowen P, et al: Changes in body weight, body composition, and energy intake in women fed high- and low-fat diets. *Am J Clin N* 1991;54:304–310.

Raphael F, Lacey J: Sociocultural aspects of eating disorders. *Ann Med* 1992;24:293–306.

Reimer L: Role of dietary fat in obesity: Fat is fattening. *J Florida M A* 1992; 79(6):382–384.

———: Obesity: A big problem. *J Florida M A* 1992;79(6):377–378.

Ross R, Leger L, Marliss E, et al: Adipose tissue distribution changes during rapid weight loss in obese adults. *Int J Obes* 1991;15:733–739.

Safai-Kutti S, Kutti J: Zinc supplementation in anorexia nervosa (letter). *Am J Clin N* 1986;44:581–582.

Schapira D: Diet, obesity, fat distribution, and cancer in women. *JAMWA* 1991; 46(4):126–131.

Smith B, Fillion T, Blass E: Orally mediated sources of calming in 1- to 3-day-old human infants. *Develop Psy* 1990;26:731–737.

Smith B, Stevens K, Torgerson W, et al: Diminished reactivity of postmature human infants to sucrose compared with term infants. *Develop Psy* 1992;28:811–820.

Stellman S, Garfinkel L: Short report: Artificial sweetener use and one-year weight changes among women. *Prev Med* 1986;15:195–202.

Thomas C, Peters J, Reed G, et al: Nutrient balance and energy expenditure during ad libitum feeding of high-fat and high-carbohydrate diets in humans. *Am J Clin N* 1992;55:934–942.

Tordoff M, Friedman M: Drinking saccharine increases food intake and preference: I. Comparison with other drinks. *Appetite* 1989;12(1):1–10.

Wadden T, Foster G, Letizia K, et al: Long-term effects of dieting on resting metabolic rate in obese outpatients. *J Am Med A* 1990;264:707–711.

Wadden T, Van Itallie T, Blackburn G: Responsible and irresponsible use of very-low-calorie diets in the treatment of obesity. *J Am Med A* 1990;263(1):83–85.

Weingarten H, Elston D: The phenomenology of food cravings. *Appetite* 1990;15 (3):231–246.

Wilterdink E, Ballor D, Keesey R: Amount of exercise per day and weeks of training: Effects on body weight and daily energy expenditure. *Med Sci Spt* 1992;24 (3):396–400.

Wing R: Weight cycling in humans: A review of the literature. *Ann Behav Med* 1992;14(2):113–119.

Wurtman J, Brzezinski A, Wurtman R, et al: Effect of nutrient intake on premenstrual depression. *Am J Obst G* 1989;161:128–134.

Yudkin J, Elsa O, Kang S, et al: Dietary sucrose affects plasma HDL-cholesterol concentration in young men. *Ann Nutr M* 1986;30:261–266.

CHAPTER EIGHT

Aharoni A, Tesler B, Paltieli Y, et al: Hair chromium content of women with gestational diabetes compared with nondiabetic pregnant women. *Am J Clin N* 1992;55:104–107.

American Academy of Pediatrics, Committee on Nutrition: Nutrition and lactation. *Pedatrics* 1981;68:435–443.

Apgar J, Everett G: Low zinc intake affects maintenance of pregnancy in guinea pigs. *J Nutr* 1991;121:192–200.

Bapurao S, Raman L, Tulpule P: Biochemical assessment of vitamin B6 nutritional status in pregnant women with orolingual manifestations. *Am J Clin N* 1982;36:581.

Barker D: The effect of nutrition of the fetus and neonate on cardiovascular disease in adult life. *P Nutr Soc* 1992;51(2):135–144.

Calcium supplementation prevents hypertensive disorders of pregnancy. *Nutr Rev* 1992;50(8):233–236.

Connor W, Neuringer M, Reisbick S: Essential fatty acids: The importance of omega-3 fatty acids in the retina and brain. *Nutr Rev* 1992;50(4):21–28.

Fenster L, Eskenazi B, Windham G, et al: Caffeine consumption during pregnancy and fetal growth. *Am J Pub He* 1991;81:458–461.

Folate deficiency and pregnancy outcome. *Nutr Rev* 1991;49(10):314–315.

Food and Nutrition Board, Institute of Medicine, National Academy of Sciences. *Nutrition During Pregnancy. Part 1: Weight Gain. Part 2: Nutrient Supplements.* Washington, DC, National Academy Press, 1990.

Funk D, Worthington-Roberts B, Fantel A: Impact of supplemental lysine or tryptophan on pregnancy course and outcome in rats. *Nutr Res* 1991;11:501–512.

Glenn F, Glenn W, Duncan R: Fluoride tablet supplementation during pregnancy for caries immunity: A study of the offspring produced. *Am J Obst G* 1982;143:560.

Hack M, Breslau N, Weissman B, et al: Effect of low birth weight and subnormal head size on cognitive abilities at school age. *N Eng J Med* 1991;325:231–237.

Heston T, Simkin P: Carbohydrate loading in preparation for childbirth. *Med Hypoth* 1991;34:97–98.

John E, Savitz D, Sandler D: Prenatal exposure to parents' smoking and childhood cancer. *Am J Epidem* 1991;133(2):123–132.

Kinsella K: Changes in life expectancy 1900–1990. *Am J Clin N* 1992;55:1196S–1202S.

Kizer K, Bankowska J, Jackson R, et al: Vitamin A—A pregnancy hazard alert. *West J Med* 1990;152:78–81.

Knight K, Keith R: Calcium supplementation on normotensive and hypertensive pregnant women. *Am J Clin N* 1992;55:891–895.

Kohrs M, Harper A, Kerr G: Effects of low-protein diet during pregnancy of the rhesus monkey. I. Reproductive efficiency. *Am J Clin N* 1976;29:136–145.

Lawrence M, McKillop F, Durnin J: Women who gain more fat during pregnancy may not have bigger babies: Implications for recommended weight gain during pregnancy. *Br J Obst G* 1991;98:254–259.

Malhotra A, Fairweather-Tait S, Wharton P, et al: Placental zinc in normal and intrauterine growth-retarded pregnancies. *Br J Nutr* 1990;63:613–621.

Marya R, Saini A, Jaswal T: Effect of vitamin D supplementation during pregnancy on the neonatal skeletal growth in the rat. *Ann Nutr Metab* 1991;35:208–212.

Massey L, Berg T: The effect of dietary caffeine on urinary excretion of calcium, magnesium, phosphorus, sodium, potassium, chloride, and zinc in healthy mice. *Nutr Res* 1985;5:1281–1284.

McCullough A, Kirksey A, Wachs T, et al: Vitamin B6 status in Egyptian mothers: Relation to infant behavior and maternal-infant interactions. *Am J Clin N* 1990; 51:1067–1074.

McGarvey S, Zinner S, Willett W, et al: Maternal prenatal dietary potassium, calcium, magnesium, and infant blood pressure. *Hypertensio* 1991;17:218–224.

MRC Vitamin Study Research Group: Prevention of neural tube defects: Results of the Medical Research Council Vitamin Study. *Lancet* 1991;338:131–137.

Murphy P: Periconceptional supplementation with folic acid: Does it prevent neural tube defects? *J Nurse-Mid* 1992;37(1):25–31.

Neggers Y, Cutter G, Acton R, et al: A positive association between maternal serum zinc concentration and birth weight. *Am J Clin N* 1990;51:678–684.

Norkus E, Rosso R: Effects of maternal intake of ascorbic acid on the postnatal metabolism of this vitamin in the guinea pig. *J Nutr* 1981;111:624.

O'Brien P, Morrison R, Pipkin F: The effect of dietary supplementation with linoleic and gamma-linolenic acids on the pressor response to angiotensin. 2. A possible role in pregnancy-induced hypertension. *Br J Cl Ph* 1985;19(3):335–342.

Ogawa H, Tominaga S, Hori K, et al: Passive smoking by pregnant women and fetal growth. *J Epidem C* 1991;45:164–168.

Oliveria S, Ellison R, Moore L, et al: Parent-child relationships in nutrient intake: The Framingham Children's Study. *Am J Clin N* 1992;56:593–598.

Reynolds R, Polansky M, Moser P: Analyzed vitamin B6 intakes of pregnant and postpartum lactating and nonlactating women. *J Am Diet A* 1984;84:1339–1334.

Roberts R, Cohan M, Forfar J: Antenatal factors in neonatal hypocalcemic convulsions. *Lancet* 1973;II:809.

Roepke J, Kirksey A: Vitamin B6 nutriture during pregnancy and lactation: I. Vitamin B6 intake levels of the vitamin in biological fluids and condition of the infant at birth. *Am J Clin N* 1979;32:2249.

Rosenfeld J: Maternal work outside the home and its effect on women and their families. *JAMWA* 1992;47(2):47–51.

Sahakian V, Rouse D, Sipes S, et al: Vitamin B6 is effective therapy for nausea and vomiting of pregnancy: A randomized double-blind placebo-controlled study. *Obstet Gyn* 1991;78:33–36.

Scholl T, Hediger M, Fischer R, et al: Anemia versus iron deficiency: Increased risk of preterm delivery in a prospective study. *Am J Clin N* 1992;55:985–988.

Shojania A: Folic acid and vitamin B12 deficiency in pregnancy and in the neonatal period. *Clin Perin* 1984;11(2):433–459.

Springer N, Bischoping K, Sampselle C, et al: Using early weight gain and other nutrition-related risk factors to predict pregnancy outcomes. *J Am Diet A* 1992;92(2):217–219.

Srisuphan W, Bracken M: Caffeine consumption during pregnancy and association with late spontaneous abortion. *Am J Obst G* 1986;154:14–20.

Suchecki D, Neto J: Prenatal stress and emotional response of adult offspring. *Physl Behav* 1991;49:423–426.

Taper L, Oliva J, Ritchey S: Zinc and copper retention during pregnancy: The adequacy of prenatal diets with and without dietary supplementation. *Am J Clin N* 1985;41:1184–1192.

Teratology Society position paper: Recommendations for vitamin A use during pregnancy. *Teratology* 1987;35(2):269–275.

Villar J, Belizan J, Fischer P: Epidemiologic observations on the relationship between calcium intake and eclampsia. *Int J Gyn O* 1983;21(4):271–278.

Wang Y, Kay H, Killam A: Decreased levels of polyunsaturated fatty acids in preeclampsia. *Am J Obst G* 1991;164:812–818.

Watkinson B, Fired P: Maternal caffeine use before, during and after pregnancy and effects upon offspring. *Neurob Tox* 1985;7:9–17.

Zeisel S: Choline: An important nutrient in brain development, liver function, and carcinogenesis. *J Am Col N* 1992;11(5):473–481.

CHAPTER NINE

Baer J, Taper J, Gwazdauskas F, et al: Diet, hormonal, and metabolic factors affecting bone mineral density in adolescent amenorrheic and eumenorrheic female runners. *J Sport Med* 1992;32:51–58.

Barnett D, Conlee R: The effects of a commercial dietary supplement on human performance. *Am J Clin N* 1984;40:586–590.

Belko A, Roe D: Exercise-riboflavin relationships. *Fed Proc* 1984;43:870.

Benson J, Allemann Y, Theintz G, et al: Eating problems and calorie intake levels in Swiss adolescent athletes. *Int J Sp M* 1990;11:249–252.

Borch-Johnsen B, Meltzer H, Stenberg V, et al: Bioavailability of daily low-dose iron supplements in menstruating women with low iron stores. *Eur J Cl N* 1990; 44:29–34.

Brilla L, Haley T: Effect of magnesium supplementation on strength training in humans. *J Am Col N* 1992;11(3):326–329.

Casoni I, Guglielmini C, Graziano L, et al: Changes of magnesium concentrations in endurance athletes. *Int J Sp M* 1990;11(3):234–237.

Cerretelli P, Marconi C: L-carnitine supplementation in humans: The effects of physical performance. *Int J Sp M* 1990;11(1):1–14.

Couzy F, LaFargue P, Guezennec C: Zinc metabolism in the athlete: Influence of training, nutrition and other factors. *Int J Sp M* 1990;11:263–266.

Cowart V: Dietary supplements: Alternatives to anabolic steroids? *Phys Sport* 1992; 20(3):189–212.

Decombaz J, Gmuender B, Sierro G, et al: Muscle carnitine after strenuous endurance exercise. *J Appl Physiol* 1992;72(2);423–427.

Devlin J, Horton E: Metabolic fuel utilization during postexercise recovery. *Am J Clin N* 1989;49:944–948.

Fern E, Bielinski R, Schutz Y: Effects of exaggerated amino acid and protein supply in man. *Experientia* 1991;47:168–171.

Flinn S, Gregory J, McNaughton L, et al: Caffeine ingestion prior to incremental cycling to exhaustion in recreational cyclists. *Int J Sp M* 1991;11:188–193.

Graham T, Spriet L: Performance and metabolic responses to a high caffeine dose during prolonged exercise. *J Appl Physiol* 1991;71(6):2292–2298.

Grandjean A: Nutritional concerns of the woman athlete. *Clin Sp Med* 1984; 3(4): 923–938.

Hickson J, Schrader J, Trischler L: Dietary intakes of female basketball and gymnastic athletes. *J Am Diet A* 1986;86:251–253.

Highet R: Athletic amenorrhoea. An update on aetiology, complications and management. *Sport Med* 1989;7:82–108.

Horton E: Metabolic fuels, utlization, and exercise. *Am J Clin N* 1989;49:931–937.

Jackson M: Muscle damage during exercise: Possible role of free radicals and protective effect of vitamin E. *P Nutr Soc* 1987;46:77–80.

Keith R, Alt L: Riboflavin status of female athletes consuming normal diets. *Nutr Res* 1991;11(7):727–734.

Keith R, O'Keeffe K, Blessing D, et al: Alternations in dietary carbohydrate, protein, and fat intake and mood state in trained female cyclists. *Med Sci Spt* 1991;23:212–216.

Kochanowski B, McMahan C: Inhibition of iron absorption by calcium in rats and dogs: Effects of mineral separation by time and enteric coating. *Nutr Res* 1990; 10:219–226.

Lampe J, Slavin J, Apple F: Poor iron status of women runners training for a marathon. *Int J Sp M* 1986;7(2):111–114.

Lemon P, Tarnopolsky M, MacDougall J, et al: Protein requirements and muscle mass/ strength changes during intensive training in novice bodybuilders. *J Appl Physiol* 1992;73(2):767–775.

Litoff D, Scherzer H, Harrison J: Effects of pantothenic acid on human exercise. *Med Sci Spt* 1985;17:287.

Lloyd T, Dolence L, Bartholomew M: Nutritional characteristics of recreational women runners. *Nutr Res* 1992;12:359–366.

Lukaski H, Hoverson B, Gallagher S, et al: Physical training and copper, iron, and zinc status of swimmers. *Am J Clin N* 1990;51:1093–1099.

Manore M, Leklem J: Effect of carbohydrate and vitamin B6 on fuel substrates during exercise in women. *Med Sci Spt* 1988;20(3):233–241.

Manore M, Leklem J, Walter M: Vitamin B6 metabolism as affected by exercise in trained and untrained women fed diets differing in carbohydrate and vitamin B6 content. *Am J Clin N* 1987;46:995–1004.

Mitchell J, Tate C, Raven P, et al: Acute response and chronic adaptation to exercise in women. *Med Sci Spt* 1992;24(6):S258–S265.

Montain S, Hopper M, Coggan A, et al: Exercise metabolism at different time intervals after a meal. *J Appl Physiol* 1991;70:882–888.

Murray R: Nutrition for the marathon and other endurance sports: Environmental stress and dehydration. *Med Sci Spt* 1992;24(9):S319–S323.

Nelson M, Meredith C, Dawson-Hughes B, et al: Hormone and bone mineral status in endurance-trained and sedentary postmenopausal women. *J Clin End* 1988; 66:927–933.

Novelli G, Bracciotti G, Falsini S: Spin-trappers and vitamin E prolong endurance to muscle fatigue in mice. *Fr Rad B* 1990;8:9–13.

Owens J, Matthews K, Wing R, et al: Can physical activity mitigate the effects of aging in middle-aged women? *Circulation* 1992;85:1265–1270.

Pascoe D, Costill D, Robergs R, et al: Effects of exercise mode on muscle glycogen restorage during repeated days of exercise. *Med Sci Spt* 1990;22:593.

Pratt C: Moderate exercise and iron status in women. *Nutr Rep* 1991;9(7):48,56.

Pryor W: Can vitamin E protect humans against the pathological effects of ozone in smog? *Am J Clin N* 1991;53:702–722.

Rehrer N, Brouns F, Beckers E, et al: Gastric emptying with repeated drinking during running and bicycling. *Int J Sp M* 1991;11:238–243.

Resina A, Fedi S, Gatteschi L, et al: Comparison of some serum copper parameters in trained runners and control subjects. *Int J Sp M* 1990;11(1):58–60.

Robertson J, Maughan R, Duthio G, et al: Increased blood antioxidant systems of runners in response to training load. *Clin Sci* 1991;80:611–618.

Seidman D, Ashkenazi I, Arnon R, et al: The effects of glucose polymer beverage ingestion during prolonged outdoor exercise in the heat. *Med Sci Spt* 1991;23:458–462.

Simonsen J, Sherman W, Lamb D, et al: Dietary carbohydrate, muscle glycogen, and power output during rowing training. *J Appl Physiol* 1991;70:1500–1505.

Staten M: The effect of exercise on food intake in men and women. *Am J Clin N* 1991;53:27–31.

Stendig-Lindberg G, Shapiro Y, Epstein Y, et al: Changes in serum magnesium concentration after strenuous exercise. *J Am Col N* 1987;6:35–40.

van Erp-Baart A, Saris W, Binkhorst R, et al: Nationwide survey on nutritional habits of elite athletes. *Int J Sp M* 1989;10:S3–S10.

Wagenmakers A, Coakley J, Edwards R: Metabolism of branched-chain amino acids and ammonia during exercise: Clues from McArdle's disease. *Int J Sp M* 1990;11:S101–S113.

Weaver C, Rajaram S: Exercise and iron status. *J Nutr* 1992;122:782–787.

Weir J, Noakes T, Myburgh K, et al: A high carbohydrate diet negates the metabolic effects of caffeine during exercise. *Med Sci Spt* 1987;19:100–105.

Wilcox A: Effects of caffeine and exercise on body fat levels in the rat. *Int J Spt M* 1985;6(6):322–324.

Williams M: Vitamin supplementation and athletic performance, in Walter P, et al (eds): Elevated dosages of vitamins. *Int J Nutr Res* 1989;163–191.

Winters L, Yoon J, Kalkwarf H, et al: Riboflavin requirements and exercise adaptation in older women. *Am J Clin N* 1992;56:526–532.

Witt E, Reznick A, Viguie C, et al: Exercise, oxidative damage and effects of antioxidant manipulation. *J Nutr* 1992;122:766–773.

Yoon S, Trebler L, Roe D: Effect of exercise on the riboflavin requirements of older women. *Fed Proc* 1987;46(4):1166.

CHAPTER TEN

Aging reduces intestinal and skeletal receptors for 1,25 dihydroxyvitamin D. *Nutr Rev* 1991;49(6):189–191.

Asche K, Heimpel H: Vitamins containing powdered drug for treatment of premenstrual and menopausal disturbances. *Ger Offen De* 1989Jul; 27:3.

Barlow D: Hormone replacement therapy and other menopause associated conditions. *Br Med B* 1992;48(2);356–365.

Bjorksten J: Longevity "A Quest." *Rejuvenation* 1981;9(3):47–52.

Bjorntorp P: Metabolic implications of body fat distribution. *Diabet Care* 1991;14:1132–1143.

Bosse T, Donald E: The vitamin B6 requirement in oral contraceptive users. I. Assessment of pyridoxal level and transferase activity in erythrocytes. *Am J Clin N* 1979; 32:1015–1023.

Chan D: The effects of dietary antioxidants on lifespan and the age-related decline in learning and memory in drosophilia melanogaster. *Age* 1985;8:145.

Covelli V, Mouton D, DeMajo V, et al: Inheritance of immune responsiveness, life span, and disease incidence in interline crosses of mice selected for high or low multi-specific antibody production. *J Immunol* 1989;142:1224–1234.

Dawson-Hughes B: Calcium supplementation and bone loss: A review of controlled clinical trials. *Am J Clin N* 1991;54:274S–280S.

Fillit H: Reversible acquired immunodeficiency in the elderly: A review. *Age* 1991; 14:83–89.

Greeley S: American women in midlife: Eating patterns and menopause. *Ann NY Acad Sci* 1989;570:162–166.

Greenstein R, Ybanez M, Zhang R, et al: Is aging preprogrammed? Observations from the brain/gut axis. *Mech Age D* 1991;61:113–121.

Harlap S: The benefits and risk of hormone replacement therapy: An epidemiological overview. *Am J Obst G* 1992;166:1986–1992.

Johnson B, Good R: Chronic dietary restriction and longevity. *Soc Exp Biol Med* 1990;193:4–5.

Katz S, Branch L, Branson M, et al: Active life expectancy. *N Eng J Med* 1983;309:1218–1224.

Keno Y, Matsuzawa Y, Tokunaga K, et al: High sucrose diet increases visceral fat accumulation in VMH-lesioned obese rates. *Int J Obes* 1991;15:205–211.

Khaw K: Epidemiology of the menopause. *Br Med B* 1992;48(2):249–261.

Kinsella K: Changes in life expectancy 1900–1990. *Am J Clin N* 1992;55:1196S–1202S.

Ley C, Lees B, Stevenson J: Sex- and menopause-associated changes in body-fat distribution. *Am J Clin N* 1992;55:950–954.

Lipschitz D, McClellan J: Impact of nutrition on the age-related decline in immune and hematologic function. *Cont Nutr* 1990;15(2):1–2.

Lobo R: The role of progestins in hormone replacement therapy. *Am J Obst G* 1992; 166:1997–2004.

Marcus R, Drinkwater B, Dalsky G, et al: Osteoporosis and exercise in women. *Med Sci Spt* 1992;24(6):S301–S307.

Masoro E: Nutrition and aging: A current assessment. *J Nutr* 1985;115(7):842–848.

McClung M: Approaches to the management of symptomatic osteoporosis. Presented at Salem Hospital, Salem, Oregon, February 1992.

Meydani M, Verdon C, Blumberg J: Effect of vitamin E, selenium, and age on lipid peroxidation events in rat cerebrum. *Nutr Res* 1985;5:1227–1236.

Monti D, Troiano L, Tropea F, et al: Apoptosis—programmed cell death: A role in the aging process? *Am J Clin N* 1992;55:1208S–1214S.

Notelovitz M: Estrogen in postmenopausal women: An opposing view. *J Fam Pract* 1989;29(4):410–415.

Owens J, Matthews K, Wing R, et al: Can physical activity mitigate the effects of aging in middle-aged women? *Circulation* 1992;85:1265–1270.

Pi-Sunyer F: Health implications of obesity. *Am J Clin N* 1991;53:1595S–1603S.

Ross M: Nutrition and longevity in experimental animals, in Winick M (ed): *Nutrition and Aging.* New York, John Wiley & Sons, 1976:43–57.

Schlemmer A, Podenphant J, Riis B, et al: Urinary magnesium in early postmenopausal women. *Magnes Tr El* 1991–92;10:34–39.

Schlettwein-Gsell D: Nutrition and the quality of life: A measure for the outcome of nutritional intervention? *Am J Clin N* 1992;55:1263S–1266S.

Schloss B: Possibilities for prolonging life in the near future. *Rejuvenation* 1981; 9(2):30–32.

Smith C, Bidlack W: Dietary concerns associated with the use of medications. *J Am Diet A* 1984;84(8):901–914.

Studd J: Complications of hormone replacement therapy in post-menopausal women. *J Roy S Med* 1992 July;85:376–378.

Tikkanen M, Juusi T, Vartianinen E, et al: Treatment of postmenopausal hypercholesterolemia with estradiol. *Act Obst Sc* 1979;88(Suppl.):83–88.

Tucker D, Penland J, Sandstead H, et al: Nutrition status and brain function in aging. *Am J Clin N* 1990;52:93–102.

Van Beresteijn E, Riedstra M, Van Der Well A, et al: Habitual dietary calcium intake and blood pressure change around the menopause: A longitudinal study. *Int J Epid* 1992;21(4):683–689.

Vellas B, Balas D, Albarede J: Effects of aging process on digestive functions. *Compr Ther* 1991;17(8):46–52.

Wahl P, Walden C, Knopp R, et al: Effect of estrogen-progestin potency on lipid/lipoprotein cholesterol. *N Eng J Med* 1983;308:862–867.

Wing R, Matthews K, Kuller L, et al: Waist to hip ratio in middle-aged women. *Arterioscle Thrombo* 1991;11:1250–1257.

Winick M (ed): *Nutrition and Aging.* New York, John Wiley & Sons, 1976.

CHAPTER ELEVEN

Allen B, Maurice P, Goodfield M, et al: The effects on psoriasis of dietary supplementation with eicosapentaenoic acid. *Br J Derm* 1985;113:777.

Craig G, Elliot C, Hughes K: Masked vitamin B12 and folate deficiency in the elderly. *Br J Nutr* 1985;54:613–619.

Evans W: Exercise, nutrition, and aging. *J Nutr* 1992;122:796–801.

Garry P, Goodwin J, Hunt W: Folate and vitamin B12 status in a healthy elderly population. *J Am Ger So* 1984;32:719–726.

Geode H, Penn N, Kelleher J, et al: Evidence of cellular zinc depletion in hospitalized but not in healthy elderly subjects. *Age Ageing* 1991;20:345–348.

Goodwin J, Hunt W, Hooper P, et al: Relationship between zinc intake, physical activity, and blood levels of high density lipoprotein cholesterol in a healthy elderly population. *Metabolism* 1985;34:519–523.

Kahin H: Laxatives: A last resort in chronic constipation. *Consultant* 1977 March:25–27.

Katahn M: Nutrition and older persons: A clinical perspective. *Nutr Rep* 1991 December;9(12):88,96.

Kennes B, Dumont I, Brohee D, et al: Effect of vitamin C supplements on cell-mediated immunity in old people. *Gerontology* 1983;29:305–310.

Klein S, Rogers R: Nutritional requirements in the elderly. *Gastro Clin* 1990 June; 19(2):473–491.

Kohrs M: New perspectives on nutritional counseling for the elderly. *Cont Nutr* 1983;8(3):1–2.

Liebman B: Nutrition and aging. *Nutr Action HealthLetter* 1992 May;19(4):1,5–7.

Lowik M, Schneijder P, Hulshop K, et al: Institutionalized elderly women have lower food intake than do those living more independently (Dutch Nutrition Surveillance System). *J Am Col N* 1992;11(4):432–440.

MacLaughlin J, Holick M: Aging decreases the capacity of human skin to produce vitamin D3. *Clin Inv* 1985;76:1536–1538.

Malasanos T, Stacpoole P: Biological effects of w-3 fatty acids in diabetes mellitus. *Diabet Care* 1991;14(12):1160–1179.

McMurtry C, Young S, Downs R, et al: Mild vitamin D deficiency and secondary hyper-parathyroidism in nursing home patients receiving adequate dietary vitamin D. *J Am Ger So* 1992;40:343–347.

Meydani M, Natiello F, Goldin B, et al: Effect of long-term fish oil supplementation on vitamin E status and lipid peroxidation in women. *J Nutr* 1991;121:484–491.

Mobarhan S, Hypert J, Friedman H: Effects of aging on beta carotene and vitamin A status. *Age* 1991;14:13–16.

Motulsky A: Nutrition and genetic susceptibility to common diseases. *Am J Clin N* 1992;55:1244S–1245S.

Munthe E, Aaseth J: Treatment of rheumatoid arthritis with selenium and vitamin E. *Sc J Rheum* 1984;S53:103.

Newton H, Schorah C, Habibzadeh N, et al: The cause and correlation of low blood vitamin C concentrations in the elderly. *Am J Clin N* 1985;42:656–659.

NIH Consensus Conference. *J Am Med A* 1984;252:799.

Pao E, Mickle S: Problem nutrients in the United States. *Food Tech* 1981; September.

Payette H, Gray-Donald K: Do vitamin and mineral supplements improve the dietary intake of elderly Canadians? *Can J Pub He* 1991 January/February;82:58–60.

The RDAs and the elderly. *Nutr MD* 1986 July;12(7):3–4.

Reddy B, Burill C, Rigotty J: Effect of diets high in omega-3 and omega-6 fatty acids on initiation and postinitiation stages of colon carcinogenesis. *Cancer Res* 1991; 51:487–491.

Ribaya-Mercado J, Russell R, Sahyoun N, et al: Vitamin B6 requirements of elderly men and women. *J Nutr* 1991;121:1062–1074.

Rosenberg I, Miller J: Nutritional factors in physical and cognitive functions of elderly people. *Am J Clin N* 1992;55:1237S–1243S.

Russell R: Changes in gastrointestinal function attributed to aging. *Am J Clin N* 1992;55:1203S–1207S.

Sager K: Senior fitness—For the health of it. *Phys Sport* 1983 October;11(10):31–36.

Tolonen M, Halme M, Sarna S: Vitamin E and selenium supplementation in geriatric patients. *Biol Tr El* 1985;7:161–168.

Tucker D, Penland J, Sandstead H, et al: Nutrition status and brain function in aging. *Am J Clin N* 1990;52:93–102.

Vellas B, Albarede J, Garry P: Diseases and aging: Patterns of morbidity with age; relationship between aging and age-associated diseases. *Am J Clin N* 1992;55:1225S–1230S.

Vellas B, Balas D, Albarede J: Effects of aging process on digestive functions. *Compr Ther* 1991;17(8):46–52.

Vitamin D supplementation in the elderly. *Lancet* 1987;I:306–307.

Vitamin E supplementation enhances immune response in the elderly. *Nutr Rev* 1991; 50(3):85–87.

Zamboni M, Armellini F, Milani M, et al: Body fat distribution in pre- and post-menopausal women: Metabolic and anthropometric variables and their inter-relationships. *Int J Obes* 1992;16:495–504.

CHAPTER TWELVE

Amable-Cuevas C, Pina-Zentella R, Wah-Laborde M: Decreased resistance to antibiotics and plasmid loss in plasmid-carrying strains of Staphylococcus aureus treated with ascorbic acid. *Mutat Res* 1991;264:119–125.

Awad A: Diet and drug interactions in the treatment of mental illness. *Can J Psych* 1984;29(7):609–613.

Benn A, Swan C, Cooke W, et al: Effect of intraluminal pH on the absorption of pteryl-monoglutamic acid. *Br Med J* 1971;1:148.

Bergman E, Massey L, Wise K, et al: Effects of dietary caffeine in renal handling of miner-als in adult women. *Life Sci* 1990;47:557–564.

Bosse T, Donald E: The vitamin B6 requirement in oral contraceptive users. I. Assessment of pyridoxal level and transferase activity in erythrocytes. *Am J Clin N* 1979; 32:1015–1023.

Bui M, Sauty A, Collet F, et al: Dietary vitamin C intake and concentration in the body fluids and cells of male smokers and nonsmokers. *J Nutr* 1992;122:312–316.

de Mesquita A, Maisonneuve P, Moerman C, et al: Lifetime consumption of alcoholic beverages, tea, and coffee and endocrine carcinoma of the pancreas: A population-based case-control study in the Netherlands. *Int J Canc* 1992;50:514–522.

Dulloo A, Miller D: Prevention of genetic fa/fa obesity with an ephedrine-methylxanthine thermogenic mixture. *Am J Physl* 1987; 252:R507–R513.

du Preez M, Lockett C: Effect of clopamide, a thiazine diuretic, on copper and zinc levels in hypertensive patients. *J Am Col N* 1991;10(1):34–37.

Dworkin B, Rosenthal W, Gordon G, et al: Diminished blood selenium levels in alcohol-ics. *Alc Clin Ex* 1984;8:535–538.

Dworkin B, Rosenthal W, Jankowski R, et al: Low blood selenium levels in alcoholics with and without advanced liver disease: Correlations with clinical and nutritional status. *Dig Dis Sci* 1985;30:838–844.

Fields M, Lewis C: Alcohol consumption aggravates copper deficiency. *Metabolism* 1990;39(6):610–613.

Franklin J, Roseberg I: Impaired folic acid absorption in inflammatory bowel disease: Effects of salicylazosulfapyridine (Azulfidine). *Gastroenty* 1973;64:517–525.

Garrison R, Somer E: *The Nutrition Desk Reference, 2d ed.* New Canaan, CT: Keats Publishing Company, 1990:p279.

Godsland I, Crook D, Wynn V, et al: Clinical and metabolic considerations of long-term oral contraceptive use. *Am J Obst G* 1992;166:1955–1963.

Golik A, Modai D, Averbukh Z, et al: Zinc metabolism in patients treated with captopril and enalapril. *Metabolism* 1990;39(7):665–667.

Goulding A, McIntosh J, Campbell D: Effect of sodium bicarbonate and 1,25 dihydroxy-cholecalciferol on calcium and phosphorus balances in the rat. *J Nutr* 1984; 114: 653–659.

Grimes D: The safety of oral contraceptives: Epidemiologic insights from the first 30 years. *Am J Obst G* 1992;166:1950–1954.

Hasling C, Sondergaard K, Charles P, et al: Calcium metabolism in postmenopausal osteoporotic women is determined by dietary calcium and coffee intake. *J Nutr* 1992; 122:1119–1126.

Hayes J, Borzelleca J: Nutrient interaction with drugs and other xenobiotics. *J Am Diet A* 1985;85:335–339.

Heimburger D, Alexander C, Birch R, et al: Improvement in bronchial squamous metaplasia in smokers treated with folate and vitamin B12. *J Am Med A* 1988; 259:1525–1530.

Hornig D, Glatthaar B: Vitamin C and smoking: Increased requirements for smokers, in Hanck A, Hornig D (eds.): Vitamins: Nutrients and Therapeutic Agents. *Int J Vit N* 1985; Suppl. 27:139.

Hoshino E, Shariff R, van Gossum A, et al: Vitamin E suppresses increased lipid peroxidation in cigarette smokers. *J Parent En* 1990;14:300–305.

Joffres M, Reed D, Yano K: Relationship of magnesium intake and other dietary factors to blood pressure: The Honolulu Heart Study. *Am J Clin N* 1987;45: 469–475.

Johansson U, Johnsson F, Joelsson B, et al: Selenium status in patients with liver cirrhosis and alcoholism. *Br J Nutr* 1986;55:227–233.

Katerndahl D, Realini J, Cohen P: Oral contraceptive use and cardiovascular disease: Is the relationship real or due to study bias? *J Fam Pract* 1992;35(20):147–157.

Klatsky A, Friedman G, Armstrong M: Coffee use prior to myocardial infarction restudied: Heavier intake may increase the risk. *Am J Epidem* 1990;132:479–488.

Leklem J: Vitamin B6 requirements and oral contraceptive use: A concern? *J Nutr* 1986; 116(3):475–477.

McEwen J: Phenylpropanolamine-associated hypertension after the use of "over-the-counter" appetite-suppressant products. *Med J Aust* 1983 July 23:71–73.

Milne D, Canfield W, Gallagher S, et al: Metabolism of ethanol in postmenopausal women fed a diet marginal in zinc. *Clin Res* 1986;34:A801.

Mohan P, Ihnen J, Levin B, et al: Effects of dehydroepiandrosterone treatment in rats with diet-induced obesity. *J Nutr* 1990;120:1103–1114.

Pacht E, Kaseki H, Mohammed J, et al: Deficiency of vitamin E in the alveolar fluid of cigarette smokers: Influence of alveolar macrophage cytotoxicity. *J Clin Inv* 1986;77:789–796.

Puccio E, McPhillips J, Barrett-Connor E, et al: Clustering of atherogenic behaviors in coffee drinkers. *Am J Pub He* 1990;80:1310–1313.

Rivera-Calimlim L: Ethanol and pantothenic acid on brain acetylcholine. *Clin Pharm* 1987;41:215.

Roe D: Drug-food and drug-nutrient interactions. *J Env P Tox* 1985;5(6):115–135.

Schectman G, Byrd J, Hoffmann R: Ascorbic acid requirements for smokers: Analysis of a population survey. *Am J Clin N* 1991;53:1466–1470.

Schenker S, Speeg K: The risk of alcohol intake in men and women: All may not be equal. *N Eng J Med* 1990;322:127–129.

Schteingart D: Effectiveness of phenylpropanolamine in the management of moderate obesity. *Int J Obes* 1992;16:487–493.

Seaborn C, Stoecker B: Effects of antacid or ascorbic acid on tissue accumulation and urinary excretion of chromium. *Nutr Res* 1990;10:1401–1407.

Seelig C: Magnesium deficiency in two hypertensive patient groups. *So Med J* 1990; 83(7):739–742.

Smith C, Bidlack W: Dietary concerns associated with the use of medications. *J Am Diet A* 1984;84(8):901–914.

Spender H, Norris C, Coffey F, et al: Effect of small amounts of antacids on calcium, phosphorus, and fluoride metabolism in man. *Gastroenty* 1975;68:990.

Subar A, Harlan L, Mattson M: Food and nutrient intake differences between smokers and non-smokers in the U.S. *Am J Pub He* 1990;80:1323–1329.

Superko H, Bortz W, Williams P, et al: Caffeinated and decaffeinated coffee effects on plasma lipoprotein cholesterol, apolipoproteins, and lipase activity: A controlled randomized trial. *Am J Clin N* 1991;54:599–605.

Susick R, Abrams G, Zurawski C, et al: Ascorbic acid and chronic alcohol consumption in the guinea pig. *Tox Appl Ph* 1986;84:329–335.

Vermaak W, Ubbink J, Barnard H, et al: Vitamin B6 nutrition status and cigarette smoking. *Am J Clin N* 1990;51:1058–1061.

Weintraub M: Long-term weight control: The National Heart, Lung, and Blood Institute funded Multimodal Intervention Study. *Clin Pharm* 1992;51(5):581–646.

Zemel M, Green J, Zemel P, et al: Effects of magnesium supplementation on erythrocyte cation transport in diuretic-treated hypertensives. *Nutr Res* 1989;9:1285–1292.

INTRODUCTION TO PART THREE

Alexander J, Peck M: Future prospects for adjunctive therapy: Pharmacologic and nutritional approaches to immune system modulation. *Crit Care Med* 1990; 18:S159.

Beisel W: History of nutritional immunology: Introduction and overview. *J Nutr* 1992;122:591–596.

Bendich A: Beta carotene and the immune response. *P Nutr Soc* 1991;50:263–274.

Block E: The chemistry of garlic and onions. *Sci Am* 1985;252:114–121.

Bogden J, Oleske J, Lavenhar M, et al: Effects of one year of supplementation with zinc and other micronutrients on cellular immunity in the elderly. *J Am Col N* 1990;9(3):214–225.

Chandra R: The role of trace elements and immune function. *Nutr Rep* 1987;5(4):24,32.
———: Excessive intake of zinc impairs immune responses. *J Am Med A* 1984; 252 (11):1443–1446.

Corman L: Effects of specific nutrients on the immune response. *Med Clin NA* 1985;69(4):759–785.

Daly J, Reynolds J, Sigel R, et al: Effect of dietary protein and amino acids on immune function. *Crit Care Med* 1990;18(2):S860.

Diplock A: Antioxidant nutrients and disease prevention. An overview. *Am J Clin N* 1991;53:189S–193S.

Fletcher M, Ziboh V: Effects of dietary supplementation with eicosapentaenoic acid or gamma linolenic acid on neutrophil phospholipid fatty acid composition and activation responses. *Inflammatio* 1990;14:585–597.

Floyd R: Role of oxygen free radicals in carcinogenesis and brain ischemia. *FASEB J* 1990;4:2587–2597.

Foote C, Denny R, Weaver L, et al: Quenching of singlet oxygen. *Ann NY Acad* 1970; 171:139–148.

Gebhard K, Gridley D, Stickney D, et al: Enhancement of immune status by high levels of dietary vitamin B6 without growth inhibition of human malignant melanoma in athymic nude mice. *Nutr Cancer* 1990;14:15–26.

Halliwell B, Gutteridge J, Cross C: Free radicals, antioxidants, and human disease: Where are we now? *J La Cl Med* 1992;119(6):598–620.

Hambridge K: The role of zinc and other trace minerals in pediatric nutrition and health. *Ped Clin NA* 1977;24:95.

Hughes G: The effects of beta-carotene on the immune system in cancer. *Nutr Rep* 1992;10(1):1,8.

Huwyler T, Hirt A, Morell A: Effect of ascorbic acid on human natural killer cells. *Immunol Let* 1985;10:173–176.

Jacob R, Kelley D, Pianalto F, et al: Immunocompetence and oxidant defense during ascorbate depletion of healthy men. *Am J Clin N* 1991;54:1302S–1309S.

Junod A: Data on oxidants and antioxidants. *B Eur Phys* 1986;22:S253–S255.

Kinsella J: Dietary polyunsaturated fatty acids affect inflammatory and immune functions. *Nutr Rep* 1990;8(10):72,80.

Kiremidjian-Schumacher L, Stotzky G: Review: Selenium and immune responses. *Envir Res* 1987;42:277–303.

Kirk S, Barbul A: Role of arginine in trauma, sepsis, and immunity. *J Parent En* 1990;14(5):S226–S229.

Kor H, Scimeca J: Influence of dietary fat replacement on immune function. *FASEB* 1991;5(5):A565, #1130.

Lau B, Tadi P, Tosk J: Allium sativum (garlic) and cancer prevention. *Nutr Res* 1990; 10:937–948.

Mai J, Sorensen P, Hansen J: High-dose antioxidant supplementation in MS patients. *Biol Tr El* 1990;24:109.

Mascio P, Murphy M, Sies H: Antioxidant defense systems: The role of carotenoids, tocopherols, and thiols. *Am J Clin N* 1991;53:194S–200S.

Meydani S, Barklund M, Liu S, et al: Vitamin E supplementation enhances cell-mediated immunity in healthy elderly subjects. *Am J Clin N* 1990;52:557–563.

Meydani S, Lichtenstein A, Cornwall S, et al: Effect of low-fat, low-cholesterol (LF-LCHL) diet enriched in N-3 fatty acids (FA) on the immune response of humans. *FASEB J* 1991;5:1449A.

Meydani S, Ribaya-Mercado J, Russel R, et al: Vitamin B6 deficiency impairs interleukin 2 production and lymphocyte proliferation in elderly adults. *Am J Clin N* 1991; 53:1275–1280.

Middleton E, Drzewiecki G: Effect of ascorbic acid and flavonoids on human basophil histamine release. *J Allerg Cl* 1992 January:278.

Nehlsen-Cannarella S, Nieman D, Balk-Lamberton A, et al: The effects of moderate exercise training on immune response. *Med Sci Spt* 1991;23(1):64–70.

Padh H: Vitamin C: Newer insights into its biochemical functions. *Nutr Rev* 1991; 49:65–70.

Pedersen B: Influence of physical activity on the cellular immune system: Mechanisms of action. *Int J Sp M* 1991;12:S23–S29.

Pocino M, Baute L, Malave I: Influence of the oral administration of excess copper on the immune response. *Fund Appl T* 1991;16:249–256.

Pryor W: Can vitamin E protect humans against pathological effects of ozone in smog? *Am J Clin N* 1991;53:702–722.

Richardson J: Vitamin C and immunosuppression. *Med Hypoth* 1986;21:383–385.

Sato K, Niki E, Shimasaki H: Free radical–mediated chain oxidation of low-density lipoprotein and its synergistic inhibition by vitamin E and vitamin C: *Arch Bioch* 1990;279:402–405.

Schleifer S, Keller S, Stein M: Stress and immunity. *Psychiatr J Univ Ottawa* 1985;10 (3):125–131.

Schmidt K: Antioxidant vitamins and beta carotene effects on immunocompetence. *Am J Clin N* 1991; 53:383S–385S.

Shilotri P, Bhat K: Effect of megadoses of vitamin C on bactericidal activity of leukocytes. *Am J Clin N* 1977;30:1077–1081.

Somer E: Immunity: A future test for nutritional status? *Nutr Rep* 1991 May:34.

————: The role of free radicals in atherogenesis: More than just speculation. *Nutr Rep* 1990 August:58.

Sword J, Pope A, Hoekstra W: Endotoxin and lipid peroxidation in vivo in selenium- and vitamin E-deficient and adequate rats. *J Nutr* 1991;121:251–257.

Teuteberg H: Food patterns in the European past. *Ann Nutr Metab* 1991;35:181–190.

Watson R: Nutrition and immunity. *Cont Nutr* 1981;6(5):1–2.

Watson R, Leonard T: Selenium and vitamins A, E, and C: Nutrients with cancer prevention and properties. *Am J Diet A* 1986;86:505–510.

Yuting C, Rongliang Z, Zhongjian J, et al: Flavonoids as superoxide scavengers and antioxidants. *Free Rad B* 1990;9:19–21.

ACQUIRED IMMUNODEFICIENCY SYNDROME (AIDS)

Baker D: Cellular antioxidant status and human immunodeficiency virus replication. *Nutr Rev* 1992;50(1):15–17.

Begin M, Das U: A deficiency of dietary gamma-linolenic acid and/or eicosapentaenoic acids may determine individual susceptibility to AIDS. *Med Hypoth* 1986;20:1–8.

Boudes P, Zittoun J, Sobel A: Folate, vitamin B12, and HIV infection. *Lancet* 1990;335 (June 9):1401–1402.

Butterworth R, Gaudreau C, Vincelette J, et al: Thiamine deficiency in AIDS. *Lancet* 1991;338 (October 26):1086.

Dworkin B, Rosenthal W, Wormser G, et al: Selenium deficiency in the acquired immunodeficiency syndrome. *J Parent En* 1986;10:405–407.

————: Abormalities of blood selenium and glutathione peroxidase activity in patients with acquired immunodeficiency syndrome and AIDS-related complex. *Biol Tr El* 1988;15:167–177.

Fauci A, Schnittman S, Poli G, et al: Immunopathogenic mechanisms in human immunodeficiency virus (HIV) infection. *Ann Int Med* 1991;114(8):678–693.

Garewal H, Ampel N, Watson R, et al: A preliminary trial of beta-carotene in subjects infected with the human immunodeficiency virus. *J Nutr* 1992;122:728–732.

Hebert J, Barone J: On the possible relationship between AIDS and nutrition. *Med Hypoth* 1988;27:51–54.

Jain V, Chandra R: Does nutritional deficiency predispose to acquired immune deficiency syndrome? *Nutr Res* 1984;4:537–543.

Keating J, Trimble K, Mulcahy F, et al: Evidence of brain methyltransferase inhibition and early brain involvement in HIB-positive patients. *Lancet* 1991;337 (April 20):935–939.

Kieburtz K, Giang D, Schiffer R, et al: Abnormal vitamin B12 metabolism in human immunodeficiency virus infection. *Arch Neurol* 1991;48:312–314.

Kotler D, Wang J, Pierson R: Body composition studies in patients with the acquired immunodeficiency syndrome. *Am J Clin N* 1985;42:1255–1265.

Manteroa E, Baum M, Morgan R, et al: Vitamin B12 in early human immunodeficiency virus-1 infection. *Arch Int Med* 1991;15(5):1019–1020.

Moseson M: Nutrition and AIDS. *Nutr Res* 1986;6:729–730.

Nutrition and HIV infection. *News* 1991;5(July):2329–2330.

Odeh M: The role of zinc in acquired immunodeficiency syndrome. *J Int Med* 1992;231:463–469.

Stall F, Ela S, Roederer M, et al: Glutathione deficiency and human immunodeficiency virus infection. *Lancet* 1992;339:909–912.

Watson R: Nutrition, immunomodulation and AIDS: An overview. *J Nutr* 1992;122:715.

ANEMIA

Bailey L: Evaluation of a new Recommended Dietary Allowance for folate. *J Am Diet A* 1992;92:463–468,471.

Borch-Johnsen B, Meltzer H, Stenberg V, et al: Bioavailability of daily low-dose iron supplements in menstruating women with low iron stores. *Eur J Cl N* 1990;44:29–34.

Borel M, Smith S, Derr J, et al: Day-to-day variation in iron-status indices in healthy men and women. *Am J Clin N* 1991;54:729–735.

Brittin H, Nossaman C: Iron content of food cooked in iron utensils. *J Am Diet A* 1986;86(7):897–901.

Craig W, Balbach L, Harris S, et al: Plasma zinc and copper levels of infants fed different milk formulas. *J Am Col N* 1984;3:183–186.

Frambach D, Bendel R: Zinc supplementation and anemia. *J Am Med A* 1991;265:869.

Gable C: Hemochromatosis and dietary iron supplementation: Implications from US mortality, morbidity, and health survey data. *J Am Diet A* 1992;92:208–212.

Hallberg L, Brune M, Erlandsson M, et al: Calcium: Effect of different amounts of nonheme- and heme-iron absorption in humans. *Am J Clin N* 1991;53:112–119.

Hallberg L, Brune M, Rossander L: The role of vitamin C in iron absorption, in Walter P, et al (eds.): *Elevated Dosages of Vitamins.* Toronto: Hans Huber Publishers, 1989,p103.

Hallberg L, Hogdahl, A, Nilsson L, et al: Menstrual blood loss: A population study. Variation at different ages and attempts to define normality. *Acta Obst Sc* 1966; 45:320–351.

Hallberg L, Norrby A, Solvell L: Oral iron with succinic acid in the treatment of iron deficiency anaemia. *Sc J Haematol* 1971;8:104.

Hallberg L, Rossander-Hulten L: Iron requirements in menstruating women. *Am J Clin N* 1991;54:1047–1058.

Hines J: Ascorbic acid and vitamin B12 deficiency. *J Am Med A* 1975;235:24.

The influence of tea on iron and aluminum bioavailability in the rat. *Nutr Rev* 1991; 49(9):287–289.

Klevay L: Changing patterns of disease: Some nutritional remarks. *J Am Col N* 1984;3(2):149–158.

Klevay L, Peck S, Barcome D: Evidence of dietary copper and zinc deficiency. *J Am Med A* 1979;241:1916.

Menta S, Pritchard M, Stegman C: Contribution of coffee and tea to anemia among NHANES II participants. *Nutr Res* 1992;12:209–222.

Morris J: Selenium deficiency in cattle associated with heinz bodies and anemia. *Science* 1984;223:491.

Narayanan M, Dawson D, Lewis M: Dietary deficiency of vitamin B12 is associated with low serum cobalamin levels in nonvegetarians. *Eur J Haema* 1991;47:115–118.

Newmark H, Scheiner J, Marcus M, et al: Stability of vitamin B12 in the presence of ascorbic acid. *Am J Clin N* 1976;29:645–649.

O'Leary M: Nutritional care of the low-birth-weight infant, in Krause M, Mahan L: *Food, Nutrition, and Diet Therapy.* Philadelphia, W.B. Saunders, 1984,pp764–765.

Ono K: Effects of large-dose vitamin E supplementation on anemia in hemodialysis patients. *Nephron* 1985;40:440–445.

Possible role of vitamin E in the conversion of cyanocobalamin to its coenzyme form. *Nutr Rev* 1979;37(10):332–333.

Siegenberg D, Baynes R, Bothwell T, et al: Ascorbic acid prevents the dose-dependent inhibitory effects of polyphenols and phytates on nonheme-iron absorption. *Am J Clin N* 1991;53:537–541.

Simmer K, Iles C, James C, et al: Are iron-folate supplements harmful? *Am J Clin N* 1987;45:122–125.

Somer E: Is the iron deficiency epidemic preventable? *Nutr Rep* 1987 July:50.

————: The case for folic acid continues. *Nutr Rep* 1991 December:90.

————: *The Essential Guide to Vitamins and Minerals.* New York, HarperCollins, 1992, p57.

Tamura T: Folic acid. *Nutr MD* 1984;10(12):1–2.

Treatment of iron-deficiency anemia complicated by scurvy and folic acid deficiency. *Nutr Rev* 1992;50(5):134–137.

Vitamin C stabilizes ferritin: New insights into iron-ascorbate interactions. *Nutr Rev* 1987;45(7):217–219.

ARTHRITIS

Belch J, Ansell D, Madhok R, et al: Effects of altering dietary essential fatty acids on requirements for non-steroidal antiinflammatory drugs in patients with rheumatoid arthritis: A double-blind placebo-controlled study. *Ann Rheum D* 1988;47:96–104.

Blake D, Merry P, Stevens C, et al: Iron free radicals and arthritis. *P Nutr Soc* 1990; 49:239–245.

Darlington L, Ramsey N, Mansfield J: Placebo-controlled, blind study of dietary manipulation therapy in rheumatoid arthritis. *Lancet* 1986;I:236–238.

Dietary fish oil alters leukotriene generation and neutrophil function. *Nutr Rev* 1986; 44:137–139.

Gough K, McCarthy C, Read A, et al: Folic acid deficiency in rheumatoid arthritis. *Br Med J* 1964;1:212–217.

Halliwell B, Wasil M, Grootveld M: Biologically significant scavenging of the myeloperoxidase-derived oxidant hypochlorous acid by ascorbic acid: Implications for antioxidant protection in the inflamed rheumatoid joint. *FEBS Letter* 1987;213:15–17.

Hanck A, Weiser H: Analgesic and anti-inflammatory properties of vitamins, in Hanck A, Hornig D (eds): *Vitamins: Nutrients and Therapeutic Agents.* Toronto, Hans Huber Publishers, 1985, pp189–205.

Helliwell M, Coombes E, Moody B, et al: Nutritional status in patients with rheumatoid arthritis. *Ann Rheum D* 1984;43:386–390.

Honkanen V, Konttinen Y, Mussalo-Rauhamaa H: Vitamins A and E, retinol binding protein and zinc in rheumatoid arthritis. *Clin Exp Rh* 1989;7:465–469.

Jacobsson L, Lindgarde F, Manthorpe R, et al: Correlation of fatty acid compositon of adipose tissue lipids and serum phosphatidylcholine and serum concentrations of micronutrients with disease duration in rheumatoid arthritis. *Ann Rheum D* 1990;49:901–905.

James M, Cleland L, Gibson R, et al: Strategies for increasing the antiinflammatory effect of fish oil. *Pros Leuk E* 1991;44:123–126.

Katz W: *Rheumatic Disease: Diagnosis and Management.* Philadelphia, J.B. Lippincott, 1977, p429.

Kjeldsen-Kragh J, Haugen M, Borchgrevink C, et al: Controlled trial of fasting and one-year vegetarian diet in rheumatoid arthritis. *Lancet* 1991;338:899–902.

Kremer J: Omega-3 fatty acids and rheumatoid arthritis: Current status. *Nutr Rev* 1988;6(5):34,36,40.

Kremer J, Bigaouette J, Timchalk M, et al: Dietary eicosapentaenoic acid (EPA) supplementation in rheumatoid arthritis (RA): A prospective blinded randomized clinical study. *Clin Res* 1985:33:A778.

Kremer J, Jubiz W, Michalek A, et al: Fish oil fatty acid supplementation in active rheumatoid arthritis. *Ann Int Med* 1987;106:497–502.

Lippiello L, Fienhold M, Grandjean C: Metabolic and intrastructural changes in articular cartilage of rats fed dietary supplements of omega-3 fatty acids. *Arth Rheum* 1990;33(7):1029.

Lovell D, Gregg D, Heubi J: Nutritional status in juvenile rheumatoid arthritis (JRA): An interim report (meeting abstract). *J Rheumatol* 1986;13(5):979.

Maddison P, Bacon P: Vitamin D deficiency, spontaneous fractures and osteopenia in rheumatoid arthritis. *Br Med J* 1974;4:433–435.

Makela A, Hyora H, Vuorinen K, et al: Trace elements (Fe, Zn, Cu, and Se) in serum of rheumatic children living in western Finland. *Sc J Rheum* 1984;S53:94.

Michalek A, Kremer J, Bigaouette J, et al: Eicosapentaenoic acid (EPA) supplementation in rheumatoid arthritis. *Am J Clin N* 1985;41:871.

Munthe E, Aaseth J: Treatment of rheumatoid arthritis with selenium and vitamin E. *Sc J Rheum* 1984;S53:103.

O'Farrell C, Price R, Fernandes L: Immune sensitization to dietary antigens associated with IgA RF in rheumatoid arthritis. *Br J Rheum* 1986;25:89.

Oldroyd K, Dawes P: Clinically significant vitamin C deficiency in rheumatoid arthritis. *Br J Rheum* 1985;24:362–363.

Panush R: Nutritional therapy for rheumatic diseases. *Ann Int Med* 1987;106(4):619–621.

Punzi L, Cavasin F, Ramonda R, et al: Retinol binding protein, zinc, and acute phase response in rheumatoid arthritis. *Clin Exp Rh* 1990;8(6):616–617.

Rheumatoid arthritis and selenium. *Nutr Rev* 1988;46:284–286.

Sanderson C, Davis R, Bayliss E: Serum pyridoxal in patients with rheumatoid arthritis. *Ann Rheum D* 1976;35:177.

Simkin P: Oral zinc sulfate in rheumatoid arthritis. *Lancet* 1976;II:539.

Tarp U, Overvad K, Hansen J, et al: Low selenium level in severe rheumatoid arthritis. *Sc J Rheum* 1985;14:97–101.

Tarp U, Overvad K, Thorling E, et al: Selenium treatment in rheumatoid arthritis. *Sc J Rheum* 1985;14:364–368.

White-O'Connor B, Sobal J, Muncie H: Dietary habits, weight history, and vitamin supplement use in elderly osteoarthritis patients. *J Am Diet A* 1989;89:378–382.

Yoshino S, Ellis E: Effect of dietary fish oil derived fatty acids on inflammation and immunological processes. *Fed Proc* 1987;46:1173.

BOWEL PROBLEMS

Hendricks K, Walker W: Zinc deficiency in inflammatory bowel disease. *Nutr Rev* 1988;46(12):401–408.

Painter N, Alameida A, Colebourne K: Unprocessed bran in treatment of diverticular disease of the colon. *Br Med J* 1972;1:137.

CANCER IN WOMEN

Adams J: Human breast cancer: Concerted role of diet, prolactin, and adrenal C19 steroids in tumorigenesis. *Int J Canc* 1992;50:854–858.

Ballard-Barbash R, Schatzkin A, Carter C, et al: Body fat distribution and breast cancer in the Framingham study. *J Nat Canc* 1990;82:286–290.

Barrett-Connor E: Hormone replacement and cancer. *Br Med B* 1992;48(2):345–355.

Basu J, Palan P, Vermund S, et al: Plasma ascorbic acid and beta carotene levels in women evaluated for HPV infection, smoking, and cervix dysplasia. *Cancer Det* 1991; 15(3):165–170.

Beaty M, Lee E, Glavert H: Influence of dietary calcium and vitamin D on colon epithelial cell proliferation and 1, 2-dimethurl-hydrazine-induced colon carcinogenesis in rats fed high fat diets. *J Nutr* 1993; 123(1):144–152.

Bingham S: Mechanisms and experimental and epidemiological evidence relating dietary fiber (non-starch polysaccharides) and starch to protection against large bowel cancer. *P Nutr Soc* 1990;49:153–171.

Borgeson C, Pardini L, Pardini R, et al: Effects of dietary fish oil on human mammary carcinoma and on lipid metabolizing enzymes. *Lipids* 1989;24(4):290–295.

Bristol J, Emmett P, Heaton K, et al: Sugar, fat, and the risk of colorectal cancer. *Br Med J* 1985;291:1467–1470.

Carrol K, Jacobson E, Eckel L, et al: Calcium and carcinogenesis of the mammary gland. *Am J Clin N* 1991;54:206S–208S.

Carroll K, Parenteau H: A suggested mechanism for effects of diet on mammary cancer. *Nutr Res* 1992;12:S159–S161.

Chen J, Geissler C, Parpia B, et al: Antioxidant status and cancer mortality in China. *Int J Epid* 1992;21(4):625–635.

Clement I: Attenuation of the anticarcinogenic action of selenium by vitamin E deficiency. *Cancer Lett* 1985;25:325–331.

Das N, Ma C, Salmon Y: The relationship of serum vitamin A, cholesterol, and triglycerides to the incidence of ovarian cancer. *Bioch Med M* 1987;37(2):213–219.

Engleman R, Day N, Chen R, et al: Calorie consumption level influences development of C3H/Ou breast adenocarcinoma with indifference to calorie source. *P Soc Exp M* 1990;193(1):23.

Edes T: Beta carotene and vitamin A: Casting separate shadows? *Nutr Rep* 1992; 10(2):9,16.

Effect of wheat fiber and vitamins C and E supplements on rectal polyps in patients at high risk for colon cancer. *Nutr Rev* 1990;48(5):218–220.

Ewertz M, Gill C: Dietary factors and breast cancer risk in Denmark. *Int J Canc* 1990; 46:779–784.

Fink D: Preventive strategies for cancer in women. *Cancer* 1987;60:1934–1941.

Garland C, Garland F, Gorham E: Can colon cancer incidence and death rates be reduced with calcium and vitamin D? *Am J Clin N* 1991;54:193S–201S.

Gerhardsson de Verdier M, Steineck G, Hagman U, et al: Physical activity and colon cancer: A case-referent study in Stockholm. *Int J Canc* 1990;46:985–989.

Graham S, Hellmann R, Marshall J, et al: Nutritional epidemiology of postmenopausal breast cancer in western New York. *Am J Epidem* 1991;134:552–566.

Heitman D: Dietary cellulose supplementation on colon cancer risk. *Nutr Rep* 1991; 9(4):65,73.

Howe G, Hirohata T, Hislop T, et al: Dietary factors and risk of breast cancer: Combined analysis of 12 case-control studies. *J Nat Canc* 1990;82(7):561–569.

Hursting S, Thornquist M, Henderson M: Types of dietary fat and the incidence of cancer at five sites. *Prev Med* 1990;19:242–253.

Ip C: Interaction of vitamin C and selenium supplementation in the modification of mammary carcinogenesis in rats. *J Nat Canc* 1986;77:299–303.

Ip C, Lisk J, Stoewsand G: Mammary cancer prevention by regular garlic and selenium-enriched garlic. *Nutr Cancer* 1992;17:279–286.

James W, Ralph A: Dietary fats and cancer: *Nutr Res* 1992;12:S147–S158.

Jones C, Schiffman M, Kurman R, et al: Elevated nicotine levels in cervical lavages from passive smoke. *Am J Pub He* 1991;81(3):378–379.

Katsouyanni K, Boyle P, Trichopoulos D: Diet and urine estrogens among postmenopausal women. *Oncology* 1991;48:490–494.

Knekt P: Serum vitamin E levels and risk of female cancers. *Int J Epid* 1988;17:281–288.

Koizumi A, Wada Y, Tsukada M, et al: Effects of energy restriction on mouse mammary tumor virus mRNA levels in mammary glands and uterus and on uterine endometrial hyperplasia and pituitary histology in C3H/SHN F1 mice. *J Nutr* 1990; 120:1401–1411.

Licciardone J, Brownson R, Change J, et al: Uterine cervical cancer risk in cigarette smokers: A meta-analytic study. *Am J Prev M* 1990;6:274–281.

Ling P, Istfan N, Lopes S, et al: Structured lipid made from fish oil and medium-chain triglycerides alters tumor and host metabolism in Yoshida sarcoma bearing rats. *Am J Clin N* 1991;53:1177–1184.

London R, Murphy L, Kitlowski K: Hypothesis: Breast cancer prevention by supplemental vitamin E. *J Am Col N* 1985;4:559–564.

Marchand L, Wilkens L, Mi M: Early-age body size, adult weight gain and endometrial cancer risk. *Int J Canc* 1991;48:807–811.

Neugut A, Johnsen C, Forde K, et al: Vitamin supplements among women with adenomatous polyps and cancer of the colon. *Dis Col Rec* 1988;31:430–432.

Newmark H, Lipkin M: Calcium, vitamin D, and colon cancer. *Cancer Res* 1992; 52:2067S–2070S.

Paganelli G, Biasco G, Brandi G, et al: Effect of vitamin A, C, and E supplementation on rectal cell proliferation in patients with colorectal adenomas. *J Nat Canc* 1992; 84(1):47–51.

Palan P, Mikhail M, Basu J, et al: Plasma levels of antioxidant beta carotene and alpha tocopherol in uterine cervix dysplasia and cancer. *Nutr Cancer* 1991;15: 13–20.

Perez R, Godwin A, Hamilton T, et al: Ovarian cancer biology. *Sem Oncol* 1991; 18(3):186–204.

Persky V, Chatterton R, Van Horn L, et al: Hormone levels in vegetarian and nonvegetarian teenage girls: Potential implications for breast cancer risk. *Cancer Res* 1992; 52:578–583.

Potter J, McMichael A: Diet and cancer of the colon and rectum: A case-control study. *J Nat Canc* 1986;76:557.

Rao A, Janezic S: The role of dietary phytosterols in colon carcinogenesis. *Nutr Cancer* 1992;18:43–52.

Reducing the risk of breast cancer. *Nutr Action Healthletter* 1988 March:4–6.

Richardson S, Gerber M, Cenee S: The role of fat, animal protein, and some vitamin consumption in breast cancer: A case control study in southern France. *Int J Canc* 1991;48:1–9.

Rose D: Dietary fiber, phytoestrogens, and breast cancer. *Nutrit* 1992;8:47–51.

Rose D, Goldman M, Connolly J, et al: High-fiber diet reduces serum estrogen concentrations in premenopausal women. *Am J Clin N* 1991;54:520–525.

Schapira D, Kumar N, Lyman G, et al: Upper-body fat distribution and endometrial cancer risk. *J Am Med A* 1991;266:1808–1811.

Schrauzer G, Molenaar T, Mead S, et al: Selenium in the blood of Japanese and American women with and without breast cancer and fibrocystic disease. *Jpn J Canc* 1985; 76:374–377.

Snowdon D: Diet and ovarian cancer. *J Am Med A* 1985;254:356.

Suzuki K, Suzuki K, Mirsuoka T: Effect of low-fat, high-fiber, and fiber-supplemented high-fat diets on colon cancer risk factors in feces of healthy subjects. *Nutr Cancer* 1992;18:63–71.

Szeluga D, Bistrian B, Mascioli E: Fish oil slows tumor growth and prolongs survival in a transplantable metastatic breast cancer model. *Am J Clin N* 1987;45(4):859.

Trock B, Lanza E, Greenwald P: Dietary fiber, vegetables, and colon cancer: Critical review and meta-analysis of the epidemiologic evidence. *J Nat Canc* 1990; 82(8):650–661.

Van T'Veer P, Kolb C, Verhoef P, et al: Dietary fiber, beta carotene and breast cancer: Results from a case-control study. *Int J Canc* 1990;45(5):825–828.

Verreault R, Chu J, Mandelson M, et al: A case-control study of diet and invasive cervical cancer. *Int J Canc* 1989;43:1050–1054.

Wald N, Boreham J, Hayward J, et al: Plasma retinol, beta carotene and vitamin E levels in relation to the future risk of breast cancer. *Br J Canc* 1984;49:321–324.

Walter C, Willett M, Meir J, et al: Relation of meat, fat, and fiber to the risk of colon cancer in a prospective study among women. *N Eng J Med* 1990;323: 1664–1672.

Welsch C: Relationship between dietary fat and experimental mammary tumorigenesis: A review and critique. *Cancer Res* 1992;52:2040S–2048S.

West D, Slattery M, Robison L, et al: Dietary intake and colon cancer: Sex- and anatomic site-specific associations. *Am J Epidem* 1989;130(5):883–894.

Willett W, Stampfer M, Colditz G, et al: Dietary fat and the risk of breast cancer. *N Eng J Med* 1987;316(1):22–28.

Wittemore A, Wu-Williams A, Lee M, et al: Diet, physical activity, and colorectal cancer among Chinese in North America and China. *J Nat Canc* 1990;82:915–926.

Yeung K, McKeown G, Li G, et al: Comparisons of diet and biochemical characteristics of stool and urine between Chinese populations with low and high colorectal cancer rates. *J Nat Canc* 1991;83:46–50.

CARDIOVASCULAR DISEASE

Abraham A, Brooks B, Eylath U: Chromium and cholesterol-induced atherosclerosis in rabbits. *Ann Nutr M* 1991;35:203–207.

Anderson R, Kozlovsky A: Chromium intake, absorption, and excretion of subjects consuming self-selected diets. *Am J Clin N* 1985;41:1177–1183.

Cara L, Armand M, Borel P, et al: Long-term wheat germ intake beneficially affects plasma lipids and lipoproteins in hypercholesterolemic human subjects. *J Nutr* 1992;122:317–326.

Cowley A, Dzau V, Buttrick P, et al: Working group on noncoronary cardiovascular disease and exercise in women. *Med Sci Spt* 1992;24(6):S277–S287.

Demirovic J, Sprifka J, Folsom A, et al: Menopause and serum cholesterol: Differences between blacks and whites. *Am J Epidem* 1992;136(2):155–164.

Douglas P, Clarkson T, Flowers N, et al: Exercise and atherosclerotic heart disease in women. *Med Sci Spt* 1992;24(6):S266–S275.

Frei B, England L, Ames B: Ascorbate is an outstanding antioxidant in human blood plasma. *P NAS US* 1989;86:6377–6381.

Gurwitz J, Col N, Avorn J: The exclusion of the elderly and women from clinical trials in acute myocardial infarction. *J Am Med A* 1992;268(11):1417–1422.

He J, Tell G, Tang Y, et al: Relation of serum zinc and copper to lipids and lipoproteins: The Yi people study. *J Am Col N* 1992;11(1):74–78.

Hennig B, Boissonneault G, Wang Y: Protective effects of vitamin E in age-related endothelial cell injury. *Int J Vit N* 1989;59:273–279.

Hennig B, Wang Y, Ramasamy S, et al: Zinc deficiency alters barrier function of cultured porcine endothelial cells. *J Nutr* 1992;122:1242–1247.

Holdsworth E, Kaufman D, Neville E: A fraction derived from brewer's yeast inhibits cholesterol synthesis by rat liver preparations in vitro. *Br J Nutr* 1991; 65:285–299.

Hoshino E, Shariff R, Van Gossum A, et al: Vitamin E suppresses increased lipid peroxidation in cigarette smokers. *J Parent En* 1990;14:300–305.

Hubbard R, Sanchez A: Oxidized cholesterol in foods you eat. *Nutr Rep* 1990;8(8):57,64.

Isles C, Hole D, Hawthorne V, et al: Relation between coronary risk and coronary mortality in women of the Renfrew and Paisley survey: Comparison with men. *Lancet* 1992;339:702–706.

Khaw K: Comments from the editor. *Br Med Bul* 1992;48(2):469–471.

Kiesewetter H, Jung F, Pindur G, et al: Effect of garlic on thrombocyte aggregation, microcirculation, and other risk factors. *Int J Cl P* 1991;29:151–155.

Koo S, Lee C, Stone W, et al: Effect of copper deficiency on the plasma clearance of native and acetylated human low-density lipoprotein. *J Nutr Bioc* 1992;3:45–50.

Kretchevsky D: Antioxidant vitamins and the prevention of cardiovascular disease. *Nutr Today* 1992;27(1):30–33.

Kuusisto P, Vapaatalo H, Manninen V, et al: Effect of activated charcoal on hypercholesterolemia. *Lancet* 1986;II:366–367.

Larsson B, Bengtsson C, Bjorntorp P, et al: Is abdominal body fat distribution a major explanation for the sex difference in the incidence of myocardial infection? *Am J Epidem* 1992;135(3):266–273.

Lau B, Lam F, Wang-Cheng R: Effect of an odor-modified garlic preparation on blood lipids. *Nutr Res* 1987;7:139–149.

Luria M: Atherosclerosis: The importance of HDL-cholesterol and prostacyclin: A role for niacin therapy. *Med Hypoth* 1990;32:21–28.

Masarei J, Rouse I, Lynch W, et al: Vegetarian diets, lipids, and cardiovascular risk. *Aust NZ J M* 1984;14:400–404.

Meade T, Berra A: Hormone replacement therapy and cardiovascular disease. *Br Med Bul* 1992;48(2):276–308.

Myers M, Basinski A: Coffee and coronary heart disease. *Arch In Med* 1992;152:1767–1772.

Nibbling diet lowers serum cholesterol. *Nutr Rev* 1990;48:288–289.

Oster O, Prellwitz W: Selenium and cardiovascular disease. *Biol Tr El* 1990;24:91–103.

1992 Heart and Stroke Facts. Dallas: American Heart Association, National Center, 7272 Greenville Avenue, Dallas, Texas, 75231–4596.

Pearson T: Decaffeinated coffee and serum LDL-cholesterol concentrations. *Am J Clin N* 1992;56:604–610.

Pi-Sunyer F: Health implications of obesity. *Am J Clin N* 1991;53:1595S–1603S.

Rees A: Lipoprotein (a): A possible link between lipoprotein metabolism and thrombosis. *Br Heart J* 1991;65:2–3.

Regnstrom J, Nilsson J, Tornvall P, et al: Susceptibility to low-density lipoprotein oxidation and coronary atherosclerosis in man. *Lancet* 1992;339:1183–1186.

Reiser S, Powell A, Yang C, et al: Effect of copper intake on blood cholesterol and its lipoprotein distribution in men. *Nutr Rep Int* 1987;36(3):641–649.

Report of the National Cholesterol Education Program Expert Panel on detection, evaluation, and treatment of high blood cholesterol in adults. *Arch Int Med* 1988;148:36–69.

Ripsin C, Keenan J, Jacobs D, et al: Oat products and lipid lowering: A meta-analysis. *J Am Med A* 1992;267(24):3317–3325.

Salonen J, Nyyssonen K, Korpela H, et al: High stored iron levels are associated with excess risk of myocardial infarction in eastern Finnish men. *Circulation* 1992;86:803–811.

Scanu A: Lipoprotein (a): A genetic risk factor for premature coronary heart disease. *J Am Med A* 1992;267(24):3326–3329.

Scanu A, Lawn R, Berg K: Lipoprotein (a) and atherosclerosis. *Ann Int Med* 1991;115(3):209–217.

Scherwitz L, Perkins L, Chesney M, et al: Hostility and health behaviors in young adults: The CARDIA study. *Am J Epidem* 1992;136:136–145.

Simopoulos A: Omega-3 fatty acids in health and disease and in growth and development. *Am J Clin N* 1991;54:438–463.

Shorey R, Day P, Willis R, et al: Effects of soybean polysaccharide on plasma lipids. *J Am Diet A* 1985;85(11):1461–1465.

Simonoff M: Chromium deficiency and cardiovascular risk. *Cardio Res* 1984;18:591–596.

Sjorgren A, Edvinsson L, Fallgren B: Magnesium deficiency in coronary artery disease and cardiac arrhythmias. *J Int Med* 1989;226:213–222.

Sklan D, Berner Y, Rabinowitch H: The effect of dietary onion and garlic on hepatic lipid concentrations and activity of antioxidative enzymes in chicks. *J Nutr Bioc* 1992;3 July:322.

Snowdon D, Phillips R, Fraser G: Meat consumption and fatal ischemic heart disease. *Prev Med* 1984;13:490–500.

Somer E: Lipoprotein (a): The missing link in heart disease? *Nutr Rep* 1991 March:18.

————: Saponins: Where diet and pharmacology meet. *Nutr Rep* 1990;8(9):66.

Steenland K: Passive smoking and the risk of heart disease. *J Am Med A* 1992; 267(1):94–99.

Superko H, Bortz W, Williams P, et al: Caffeinated and decaffeinated coffee effects on plasma lipoprotein cholesterol, apolipoproteins, and lipase activity: A controlled, randomized trial. *Am J Clin N* 1991;54:599–605.

Ulbricht T, Southgate D: Coronary heart disease: Seven dietary factors. *Lancet* 1991; 338:985–992.

Wenger N: Exclusion of the elderly and women from coronary trials: Is their quality of care compromised? *J Am Med A* 1992;268(11):1460–1461.

Woods K, Fletcher S, Roffe C, et al: Intravenous magnesium sulphate in suspected acute myocardial infarction: Results of the second Leicester Intravenous Magnesium Intervention Trial (LIMIT-2). *Lancet* 1992;339:1553–1558.

Yudkin J: Diet and coronary heart disease: Why blame fat? *J Roy S Med* 1992; 85(9):515–516.

CARPAL TUNNEL SYNDROME

Amadio P: Pyridoxine and carpal tunnel syndrome. *Nutr Rep* 1988;6:65,72.

Bassler K: Use and abuse of high dosages of vitamin B6, in Walter P, et al. (eds.): *Elevated Dosages of Vitamins.* Toronto, Hans Huber Publishers, 1989,pp120–126.

Byers C, DeLisa J, Franket K, et al: Pyridoxine metabolism in carpal tunnel syndrome with and without peripheral neuropathy. *Arch Phys M* 1983;64:125.

Del Tredici A, Bernstein A, Chinn K: Vitamin B6 therapy for carpal tunnel syndrome. *Fed Proc* 1985;44:775.

Driskell J, Wesley R, Hess I: Effectiveness of pyridoxine hydrochloride treatment of carpal tunnel syndrome patients. *Nutr Rep In* 1986;34:1031–1040.

Ellis J: The treatment of carpal tunnel syndrome with vitamin B6. *South Med J* 1986;79:15.

————: Tenosynovitis including carpal tunnel syndrome (CTS) responsive to vitamin B6. *FASEB J* 1988;2:A439.

Ellis J, Filkers K, Watanbe T, et al: Clinical results of a crossover treatment with pyridoxine and placebo of the carpal tunnel syndrome. *Am J Clin N* 1979;32:2040–2046.

Friedman M, Resnick J, Baer R: Subepidermal vesicular dermatosis and sensory peripheral neuropathy caused by pyridoxine abuse. *J Am Acad D* 1986;14:915–917.

Podell R: Nutritional supplementation with megadoses of vitamin B6. *Postgr Med* 1985;77(3):113–116.

Shirukuishi S, Nishii S, Ellis J, et al: The carpal tunnel syndrome as a probable primary deficiency of vitamin B6 rather than a deficiency of dependency state. *Bioc Biop R* 1980;95:1126–1130.

Vitamin B6 toxicity: A new megavitamin syndrome. *Nutr Rev* 1984;42(2):44–46.

CERVICAL DYSPLASIA

Basu J, Palan P, Vermund S, et al: Plasma ascorbic acid and beta carotene levels in women evaluated for PHV infection, smoking, and cervix dysplasia. *Cancer Det* 1991; 15(3):165–170.

Buckley D, McPherson S, North C, et al: Dietary micronutrients and cervical dysplasia in southwestern American Indian women. *Nutr Cancer* 1992;17:179–185.

Butterworth C: New concepts in nutrition and cancer: Implications for folic acid. *Cont Nutr* 1980;5(12):1–2.

Butterworth C, Hatch K, Macaluso M, et al: Folate deficiency and cervical dysplasia. *J Am Med A* 1992;267:528–533.

Butterworth C, Hatch K, Gore H, et al: Improvement in cervical dysplasia associated with folic acid therapy in users of oral contraceptives. *Am J Clin N* 1982;35:73–82.

Butterworth C, Hatch K, Soong S, et al: Oral folic acid supplementation for cervical dysplasia: A clinical intervention trial. *Am J Obst G* 1992;166:803–809.

Folate deficiency, parenteral caffeine, and cytogenetic damage in mice. *Nutr Rev* 1991;49(9):285–287.

Kirby A, Spiegelhalter D, Day N, et al: Conservative treatment of mild/moderate cervical dyskaryosis: Long-term outcome. *Lancet* 1992;339:828–831.

Palan P, Mikhail M, Basu J, et al: Plasma levels of antioxidant beta carotene and alpha tocopherol in uterine cervix dysplasias and cancer. *Nutr Cancer* 1991;15:13–20.

Sunderstrom H, Vrjonheikki E: Low serum selenium concentration in patients with cervical or endometrial cancer. *Int J Gyn O* 1984;22:35–40.

CHRONIC FATIGUE SYNDROME

Cox I, Campbell J, Dowson D: Red blood cell magnesium and chronic fatigue syndrome. *Lancet* 1991;337:757–760.

Gin W, Christiansen F, Peter J: Immune function and the chronic fatigue syndrome. *Med J Aust* 1989;151:117–118.

Immunological abnormalities in the chronic fatigue syndrome. *Med J Aust* 1990; 152:50–51.

Hales D: Why are you so tired? *Am Health* 1987 May:54–60.

Katon W, Russo J: Chronic fatigue syndrome criteria. *Arch In Med* 1992;152:1604–1609.

Kroenke K: Chronic fatigue syndrome: Is it real? *Postgr Med* 1991;89(2):44–55.

Milton J, Clements G, Edwards R: Immune responsiveness in chronic fatigue syndrome. *Postg Med J* 1991;67:532–537.

Stoner B, Corey G: Chronic fatigue syndrome: A practical approach. *NC Med J* 1992; 53(6):267–270.

Straus S: Defining chronic fatigue syndrome. *Arch In Med* 1992;152:1569–1570.

THE COMMON COLD

Chandra R: Excessive intake of zinc impairs immune responses. *J Am Med A* 1984; 252:1443–1446.

Duchateau J, Delepesse G, Vrijens R, et al: Beneficial effects of oral zinc supplementation on the immune response of old people. *Am J Med* 1981;70:1001.

Eby G, Davis D, Halcomb W: Reduction in duration of common colds by zinc gluconate lozenges in a double-blind study. *Antim Ag Ch* 1984;25(1):20–24.

Hemila H: Vitamin C and the common cold. *Br J Nutr* 1992;67:3–16.

Pudh H: Vitamin C: Newer insights into its biochemical functions. *Nutr Rev* 1991; 49:65–70.

Rivers J: Safety of high-level vitamin C ingestion, in Walter P, et al (eds): *Elevated Dosages of Vitamins.* Toronto, Hans Huber Publishers, 1989,pp95–102.

Siegel B: Enhanced interferon response to murine leukemia virus by ascorbic acid. *Infect Immun* 1974;10:409.

Yuting C, Rongliang Z, Zhongjian J, et al: Flavonoids as superoxide scavengers and anti-oxidants. *Free Rad B* 1990;9:19–21.

CUTS, SCRATCHES, BRUISES, AND BURNS

Agren M, Stromberg H, Rindby A, et al: Selenium, zinc, iron, and copper levels in serum of patients with arterial and venous leg ulcers. *Act Der-Ven* 1986;66:237–240.

Bieri J, Corash L, Hubbard V: Medical uses of vitamin E. *N Eng J Med* 1983; 308(18):1063–1071.

Black M, Medeiros D, Brunett E, et al. Zinc supplements and serum lipids in young adult white males. *Am J Clin N* 1988;47:970–975.

Block E: The chemistry of garlic and onions. *Sci Am* 1985;252:114–119.

Boosalis M, Solem L, Cerra F, et al: Increased urinary zinc excretion after thermal injury. *J La Cl Med* 1991;118:538–545.

Brown C, Bechtel P, Forbes R, et al: Bioavailability of zinc derived from beef and the effect of low dietary zinc intake on skeletal muscle zinc concentrations. *Nutr Res* 1985;5:117–122.

Cheraskin E: The prevalence of hypovitaminosis C. *J Am Med A* 1985;254:2894.

Gibson R: Trace element deficiencies in humans. *Can Med A J* 1991;145:231.

Goldstein R, Augustine A, Purucker E, et al: Effect of vitamin E and allopurinol on lipid peroxide and glutathione level in acute skin graphs. *J Inves Der* 1990;95:470.

Kurolwa K, Nelson J, Boyce S, et al: Metabolic and immune effect of vitamin E supplementation after burn. *J Parent En* 1991;51:22–26.

Padh H: Vitamin C: Newer insights into its biochemical functions. *Nutr Rev* 1991;49:65–70.

Sandstead H: Zinc deficiency: A public health problem? *Am J Dis Ch* 1991;145:853–859.

Shelton R: Aloe vera: Its chemical and therapeutic properties. *Int J Derm* 1991;30(10):679–683.

Sugden P, Fuller S: Regulation of protein-turnover in skeletal and cardiac-muscle (Review). *Biochem J* 1991;273:21–37.

Vaxman F, Chalkiadakis G, Maldonade H, et al: Pantothenic acid and wound healing process: Strength improvements in colonic anastomosis. *Dig Dis Sci* 1986;31:469S.

DIABETES

Abraham A, Brooks B, Eylath U: The effects of chromium supplementation on serum glucose and lipids in patients with and without non-insulin-dependent diabetes. *Metabolism* 1992;41(7):768–771.

Anderson R: Chromium, glucose tolerance, and diabetes. *Biol Tr El Res* 1992;32:19–24.

Anderson R, Polansky M, Bryden N, et al: Supplemental chromium effects on glucose, insulin, glucagon, and urinary chromium losses in subjects consuming controlled low-chromium diets. *Am J Clin N* 1991;54:909–916.

Bierenbaum M, Noon F, Machlin L, et al: The effect of supplemental vitamin E on serum parameters in diabetic, post coronary and normal subjects. *Nutr Rep In* 1985;31:1171–1180.

Boyden J, Starich G, Lardinois C: Dietary enrichment with omega 3 fatty acids leads to their incorporation into the pancreatic islet and skeletal muscle phospholipid membranes. *Clin Res* 1987;35:A164.

Brand J, Colagiuri S, Crossman S, et al: Low-glycemic index foods improve long-term glycemic control in NIDDM. *Diabet Care* 1991;14(2):95–101.

Brazg R, Duell P, Gilmore M, et al: Effects of dietary antioxidants on LDL oxidation in noninsulin-dependent diabetics. *Clin Res* 1992;40:103A.

Cunningham J, Ellis S, McVeigh K, et al: Reduced mononuclear leukocyte ascorbic-acid content of adults with insulin-dependent diabetes mellitus consuming adequate dietary vitamin C. *Metabolism* 1991;40:146–149.

Elamin A, Tuvemo T: Magnesium and insulin-dependent diabetes mellitus. *Diabet Re C* 1990;10:203–209.

Faure P, Roussel A, Coudray C, et al: Zinc and insulin sensitivity. *Biol Tr El* 1992;32: 305.

Garg A, Benanome A, Grundy S, et al: Comparison of a high-carbohydrate diet with a high-monounsaturated fat diet in patients with non–insulin dependent diabetes mellitus. *N Eng J Med* 1988;319:829–834.

Gisinger C, Watanabe J, Colwell J: Vitamin E and platelet eicosanoids in diabetes mellitus. *Prost Leuk E* 1990;40(3):169–176.

Havivi E, On H, Reshef A, et al: Vitamins and trace metals status in non–insulin dependent diabetes mellitus. *Int J Vit N* 1991;61:328–333.

Kuligowski J, Halperin K: Stainless steel cookware as a significant source of nickel, chromium, and iron. *Arch Env C* 1992;23(2):211–215.

Malasanos T, Stacpoole P: Biological effects of omega-3 fatty acids in diabetes mellitus. *Diabetes Care* 1991;14(12):1160–1179.

Mooradian A, Morley J: Micronutrient status in diabetes mellitus. *Am J Clin N* 1987; 45:877–895.

Paolisso G, Sgambato S, Gambardella A, et al: Daily magnesium supplements improve glucose tolerance in elderly subjects. *Am J Clin N* 1992;55:1161–1167.

Roongpisuthipong C, Karnajanachumpon S: Vitamin status in elderly diabetic subjects. *FASEB J* 1991;5:1299A.

Simonoff M: Chromium deficiency and cardiovascular risk: A review. *Cardio Res* 1984;18:591–596.

Sinclair A, Girling A, Gray L, et al: Disturbed handling of ascorbic acid in diabetic patients with and without microangiopathy during high-dose ascorbate supplementation. *Diabetolog* 1991;34:171–175.

Tagliaferro V, Cassader M, Bozzo C, et al: Moderate guar gum addition to usual diet improves peripheral sensitivity to insulin and lipaemic profile in NIDDM. *Diabete Met* 1985;11:383–385.

Vague P, Vialettes B, Lassmann-Vague V, et al: Nicotinamide may extend remission phase of insulin-dependent diabetics. *Lancet* 1987;I:619–620.

Vorster H, Lotter A, Odendaal I: Effects of an oats fibre tablet and wheat bran in healthy volunteers. *S Afr Med J* 1986;69:435–438.

ENDOMETRIOSIS

Apgar B: Endometriosis. *Postgr Med* 1992;92(1):283–298.

Covens A, Christopher P, Casper R: The effect of dietary supplementation with fish oil fatty acids on surgically induced endometriosis in the rabbit. *Fert Steril* 1988;49:698–703.

Cramer D, Wilson E, Stillman R, et al: The relation of endometriosis to menstrual characteristics, smoking, and exercise. *J Am Med A* 1986;255:1904–1908.

Farley T, Rosenberg M, Rowe P, et al: Intrauterine devices and pelvic inflammatory disease: An international perspective. *Lancet* 1992;339:785–788.

Gleicher N, El-Roeiy A, Confino E, et al: Is endometriosis an autoimmune disease? *Obstet Gyn* 1987;70(1):115–122.

Kirshon B, Poindexter A: Contraception: A risk factor for endometriosis. *Obstet Gyn* 1988;71:829–831.

Oosterlynck D, Cornillie F, Waer M, et al: Women with endometriosis show a defect in natural killer activity resulting in a decreased cytotoxicity to autologous endometrium. *Fert Steril* 1991;56(1):45.

Rawson J: Prevalence of endometriosis in asymptomatic women. *J Repro Med* 1991; 36(7):513–517.

EYES AND VISION

Bode A: An enzymatic system for maintaining ascorbic acid in its reduced form in ocular tissues. *Inv Ophth V* 1991;32(4):1101.

Bode A, Vanderpool S, Carlson E, et al: Ascorbic acid uptake and metabolism by corneal endothelium. *Inv Ophth V* 1991;32(8):2266–2271.

Connor W, Neuringer M, Reisbick S: Essential fatty acids: The importance of n-3 fatty acids in the retina and brain. *Nutr Rev* 1992;50(4):21–29.

Devamanoharan P, Henein M, Morris S, et al: Prevention of selenite cataract by vitamin C. *Exp Eye Res* 1991;52:563–568.

Devamanoharan P, Morris S, Henein M, et al: Prevention of selenite cataract by vitamin C. *Inv Ophth V* 1991;32(4):724.

Eye disease and nutrition: The missing link? *Nestle Worldview* 1991;3(1):2.

Garland D: Ascorbic acid and the eye. *Am J Clin N* 1991;54:1198S–1202S.

Goldberg J, Flowerdew G, Smith E, et al: Factors associated with age-related macular degeneration. *Am J Epidem* 1988;128:700–710.

Hankinson S, Stampfer M, Seddon J, et al: Nutrient intake and cataract extraction in women: A prospective study. *Br Med J* 1992;305:335–339.

Hankinson S, Willett W, Colditz G, et al: A prospective study of cigarette smoking and risk of cataract surgery in women. *J Am Med A* 1992;268(8):994–998.

Jacques P, Chylack L: Epidemiological evidence of a role for the antioxidant vitamins and carotenoids in cataract prevention. *Am J Clin N* 1991;53:352S–355S.

Jacques P, Chylack L, McGandy R, et al: Antioxidant status in persons with and without senile cataracts. *Arch Ophth* 1988;106:337–340.

Jamall I, Roque H: Cadmium-induced alterations in ocular trace elements. *Biol Tr El* 190;23:55–63.

Mares-Perlman J, Klein B, Klein R, et al: Relationship between diet and cataract prevalence. *Inv Ophth V* 1991;32(4):723.

Robertson J, Donner A, Trevithick J: A possible role for vitamins C and E in cataract prevention. *Am J Clin N* 1991;53:346S–351S.

————: Vitamin E intake and risk of cataracts in humans. *Ann NY Acad* 1989;570:372–382.

Runge P, Munner D, McAllister J, et al: Oral vitamin E supplements can prevent the retinopathy of abetalipoproteinaemia. *Br J Ophth* 1986;70:166–173.

Taylor A, Jacques P, Nadler D, et al: Relationship between ascorbic acid intake and levels of total and reduced ascorbic acid in human lens. *Inv Ophth V* 1991;32(4):723.

Taylor A, Jahngen-Hodge J, Huang L, et al: Aging in the eye lens: Roles for proteolysis and nutrition in formation of cataract. *Age* 1991;14:65–71.

Torii H, Okada H, Majima Y, et al: Effect of vitamin E–containing liposome on the development of an in vitro xylose cataract. *Inv Ophth V* 1991;32(4):749.

Varma S: Scientific basis for medical therapy of cataracts by antioxidants. *Am J Clin N* 1991;53:335S–345S.

Vitale S, West S, Hallfrisch J, et al: Plasma vitamin C, E, and beta carotene levels and risk of cataract. *Inv Ophth V* 1991;32(4):723.

Wu S, Leske M, Chylack L, et al: The lens of opacities case-control study: II. Biochemical risk factors. *Inv Ophth V* 1991;32(4):723.

Zinc and macular degeneration. *Nutr Rev* 1990;48(7):285–287.

FATIGUE

Cheraskin E, Ringsdorf W, Medford F: Daily vitamin C consumption and fatigability. *J Am Ger So* 1976;24:136–137.

Lione A, Allen P, Smith J: Aluminum coffee percolators as a source of dietary aluminum. *Food Chem T* 1984;22:265–268.

FERTILITY

Alexander M, Lazan K, Rasmussen K: Effect of chronic protein-energy malnutrition on fecundability, fecundity, and fertility in rats. *J Nutr* 1988;118:883–887.

Baer J, Taper J, Gwazdauskas F, et al: Diet, hormonal, and metabolic factors affecting bone mineral density in adolescent amenorrheic and eumenorrheic female runners. *J Sport Med* 1992;32:51–58.

Dawson D, Sauers A: Infertility and folate deficiency. Case reports. *Br J Obst G* 1982; 89:678–680.

Evans H, Bishop K: Existence of a hitherto unknown dietary factor essential for reproduction. *J Am Med A* 1923;81:889–892.

Kemmann E, Pasquale S, Skaf R: Amenorrhea associated with carotenemia. *J Am Med A* 1983;249:926–929.

Loucks A, Horvath S: Athletic amenorrhea: A review. *Med Sci Spt* 1985;17(1):56–72.

Loucks A, Vaitukaitis J, Cameron J, et al: The reproductive system and exercise in women. *Med Sci Spt* 1992;24(6):S288–S293.

MRC Vitamin Study Research Group: Prevention of neural tube defects: Results of the Medical Research Council Vitamin Study. *Lancet* 1991;338:131–137.

Murphy P: Periconceptional supplementation with folic acid: Does it prevent neural tube defects? *J Nurse-Mid* 1992;37(1):25–31.

Pasquali R, Antenucci D, Casimirri F, et al: Clinical and hormonal characteristics of obese amenorrheic hyperandrogenic women before and after weight loss. *J Clin En* 1989;68:173.

Pirke K, Schweiger U, Laessle R, et al: Dieting influences the menstrual cycle: Vegetarian versus nonvegetarian diet. *Fert Steril* 1986;46(6):1083–1088.

Prior J, Vigna Y, McKay D: Reproduction for the athletic woman. *Sport Med* 1992; 14(3):190–199.

Somer E: *The Essential Guide to Vitamins and Minerals.* New York, HarperCollins, 1991,pp109, 116.

FIBROCYSTIC BREAST DISEASE

Arthur J, Ellis I, Flowers C, et al: The relationship of "high risk" mammographic patterns to histological risk factors for development of cancer in the human breast. *Br J Radiol* 1990;63:845–849.

Brinton L: Relationship of benign breast disease to breast cancer. *Ann NY Acad* 1990; 586:266–271.

Devitt J, To T, Miller A: Risk of breast cancer in women with breast cysts. *Can Med A J* 1992;147(1):45.

Gibson W: The relationship of fibrocystic disease to breast carcinoma. *JMSMA* 1988 May:137–139.

Is "fibrocystic disease" of the breast precancerous? *Arch Path L* 1986;110:171–173.

London S, Connolly J, Schmitt S, et al: A prospective study of benign breast disease and the risk of breast cancer. *J Am Med A* 1992;267(7):941–944.

Lubin F, Ron E, Wax Y, et al: A case-controlled study of caffeine and methylxanthines in benign breast disease. *J Am Med A* 1985;253:2388–2392.

Lubin F, Wax Y, Ron E, et al: Nutritional factors associated with benign breast disease etiology: A case-control study. *Am J Clin N* 1989;50(3):551–556.

Meyer E, Sommers D, Reitz C, et al: Vitamin E and benign breast disease. *Surgery* 1990;107:549–551.

Minton J, Foecking M, Webster D, et al: Caffeine, cyclic nucleotides, and breast disease. *Surgery* 1979;86:105–109.

————: Response of fibrocystic disease to caffeine withdrawal and correlation of cyclic nucleotides with breast disease. *Am J Obst G* 1979;135(1):157–158.

Molina R, Filella X, Herranz M, et al: Biochemistry of cyst fluid in fibrocystic disease of the breast. *Ann NY Acad* 1990;586:29–41.

Newell G, Ellison N (eds): *Nutrition and Cancer: Etiology and Treatment.* New York, Raven Press, 1981,pp93–110.

Norwood S: Fibrocystic breast disease: An update and review. *JOGNN* 1990 March/April:116–121.

Page D, Dupont W: Benign breast disease: Indicators of increased breast cancer risk. *Cancer Det* 1992;16(2):93–97.

Rohan T, Cook M, McMichael A: Methylxanthines and benign proliferative epithelial disorders of the breast in women. *Int J Epid* 1989;18(3):626–633.

Rose D, Boyer A, Haley N, et al: Low fat diet in fibrocystic disease of the breast with cyclical mastalgia. A feasibility study. *Am J Clin N* 1985;41:856.

Simard A, Vobecky J, Vobecky J: Nutrition and lifestyle factors in fibrocystic disease and cancer of the breast. *Cancer Det* 1990;14(5):567–572.

Skidmore F: The epidemiology of breast cyst disease in two British populations and the incidence of breast cancer in these groups. *Ann NY Acad* 1990;586:276–283.

Vorherr H: Vitamin E as an adjunct for treatment of fibrocystic disease. *Vitamin E Seminar* April 28–May 2, 1986. LaGrange, IL. VERIS.

FLUID RETENTION

Horrobin D: The role of essential fatty acids and prostaglandins in the premenstrual syndrome. *J Repro Med* 1983;28(7):465–468.

London R, Sundarom G, Murphy L, et al: The effect of alpha tocopherol on premenstrual symptomatology: A double-blind study. *J Am Col N* 1983;2:115.

Muenter M, Perry H, Ludwig J: Chronic vitamin A intoxication in adults. Hepatic, neurologic and dermatologic complications. *Am J Med* 1971;50(1):129–136.

Williams M, Harris R, Dean B, et al: Controlled trial of pyridoxine in the premenstrual syndrome. *J Int Med R* 1985;13:174–179.

FOOD INTOLERANCE

Bahna S: Critique of various dietary regimens in the management of food allergy. *Ann Allergy* 1986;57(1):48–52.

Butkus S, Mahan L: Food allergies: Immunological reactions to food. *J Am Diet A* 1986;86:601–608.

Chandra R: Food allergy: 1992 and beyond. *Nutr Res* 1992;12:93–99.

The continuing sulfite story. *Nutr MD* 1986;12:2–3.

Cornwell N, Clarke L, van Nunen S: Intolerance to dietary chemicals in recurrent idiopathic headache. *Clin Pharm* 1987;11(2):201.

Ferguson A: Food sensitivity or self-deception? *N Eng J Med* 1990;323:476–478.

Food sensitivity and dairy products. *Dairy Council Digest* 1989;60(5):25–30.

The Institute of Food Technologists' Expert Panel on Food Safety and Nutrition: Food allergies and other food sensitivities. *Cont Nutr* 1985;10(11):1–2.

Jewett D, Phil D, Fein G: A double-blind study of symptoms provocation to determine food sensitivity. *N Eng J Med* 1990;323:429,476.

Pearson D: Pseudo food allergy. *Br Med J* 1986;292:221.

Reactions to food additives. *J Roy S Med* 1992;85:513–515.

Swain A, Soutter V, Loblay R, et al: Salicylates, oligoantigenic diets and behavior. *Lancet* 1985;II:41–42.

HAIR

Gummer C: Diet and hair loss. *Sem Dermat* 1985;4:35.

Hodges R: How nutrition affects the skin. *Prof Nutr* 1979;Fall:1–5.

Krehl W: Nutrition and diseases of the skin, in Goodhart R, Shils E (eds): *Modern Nutrition in Health and Disease,* 5th ed. Philadelphia, Lea and Febiger, 1973,pp941–949.

Marlow M, Cossairt A, Stellern J, et al: Decreased magnesium in the hair of autistic children. *J Orthomol Psych* 1983;13(2):117–122.

Marlowe M, Moon C, Errera J, et al: Hair mineral content as a predictor of mental retardation. *J Orthomol Psych* 1983;12(1):26–33.

Smith B: Cardiovascular risk as related to an element pattern in hair. *Tr Elem Med* 1987;4(3):131–133.

HEADACHES

Benedittis G, Lorenzetti A: Minor stressful life events (daily hassles) in chronic primary headache: Relationship with MMPI personality patterns. *Headache* 1992; 32:330–332.

Bernstein A: Vitamin B6 and clinical neurology. *Ann NY Acad* 1990;585:250–260.

Corbett J, Selhorst J, Waybright E, et al: Liver lover's headache: Pseuodotumor cerebri and vitamin A intoxication. *J Am Med A* 1984;252:3365.

Cornwell N, Clarke L, VanNunen S: Intolerance to dietary chemicals in recurrent idiopathic headache. *Clin Pharm* 1987;41:201.

deBelleroche J, Cook G, Das E, et al: Erythrocyte choline concentration and cluster headaches. *Br Med J* 1984;288:268–270.

Diamond S: Diet and headache. *Nutr Rep* 1987;5:12–13.

Glueck C, McCarren T, Hitzemann R, et al: Amelioration of severe migraine with omega-3 fatty acids: A double-blind, placebo-controlled clinical trial. *Am J Clin N* 1986;43:710.

Koehler S, Glaros A: The effect of aspartame on migraine headache. *Headache* 1988; 28:10–13.

Harrison D: Copper as a factor in the dietary precipitation of migraine. *Headache* 1986;26:248–250.

Hughes E, Gott P, Weinstein R, et al: Migraine: A diagnostic test for etiology of food sensitivity by a nutritionally supported fast and confirmed by long-term report. *Ann Allergy* 1985;55:28–32.

Leonard T, Watson R, Mohs M: The effects of caffeine on various body systems: A review. *J Am Diet A* 1987;87:1048–1053.

Lipton R, Newman L, Cohen J, et al: Aspartame as a dietary trigger of headache. *Headache* 1989;29:90–92.

Mader R, Deutsch H, Siebert G, et al: Vitamin status of inpatients with chronic cephalgia and dysfunction pain syndrome and effects of a vitamin supplementation. *Int J Vit N* 1988;58:436–441.

McCarron T, Hitzemann R, Smith R, et al: Amelioration of severe migraine by fish oil (omega-3) fatty acids. *Am J Clin N* 1985;41:874.

National Research Council, *Recommended Dietary Allowances, Tenth edition.* Washington, DC, National Academy Press, 1989,pp87–88.

Winsor A, Strongin E: A study of the development of tolerance for caffeinated beverages. *J Exp Psy* 1933;135:725–744.

Zeisel S, DaCosta K, Franklin P, et al: Choline: An essential nutrient for humans. *FASEB J* 1991;5:2093–2098.

HYPERTENSION

Abraira C, Henderson W, Mehta S: Systolic blood pressure (BP) enhancing effect of dietary sucrose (S) in humans. *J Am Col N* 1987;6:79.

Anderson J: High-fiber, hypocalorie versus very-low-calorie diet effects on blood pressure of obese men. *Clin Res* 1986;34:A792.

Basta L: Regression of atherosclerotic stenosing lesions of the renal arteries and spontaneous cure of systemic hypertension through control of hyperlipidemia. *Am J Med* 1976;61:420–421.

Bell R, Eldrid M, Watson F: The influence of NaCl and KCl on urinary calcium excretion in healthy, young women. *Nutr Res* 1992;12:17–26.

Betts N, Foote D: Nutrient intake and hypertension risk factors among blue collar workers. *Nutr Rep In* 1985;32:1163–1169.

Burr M, Sweetnam P, Barasi M: Dietary fibre, blood pressure, and plasma cholesterol. *Nutr Res* 1985;5:465–472.

Elliott P: Observational studies of salt and blood pressure. *Hypertensio* 1991;17(Suppl. I):3–8.

Flynn M, Gibney M: Obesity and health: Why slim? *P Nutr Soc* 1991;50:413–432.

Giles T, Chobanian A: *Magnesium Deficiency: A New Cardiovascular Risk Factor.* Fort Lee, NJ, Health Care Communications, Inc., 1990.

Gilliland M, Zawada E, McClung D, et al: Preliminary reports: Natriuretic effects of calcium supplementation in hypertensive women over 40. *J Am Col N* 1987; 6(2):139–143.

Hamet P, Mongeau E, Lambert J, et al: Interaction among calcium, sodium, and alcohol intake as determinants of blood pressure. *Hypertensio* 1991;17(1):1150–1154.

Itoh R, Oka J, Echizen H, et al: The interrelation of urinary calcium and sodium intake in healthy elderly Japanese. *Int J Vit N* 1991;61:159–165.

Jones K: The thrill of victory: Blood pressure variability and the Type A behavior pattern. *J Behav Med* 1985;8:277.

Knight K, Keith R: Calcium supplementation on normotensive and hypertensive pregnant women. *Am J Clin N* 1992;55:891–895.

Langford H: Sodium-potassium interaction in hypertension and hypertensive cardiovascular disease. *Hypertensio* 1991;17 (Suppl. I): 155–157.

Lawton W, Fitz A, Anderson E, et al: Effect of dietary potassium on blood pressure, renal function, muscle sympathetic nerve activity, and forearm vascular resistance and flow in normotensive and borderline hypertensive humans. *Circulation* 1990;81: 173–184.

Margolin G, Huster G, Glueck C, et al: Blood pressure lowering in elderly subjects: A double-blind crossover study of omega-3 and omega-6 fatty acids. *Am J Clin N* 1991;53:562–572.

McCarron D, Reusser M: The integrated effects of electrolytes on blood pressure. *Nutr Rep* 1991;9(8):56,64.

Osilesi O, Trout D, Ogunwole J, et al: Blood pressure and plasma lipids during ascorbic acid supplementation in borderline hypertensive and normotensive adults. *Nutr Res* 1991;11:405–412.

Pi-Sunyer F: Health implications of obesity. *Am J Clin N* 1991;53:1595S–1603S.

Radack K, Deck C, Huster G: The effects of low doses of n-3 fatty acid supplementation on blood pressure in hypertensive subjects. *Arch In Med* 1991;151:1173–1180.

Ruppert M, Diehl J, Kolloch R, et al: Short-term dietary sodium restriction increases serum lipids and insulin in salt-sensitive and salt-resistant normotensive adults. *Klin Woch* 1991;69 (Suppl. XXV):51–57.

Sagnella G, MacGregor G: Characteristics of an ATPase inhibitor in extracts of tea. *Am J Clin N* 1984;40:36–41.

Simopoulos A: Omega-3 fatty acids in health and disease and in growth and development. *Am J Clin N* 1991;54:438–463.

Singh B, Hollenberg N, Poole-Wilson P, et al: Diuretic-induced potassium and magnesium deficiency: Relation to drug-induced QT prolongation, cardiac arrhythmias and sudden death. *J Hypertens* 1992;10:301–316.

Singh R, Sircar A, Rastogi S, et al: Dietary modulators of blood pressure in hypertension. *Eur J Clin N* 1990;44:319–327.

Sowers M, Wallace R, Lemke J: The association of intakes of vitamin D and calcium with blood pressure among women. *Am J Clin N* 1985;42:135.

Trevisan M: Relationship between total and varied sources of dietary calcium intake and blood pressure. *Am J Epidem* 1986;124:507.

Vitamin C and lowering of blood pressure: Need for intervention trials? *J Hypertens* 1991;9(11):1076–1077.

Weder A, Egan B: Potential deleterious impact of dietary salt restriction on cardiovascular risk factors. *Klin Woch* 1991:69(Suppl. XXV):45–50.

Whang R, Whang D, Ryan M: Refractory potassium repletion. *Arch Int Med* 1992;152:40–45.

Whelton P, Klag M: Magnesium and blood pressure: Review of the epidemiological and clinical trial experience. *Am J Card* 1989;63(14):26G–30G.

White W, Schulman P, McCabe E, et al: Average daily blood pressure, not office blood pressure, determines cardiac function in patients with hypertension. *J Am Med A* 1989;261:873–877.

Wise K, Bergman E, Massey L: Effects of caffeine on urinary calcium excretion in hypertensive and normotensive humans. *Fed Proc* 1986;45:373.

HYPOGLYCEMIA

Anderson R: The role of chromium in the control of high and low blood sugar. *Nutr Rep* 1988;6:41,48.

Anderson R, Polansky M, Bryden N, et al: Effect of chromium supplementation on insulin, insulin binding and C-peptide values of hypoglycemic human subjects. *Am J Clin N* 1985;41:841.

Bell L, Tiglio L, Fairchild M: Dietary strategies in the treatment of reactive hypoglycemia. *J Am Diet A* 1985;85(9):1141–1143.

Campbell P, Gerich J: Mechanisms for prevention, development and reversal of hypoglycemia. *Adv Intern Med* 1988;33:205–230.

Danowski T, Nolan S, Stephan T: Hypoglycemia. *World Rev Nutr Dietetics* 1975;22: 288–303.

Guar gum and hypoglycemia in the rat. *Nutr Rev* 1989;47(1):28–31.

Hofeldt F, Dippe S, Forsham P: Diagnosis and classification of reactive hypoglycemia based on hormonal changes in response to oral and intravenous glucose administration. *Am J Clin N* 1972;25:1193–1201.

Wolever T: Relationship between dietary fiber content and composition in foods and the glycemic index. *Am J Clin N* 1990;51:72–75.

INSOMNIA

Dakshinamurti K, Sharma S, Bonke D: Influence of B vitamins on binding properties of serotonin receptors in the CNS of rats. *Klin Woch* 1990;68:142–145.

Ohta T, Ando K, Iwata T, et al: Treatment of persistent sleep-wake schedule disorders in adolescents with methylcobalamin (vitamin B12). *Sleep* 1991;14(5):414–418.

Okawa A, Mishima K, Nanami T, et al: Vitamin B12 treatment for sleep-wake rhythm disorders. *Sleep* 1990;13(1):15–23.

Penland J: Effects of trace element nutrition on sleep patterns in adult women. *FASEB J* 1988;2:A434.

Pollet P, Leathwood P: The influence of tryptophan on sleep in man. *Int J Vit N* 1983; 53:223.

Sandyk R, Consroe P, Iacono R, et al: L-tryptophan in drug-induced movement disorders with insomnia. *N Eng J Med* 1986;314:1257.

Shukla A, Agarwal K, Chansuria J, et al: Effect of latent iron deficiency on 5-hydroxytryptamine metabolism in rat brain. *J Neurochem* 1989;52:730–735.

MOOD AND EMOTIONS

Abou-Saleh M, Coppen A: The biology of folate in depression: Implications for nutritional hypotheses of the psychoses. *J Psych Res* 1986;29(2):91–101.

Bell I: Vitamin B12 and folate in acute geropsychiatric inpatients. *Nutr Rep* 1991; 9(1):1,8.

Bell I, Edman J, Morrow F, et al: Brief communication: Vitamin B1, B2, and B6 augmentation of tricyclic antidepressant treatment in geriatric depression with cognitive dysfunction. *J Am Col N* 1992;11(2):159–163.

————: B complex vitamin patterns in geriatric and young adult inpatients with major depression. *J Am Ger So* 1991;39:252–257.

Benton D, Cook R: The impact of selenium supplementation on mood. *Biol Psychi* 1991;29:1092–1098.

Blum I, Vered Y, Graff E, et al: The influence of meal composition on plasma serotonin and norepinephrine concentrations. *Metabolism* 1992;41(2):137–140.

Carney M: Vitamin deficiency and mental symptoms. *Br J Psychi* 1990;156:878–882.

Christensen L: The roles of caffeine and sugar in depression. *Nutr Rep* 1991;9(3):16,24.

Eipper B, Mains R: The role of ascorbate in the biosynthesis of neuroendocrine peptides. *Am J Clin N* 1991;54:1153S–1156S.

Godfrey P, Toone B, Carney M, et al: Enhancement of recovery from psychiatric illness by methylfolate. *Lancet* 1990 August;18:392–395.

Hancock M, Hullin R, Aylard P, et al: Nutritional state of elderly women on admission to mental hospital. *Br J Psychi* 1985;147:404–407.

Kehoe P, Blass E: Behaviorally functional opioid systems in infant rats: II. Evidence for pharmacological, physiological, and psychological mediation of pain and stress. *Behav Neuro* 1986;100:624–630.

Kretsch M, Sauberlich H, Newbrun E: Electroencephalographic changes and periodontal status during short-term vitamin B6 depletion of young, nonpregnant women. *Am J Clin N* 1991;53:1266–1274.

Lieberman H, Corkin S, Spring B, et al: Mood, performance, and pain sensitivity: Changes induced by food constituents. *J Psych Res* 1982/1983:17:135–145.

Lozoff B, Jimenez E, Wolf A: Long-term developmental outcome of infants with iron deficiency. *N Eng J Med* 1991;325:687–694.

Matchar D, Feussner J, Watson D, et al: Significance of low serum vitamin B12 levels in the elderly. *J Am Ger So* 1986;34:680–681.

McCullough A, Kirksey A, Wachs T, et al: Vitamin B6 status of Egyptian mothers: Relation to infant behavior and maternal-infant interactions. *Am J Clin N* 1990; 51:1067–1074.

Morris D, Lubin A: A review of the symposium: Diet and behavior—A multidisciplinary evaluation. *Cont Nutr* 1985;10(5):1–2.

Rapoport J, Kruesi M: Behavior and nutrition: A mini review. *Cont Nutr* 1983;8(10):1–2.

Roufs J: Review of L-tryptophan and eosinophilia-myalgia syndrome. *J Am Diet A* 1992;92:844–850.

Sandstead H: Nutrition and brain function: Trace elements. *Nutr Rev* 1986;44:37–41.

Smith B, Fillion T, Blass E: Orally mediated sources of calming in 1- to 3-day-old human infants. *Develop Psy* 1990;26:731–737.

Smith B, Stevens K, Torgerson W, et al: Diminished reactivity of postmature human infants to sucrose compared with term infants. *Develop Psy* 1992;28:811–820.

Soemantri A, Pollitt E, Kim I: Iron deficiency anemia and educational achievement. *Am J Clin N* 1986;42:1221.

Somer E: *The Essential Guide to Vitamins and Minerals.* New York, HarperCollins, 1992,pp181–182.

Tucker D, Penland J, Sandstead H, et al: Nutrition status and brain function in aging. *Am J Clin N* 1990;52:93–102.

Tucker D, Sandstead H, Penland J, et al: Iron status and brain function: Serum ferritin levels associated with asymmetries of cortical electrophysiology and cognitive performance. *Am J Clin N* 1984;39:105–113.

Wurtman J: The involvement of brain serotonin in excessive carbohydrate snacking by obese carbohydrate cravers. *J Am Diet A* 1984;84(9):1004–1007.

Wurtman R, Wurtman J: Carbohydrates and depression. *Sci Am* 1989 January:68–75.

Young S: Some effects of dietary components (amino acids, carbohydrate, folic acid) on brain serotonin synthesis, mood, and behavior. *Can J Physl* 1991;69:893–903.

MUSCLE CRAMPS

Bray T, Bettger W: The physiological role of zinc as an antioxidant. *Free Rad B* 1990; 8:281–291.

Bye A, Kan A: Cramps following exercise. *Aust Paediatr J* 1988;24:258–259.

Casoni I, Guglielmini C, Graziano L, et al: Changes of magnesium concentrations in endurance athletes. *Int J Sp Med* 1990;11(3):234–237.

Fishman R: Neurological aspects of magnesium metabolism. *Arch Neurol* 1965;12: 562–569.

Fourman P: The tetany of potassium deficiency. *Lancet* 1954 September;11:525–526.

Hammar M, Berg G, Solheim F, et al: Calcium and magnesium status in pregnant women. A comparison between treatment with calcium and vitamin C in pregnant women with leg cramps. *Int J Vit N* 1987;57:179–183.

Jansen P, Joosten E, Vingerhoets H: Muscle cramp: Main theories as to aetiology. *Arch Psychiatr Neurol Sci* 1990;239:337–342.

Joborn H, Hjemdahl P, Larsson P, et al: Effects of prolonged adrenalin infusion and of mental stress on plasma minerals and parathyroid hormone. *Clin Phys B* 1990;10:37–53.

Keen C, Lowney P, Gershwin M, et al: Dietary magnesium intake influences exercise capacity and hematologic parameters in rats. *Metabolism* 1987;36(8):788–793.

Lawton W, Fitz A, Anderson E, et al: Effect of dietary potassium on blood pressure, renal function, muscle sympathetic nerve activity, and forearm vascular resistance and flow in normotensive and borderline hypertensive humans. *Circulation* 1990; 81:173–184.

Novelli G, Bracciotti G, Falsini S: Spin-trappers and vitamin E prolong endurance to muscle fatigue in mice. *Free Rad B* 1990;8:9–13.

Pennington J: Nutritional elements of the Total Diet Study. *Nutr Rep* 1992;10(5): 33,40.

Safran M, Garret W, Seaber A, et al: The role of warmup in muscular injury prevention. *Am J Sp Med* 1988;16:123–129.

Seelig M: Cardiovascular consequences of magnesium deficiency and loss: Pathogenesis, prevalence and manifestations—Magnesium and chloride loss in refractory potassium repletion. *Am J Card* 1989;63:4G–21G.

Seelig M: Magnesium requirements in human nutrition. *Cont Nutr* 1982;7(1):1–2.

Somer E: *The Essential Guide to Vitamins and Minerals.* New York, HarperCollins, 1992,pp80–81.

Stendig-Lindberg G, Shapiro Y, Epstein Y, et al: Changes in serum magnesium concentration after strenuous exercise. *J Am Col N* 1987;6:35–40.

Wilkinson R, Lucas G, Heath D, et al: Hypomagnesaemic tetany associated with prolonged treatment with aminoglycosides. *Br Med J* 1986;292:818–820.

OSTEOPOROSIS

Abraham G, Grewal H: A total dietary program emphasizing magnesium instead of calcium. *J Repro Med* 1990;35(5):503–506.

Andon M, Smith K, Bracker M, et al: Spinal bone density and calcium intake in healthy postmenopausal women. *Am J Clin N* 1991;54:927–929.

Bergman E, Erickson M, Boyungs J: Caffeine knowledge, attitudes, and consumption in adult women. *J Nutr Ed* 1992;24:179–184.

Brautbar N, Gruber H: Magnesium and bone disease. *Nephron* 1986;44(1):1–7.

Calcium supplementation and bone loss in postmenopausal women. *Nutr Rev* 1991; 49(6):184–187.

Charles P: Calcium absorption and calcium bioavailability. *J Int Med* 1992;231:161–168.

Compston J: HRT and osteoporosis. *Br Med B* 1992;48(2):309–344.

Cooper C, Atkinson E, Wahner H, et al: Is caffeine consumption a risk factor for osteoporosis? *J Bone Min* 1992;7(4):465–471.

Dawson-Hughes B: Calcium supplementation and bone loss: A review of controlled clinical trials. *Am J Clin N* 1991;54:274S–280S.

Dawson-Hughes B, Dallal G, Krall E, et al: Effect of vitamin D supplementation on wintertime and overall bone loss in healthy postmenopausal women. *Ann Int Med* 1991;115(7):505–511.

DePriester J, Cole T, Bishop N: Bone growth and mineralisation in children aged 4 to 10 years. *Bone Miner* 1991;12:57–65.

Estrogen therapy for osteoporisis—even in the elderly. *Ann Int Med* 1992;117(1):85–86.

Fehily A, Coles R, Evans W, et al: Factors affecting bone density in young adults. *Am J Clin N* 1992;56:579–586.

Fluoride and osteoporosis. *Nutr MD* 1979;5:5.

Freudenheim J, Johnson N, Smith E: Relationships between usual nutrient intake and bone-mineral content of women 35 to 65 years of age: Longitudinal and cross-sectional analysis. *Am J Clin N* 1986;44:863–876.

Fujita T: Vitamin D in the treatment of osteoporosis. *P Soc Exp M* 1992;199:394–399.

Harvey J, Kenny P, Poindexter J, et al: Superior calcium absorption from calcium citrate than calcium carbonate using external forearm counting. *J Am Col N* 1990; 9:583–587.

Heaney R: Calcium in the prevention and treatment of osteoporosis. *J Int Med* 1992; 231:169–180.

Itoh R, Oka J, Echizen H, et al: The interrelation of urinary calcium and sodium intake in healthy elderly Japanese. *Int J Vit N* 1991;61:159–165.

Licata A, Jones-Gall D: Effects of supplemental calcium on serum and urinary calcium in osteoporotic patients. *J Am Col N* 1992;11(2):164–167.

Lindsay R: The effect of sex steroids on the skeleton in premenopausal women. *Am J Obst G* 1992;166:1993–1996.

Marcus R, Drinkwater B, Dalsky G, et al: Osteoporosis and exercise in women. *Med Sci Spt* 1992;24(6):S301–S307.

Matkovic V: Calcium and peak bone mass. *J Int Med* 1992;231:151–160.

Miller J, Smith D, Flora L, et al: Calcium absorption from calcium carbonate and a new form of calcium (CCM) in healthy male and female adolescents. *Am J Clin N* 1988;48:1291–1294.

Mosekilde L: Osteoporosis and calcium. *J Int Med* 1992;231:145–149.

Prince R, Smith M, Dick I, et al: Prevention of postmenopausal osteoporosis. *N Eng J Med* 1991;325(17):1189–1195.

Schapira D: Alcohol abuse and osteoporosis. *Sem Arth Rh* 1990;19(6):371–376.

Seelig M: Cardiovascular consequences of magnesium deficiency and loss: Pathogenesis, prevalence and manifestations—magnesium and chloride loss in refractory potassium repletion. *Am J Card* 1989;63:4G-21G.

Somer E: Calcium, vitamin D, and osteoporosis: Three's the charm. *Nutr Rep* 1992; May:34.

Strause L, Hegenauer J, Saltman P, et al: Effects of long-term dietary manganese and copper deficiency on rat skeleton. *J Nutr* 1986;116:135–141.

Thomas M, Simmons D, Kidder L, et al: Calcium metabolism and bone mineralization in female rats fed diets marginally sufficient in calcium: Effects of increased dietary calcium intake. *Bone Miner* 1991;12:1–14.

Villareal D, Civitelli R, Chines A, et al: Subclinical vitamin D deficiency in postmenopausal women with a low vertebral bone mass. *J Clin End* 1991;72:628–634.

Walden O: The relationship of dietary and supplemental calcium intake to bone loss and osteoporosis. *J Am Diet A* 1989;89:397–400.

PREMENSTRUAL SYNDROME

Abraham G: Premenstrual tension. *Curr P Obst Gyn* 1980;3:5–8.

————: Nutritional factors in the etiology of the premenstrual tension syndromes. *J Repro Med* 1983;28:446.

Abraham G, Hargrove J: Effect of vitamin B6 on premenstrual symptomatology in women with premenstrual tension syndromes: A double-blind crossover study. *Infertil* 1980;3:155–165.

Abraham G, Rumley R: Role of nutrition in managing the premenstrual tension syndrome. *J Repro Med* 1987;32:405.

Barr W: Pyridoxine supplements in premenstrual syndrome. *Practition* 1984; 228: 425–427.

Berger A, Schaumburg H, Schroeder C, et al: Dose response, coasting, and differential fiber vulnerability in human toxic neuropathy: A prospective study of pyridoxine neurotoxicity. *Neurology* 1992;42(7):1367–1370.

Chuong C, Dawson E, Smith E: Vitamin E levels in premenstrual syndrome. *Am J Obst G* 1990;163:1591–1595.

Dalvit S: The effect of the menstrual cycle on patterns of food intake. *Am J Clin N* 1981;34:1811.

Horrobin D: The role of essential fatty acids and prostaglandins in the premenstrual syndrome. *J Repro Med* 1983;28:465–468.

Kendall K, Schnurr P: The effects of vitamin B6 supplementation on premenstrual symptoms. *Obstet Gyn* 1987;70:145–149.

Lee K, Rittenhouse C: Prevalence of perimenstrual symptoms in employed women. *Women Heal* 1991;17(3):17–32.

Lissner L, Stevens J, Levitsky D, et al: Variation in energy intake during the menstrual cycle: Implications for food intake research. *Am J Clin N* 1988;48:956.

London R, Sundaram G, Murphy L, et al: The effect of alpha-tocopherol on premenstrual symptomatology: A double-blind study. *J Am Col N* 1983;2:115.

Mills J: Is it my period or is it my life? *Shape* 1991 November:86–90.

Mira M, Stewart P, Abraham S: Vitamin and trace element status in premenstrual syndrome. *Am J Clin N* 1988;47:636–641.

Moos R: The development of a menstrual distress questionnaire. *Psychos Med* 1968; 30:853.

Reid R: Premenstrual syndrome. *New Eng J Med* 1991;324(17):1208–1210.

————: Premenstrual syndrome: A time for introspection. *Am J Obst G* 1986;155:921.

Rossignol A: Caffeine-containing beverages and premenstrual syndrome in young women. *Am J Pub He* 1985;75:1335.

Sherwood R, Rocks B, Stewart A, et al: Magnesium and the premenstrual syndrome. *Ann Clin Bi* 1986;23:667–670.

Smith S, Sauder C: Food cravings, depression, and premenstrual problems. *Psychos Med* 1969;31:281.

Tomelleri R, Granulate K: Menstrual cycle and food cravings in young college women. *J Am Diet A* 1987;87(3):311–315.

Webb P: 24-hour energy expenditure and the menstrual cycle. *Am J Clin N* 1986;44:614.

Williams M, Harris R, Dean B, et al: Controlled trial of pyridoxine in the premenstrual syndrome. *J Int Med Res* 1985;13:174.

Wurtman J, Brzezinski A, Wurtman R, et al: Effect of nutrient intake on premenstrual depression. *Am J Obst G* 1989;161:1228–1234.

SEXUALLY TRANSMITTED DISEASES (STD)

Algert S, Stubblefield N, Grasse B, et al: Assessment of dietary intake of lysine and arginine in patients with herpes simplex. *J Am Diet A* 1987;87:1560–1561.

Armstrong E, Elenbass J: Lysine for herpes simplex virus. *Drug Intel Clin Pha* 1983; 39:186.

Griffith R, Norins A, Kagan C: A multicentered study of lysine therapy in herpes simplex infection. *Dermatolog* 1978;156:257–267.

Kagan C: Failure of lysine (letter). *Arch Dermat* 1985;121(1):21.

McCune M, Perry H, Muller S, et al: Treatment of recurrent herpes simplex infections with L-lysine monohydrochloride. *Cutis* 1984;34:366–373.

Milman N, Scheibel N, Jessen O: Lysine prophylaxis in recurrent herpes simplex labialis. *Act Der-Ven* 1980;60(1):85–87.

Seidman S, Mosher W., Aral S: Women with multiple sexual partners: United States,

1988. *Am J Pub He* 1992;82(10):1388–1394.

Simon C, VanMelle G, Ramelet A: Failure of lysine in frequently recurrent herpes simplex infection (letter). *Arch Dermat* 1985;121(2):167.

Terezhalmy G, Bottomly W, Pelleu G: The use of water-soluble bioflavonoid–ascorbic acid complex in the treatment of recurrent herpes labialis. *Oral Surg O* 1978; 45(1):56–62.

Thein D, Hurt W: Lysine as a prophylactic agent in the treatment of recurrent herpes simplex labialis. *Oral Surg O* 1984;58:659–666.

Walsh D, Griffith R, Behforooz A: Subjective response to lysine in the therapy of herpes simplex. *J Antimicro* 1983;12:489–496.

White L, Freeman C, Forrester B, et al: In vitro effect of ascorbic acid on infectivity of herpes viruses and paramyxoviruses. *J Clin Micr* 1986;527–531.

SKIN

Allen B, Maurice P, Goodfiled M, et al: The effects on psoriasis of dietary supplementation with eicosapentaenoic acid. *Br J Derm* 1985;113:777.

Bark K, Combs G, Gross E, et al: The effects of topical and oral L-selenomethionine on pigmentation and skin cancer induced by ultraviolet irradiation. *Nutr Cancer* 1992;17:123–137.

Cancer Facts & Figures, 1992. Atlanta, GA: American Cancer Society, 1599 Clifton Road, N.E., Atlanta, GA 30329–4217.

Czarnecki D, Collins N, Meehan C, et al: The skin cancer epidemic: Will it be worse than we think? *Int J Derm* 1991;30(10):695.

Danilevicius V: Dermatology: More than skin deep. *J Am Med A* 1977 April;4:1469–1470.

Darr D, Combs S, Dunstan S, et al: Topical vitamin C protects porcine skin from ultraviolet radiation–induced damage. *Br J Derm* 1992;127:247–253.

Dyall-Smith D, Scurry J: Mercury pigmentation and high mercury levels from the use of a cosmetic cream. *Med J Aust* 1990;153:409–415.

Eichner R, Kahn M, Capetola R, et al: Effects of topical retinoids on cytoskeletal proteins: Implications for retinoid effects on epidermal differentiation. *J Inves Der* 1992; 98:154–161.

Engel A, Johnson M, Haynes S: Health effects of sunlight exposure in the United States. *Arch Dermat* 1988;124:72–79.

Fraser M, Hartge P, Tucker M: Melanoma and nonmelanoma skin cancer: Epidemiology and risk factors. *Sem Onc Nurs* 1991;7(1):2–12.

Gardner S, Weiss J: Clinical features of photodamage and treatment with topical tretinoin. *J Derm Surg* 1990;16:925–931.

Gensler H, Magdaleno M: Topical vitamin E inhibition of immunosuppression and tumorigenesis induced by ultraviolet irradiation. *Nutr Cancer* 1991;15:97–106.

Greaves M: Itching—research has barely scratched the surface. *N Eng J Med* 1992; 326(15):1016–1017.

Kornhauser A, Wamer W, Giles A: Effect of dietary beta carotene on psoralen-induced phototoxicity. *Ann NY Acad* 1985;453:91–104.

Lowe N: Sunscreens and the prevention of skin aging. *J Derm Surg* 1990;16:936–938.

Matarasso S, Salman S, Glogau R, et al: The role of chemical peeling in the treatment of photodamaged skin. *J Derm Surg* 1990;16:945–954.

Neild V, Marsden R, Bailes J, et al: Egg and milk exclusion diets in atopic eczema. *Br J Derm* 1986;114:117–123.

Rebello T, Atherton D, Holden C: The effect of oral zinc administration on sebum-free fatty acids in acne vulgaris. *Act Der-Ven* 1986;66:305–310.

Record I, Dreosti I, Konstantinopoulos M, et al: The influence of topical and systemic vitamin E on ultraviolet light–induced skin damage in hairless mice. *Nutr Cancer* 1991;16:219–225.

Shupack J, Haber R, Stiller M: The future of topical therapy for cutaneous aging. *J Derm Surg* 1990;16:941–944.

Takamoto S, Onishi T, Morimoto S, et al: Effect of 1-alpha hydroxycholecalciferol on psoriasis vulgaris: A pilot study. *Calcif Tis* 1986;39:360–364.

Vargo N: Basal and squamous cell carcinomas: An overview. *Sem Oncol Nurs* 1991; 7(1):13–25.

Vitamin D and psoriasis. *Nutr Rev* 1992;50(5):138–140.

White W, Roe D: Effect of in vivo irradiation on plasma levels of carotenoids and vitamin A. *Fed Proc* 1986;45:831.

Wright S: Essential fatty acids and the skin. *Br J Derm* 1991;125:503–515.

Ziboh V, Miller C, Kragballe K, et al: Effects of an 8-week dietary supplementation of eicosapentaenoic acid in serum PMNs and epidermal fatty acids of psoriatic subjects. *J Inves Der* 1985;84:300.

STRESS

Bender D: B vitamins and the nervous system. *Neurochem I* 1984;6(3):297–321.

Burchfield S, Holmes T, Harrington R: Personality differences between sick and rarely sick individuals. *Soc Sci Med* 1981;15E:145–148.

Christiansen L, Kreitsch K, White B, et al: Impact of a dietary change on emotional distress. *J Abn Psych* 1985;94:565–579.

Chrousos G, Gold P: The concepts of stress and stress system disorders. *J Am Med A* 1992;267(9):1244–1251.

Classen H: Stress and magnesium. *Artery* 1981;9(3):182–189.

Couzy F, Lafargue P, Guezennec C: Zinc metabolism in the athlete: Influence of training, nutrition and other factors. *Int J Sp M* 1990;11(4):263–266.

DiPalma J: Magnesium replacement therapy. *Am Fam Phys* 1990;42(1):173–176.

Ericsson Y, Angmar-Mansson B, Flores M: Urinary mineral ion loss after sugar ingestion. *Bone Miner* 1990;9:233–237.

Fawaz F: Zinc deficiency in surgical patients: A clinical study. *J Parent En* 1985;9:364–369.

Fine K, Santa Ana C, Porter J, et al: Intestinal absorption of magnesium from food and supplements. *J Clin Inv* 1991;88:396–402.

Hill P: It is not what you eat, but how you eat it: Digestion, lifestyle, nutrition. *Nutrit* 1991;7(6):385–395.

Irvin M, Hutchins B: A conspectus of research on vitamin C requirements of man. *J Nutr* 1976;106:823–879.

Joborn H, Hjemdahl P, Larsson P, et al: Effects of prolonged adrenaline infusion and of mental stress on plasma minerals and parathyroid hormone. *Clin Physl* 1990;10:37–53.

Kallner A: Influence of vitamin C status on the urinary excretion of catecholamines in stress. *Human Nutr: Clin Nutr* 1983;37:405.

Kipp D: Stress and nutrition. *Cont Nutr* 1984;9(7):1–2.

Lampe J, Slavin J, Apple F: Poor iron status of women runners training for a marathon. *Int J Sp M* 1986;7:111–114.

Lloyd R: Possible mechanisms of psychoneuroimmunological interaction. *Advances* 1984;1(2):43–51.

Parker C: Environmental stress and immunity: Possible implications for IgE-mediated allergy. *Persp Biol* 1991;34(2):197–212.

Pratt C: Moderate exercise and iron status in women. *Nutr Rep* 1991;9(7):48,56.

Pryor W: Can vitamin E protect humans against the pathological effects of ozone in smog? *Am J Clin N* 1991;53:702–722.

Resina A, Fedi S, Gatteschi L, et al: Comparison of some serum copper parameters in trained runners and control subjects. *Int J Sp M* 1990;11:58–60.

Rubinow D: Brain, behavior, and immunity: An interactive system. *J Nat Canc Monogr* 1990;10:79–82.

Schliefer S, Keller S, Stein M: Stress effects on immunity. *Psychiat J* 1985;10(3):125–131.

Seelig M: Cardiovascular consequences of magnesium deficiency and loss: Pathogenesis, prevalence, and manifestations—Magnesium and chloride loss in refractory potassium repletion. *Am J Card* 1989;63:4G–21G.

Singh A, Smoak B, Patterson K, et al: Biochemical indices of selected trace minerals in men: Effects of stress. *Am J Clin N* 1991;53:126–131.

Somer E: *The Essential Guide to Vitamins and Minerals.* New York, HarperCollins, 1992,p222.

Swarth, J: *Stress and Nutrition.* San Diego, CA, Health Media of America, 1988.

URINARY TRACT INFECTIONS

Johnson J, Stamm W: Urinary tract infections in women: Diagnosis and treatment. *Ann Int Med* 1989;111:906–917.

Taylor W: Renal calculi and self-medication with multivitamin preparations containing vitamin D. *Clin Sci* 1972;42(4):515–522.

YEAST INFECTIONS

Almekinders L, Greene W: Vertebral Candida infections: A case report and review of the literature. *Clin Orthop* 1991;267:174–178.

Edman J, Sobel J, Taylor M: Zinc status in women with recurrent vulvovaginal candidiasis. *Am J Obst G* 1986;155:1082.

Galland L: Nutrition and Candida albicans, in Bland J (ed): *A Year in Nutritional Medicine, 1986, ed 2.* New Canaan, CT, Keats Publishing, 1986,pp203–238.

Golden B, Gorbach S: The effect of milk and lactobacillus feeding on human intestinal bacterial enzyme activity. *Am J Clin N* 1984;39:756–761.

————: Effect of Lactobacillus acidophilus dietary supplements on 1,2 dimethylhydrazine dihydrochloride-induced intestinal cancer in rats. *J Nat Canc* 1980;64: 263–265.

Hilton E, Isenberg H, Alperstein P, et al: Ingestion of yogurt containing Lactobacillus acidophilus as prophylaxis for Candida vaginitis. *Ann Int Med* 1992;116 (5):353–357.

Kalo-Klein A, Witkin S: Regulation of the immune response of Candida albicans by monocytes and progesterone. *Am J Obst G* 1991;164:1351–1354.

————: Candida albicans: Cellular immune system interactions during different stages of the menstrual cycle. *Am J Obst G* 1989;161:1132–1136.

McKenzie H, Main J, Pennington C, et al: Antibody to selected strains of Saccharomyces cerevisiae (baker's and brewer's yeast) and Candida albicans in Crohn's disease. *Gut* 1990;31(5):536–538.

Montes L, Krumdieck C, Cornwell P: Hypovitaminosis A in patients with mucocutaneous candidiasis. *J Infect Dis* 1973;128:227–230.

Reed B, Slattery M, French T: The association between dietary intake and reported history of Candida vulvovaginitis. *J Fam Prac* 1989;29(5):509–515.

Witkin S, Yu L, Ledger W: Inhibition of Candida albicans–induced lymphocyte proliferation by lymphocytes and sera from women with recurrent vaginitis. *Am J Obst G* 1983;147:809–811.

Yogurt: Its nutritional and health benefits. *Dairy Council Digest* 1990;61(2):7–12.

INDEX

Page numbers in **bold print** refer to figures and tables.